Congenital Heart Disease

METHODS IN MOLECULAR MEDICINE™

John M. Walker, Series Editor

METHODS IN MOLECULAR MEDICINE™

Congenital Heart Disease

Molecular Diagnostics

Edited by

Mary Kearns-Jonker

Transplantation Biology Research Lab
Division of Cardiothoracic Surgery
Children's Hospital of Los Angeles
Los Angeles, CA

HUMANA PRESS ✳ TOTOWA, NEW JERSEY

© 2006 Humana Press Inc.
999 Riverview Drive, Suite 208
Totowa, New Jersey 07512

www.humanapress.com

This publication is printed on acid-free paper. ∞
ANSI Z39.48-1984 (American Standards Institute) Permanence of Paper for Printed Library Materials.

Production Editor: Melissa Caravella

Cover design by Patricia F. Cleary

Cover illustration: Cover artwork by Alexa Jonker. We thank Irina Shulkin for assistance with the graphic layout.

For additional copies, pricing for bulk purchases, and/or information about other Humana titles, contact Humana at the above address or at any of the following numbers: Tel.: 973-256-1699; Fax: 973-256-8341; E-mail: orders@humanapr.com; or visit our Website: www.humanapress.com

Printed in the United States of America. 10 9 8 7 6 5 4 3 2 1

eISBN 1-59745-088-X

ISSN 1543-1894

Library of Congress Cataloging in Publication Data

Congenital heart disease : molecular diagnostics / edited by Mary Kearns-Jonker.
    p. ; cm. -- (Methods in molecular medicine ; 126)
  Includes bibliographical references and index.
  ISBN 1-58829-375-0 (alk. paper)
  1. Congenital heart disease--Molecular diagnosis. 2. Congenital heart
disease--Genetic aspects. 3. Heart--Diseases--Molecular diagnosis.
4. Heart--Diseases--Genetic aspects. 5. Molecular diagnosis.
  I. Kearns-Jonker, Mary. II. Series.
  [DNLM: 1. Heart Defects, Congenital--diagnosis. 2. Diagnostic
Techniques, Cardiovascular. 3. Heart Defects, Congenital--genetics.
4. Molecular Biology--methods.   WG 220 C7543 2006]
  RC687.C666 2006
  616.1'042--dc22   2005026174

Preface

The *Methods in Molecular Medicine*™ series is noted for providing clinicians, research scientists, and interested individuals with detailed experimental procedures that are written by leading experts in the field. *Congenital Heart Disease: Molecular Diagnostics* introduces a series of techniques that are currently used to identify the molecular basis for cardiovascular disease. New knowledge gained from the application of molecular genetics to medicine has had a significant impact in biomedical research. The chapters in this book update the reader on new developments in the field and introduce the technology currently used to define the molecular genetic basis for congenital malformations of the heart, cardiomyopathies, cardiac tumors, and arrythmias in human patients. In addition, the limitations to identifying patients with congenital heart disease using this information during both pre- and postnatal periods is discussed in this volume. The experimental techniques are presented in sufficient detail to ensure that the procedures can be reproduced in any laboratory, irrespective of the level of experience of the investigators. The notes section included at the end of each chapter provides valuable insight for troubleshooting, experimental design, and data analysis that come from the benefit of the expertise of the authors who are all renowned and well-respected in the field. It is my hope that *Congenital Heart Disease: Molecular Diagnostics* will be a valuable resource for medical personnel, researchers, patients, and their families.

I would like to express my gratitude to the authors of this volume for their enthusiasm for the work and thoughtful input into each chapter. I would also like to thank the series editor, Professor John Walker, for his guidance and endless patience during the preparation of this volume.

This book is dedicated to my mom, Lillian Kearns, and to my family for their continuous love and support.

Mary Kearns-Jonker

Contents

Contributors

ARISTOTELIS ASTRINIDIS • *Department of Medical Oncology, Fox Chase Cancer Center, Philadelphia, PA*

J. DAVID BARRANS • *Department of Medicine, Brigham and Women's Hospital, Boston, MA*

CRAIG T. BASSON • *Greenberg Cardiology Division, Department of Medicine, Weill Medical College of Cornell University, New York, NY*

D. WOODROW BENSON • *Division of Cardiology, Department of Pediatrics, Cincinnati Children's Hospital Medical Center, Cincinnati, OH*

ZAHURUL A. BHUIYAN • *Department of Clinical Genetics, Academic Medical Center, Amsterdam, The Netherlands*

HENNIE BIKKER • *Department of Clinical Genetics, Academic Medical Center, Amsterdam, The Netherlands*

PAUL COUCKE • *Department of Medical Genetics, Ghent University Hospital, Ghent, Belgium*

ANNE DE PAEPE • *Department of Medical Genetics, Ghent University Hospital, Ghent, Belgium*

DEBORAH A. DRISCOLL • *Division of Reproductive Genetics, Department of Obstetrics and Gynecology, University of Pennsylvania Medical Center, Philadelphia, PA*

NAVARATNAM ELANKO • *Genetics Unit, St. George's Hospital, London, United Kingdom*

ELIZABETH GOLDMUNTZ • *The Division of Cardiology, Abramson Research Center, The Children's Hospital of Philadelphia, Philadelphia, PA*

CATHY J. HATCHER • *Greenberg Cardiology Division, Department of Medicine, Weill Medical College of Cornell University, New York, NY*

ELIZABETH PETRI HENSKE • *Department of Medical Oncology, Fox Chase Cancer Center, Philadelphia, PA*

STEVE JEFFERY • *Division of Medical Genetics, Department of Clinical Developmental Sciences, St. George's University of London, London, United Kingdom*

ANN M. JOSEPH-GEORGE • *Genetics and Genomic Biology, The Hospital for Sick Children, Toronto, Ontario, Canada*

MARY KEARNS-JONKER • *Transplantation Biology Research Lab, Division of Cardiothoracic Surgery, Children's Hospital of Los Angeles, Los Angeles, CA*

CHOONG-CHIN LIEW • *Department of Medicine, Brigham and Women's Hospital, Boston, MA*

DEBORAH A. MCDERMOTT • *Greenberg Cardiology Division, Department of Medicine, Weill Medical College of Cornell University, New York, NY*

ELIZABETH MOORE • *Division of Human Genetics, The Children's Hospital of Philadelphia, Abramson Research Center, Philadelphia, PA*

LUCY R. OSBORNE • *Department of Medicine, The University of Toronto, Toronto, Ontario, Canada*

MASSIMO PANDOLFO • *Service de Neurologie, Université Libre de Bruxelles-Hôpital Erasme, Bruxelles, Belgium*

ALEX V. POSTMA • *Experimental and Molecular Cardiology Group, Academic Medical Center, Amsterdam, The Netherlands*

STEPHEN W. SCHERER • *Genetics and Genomic Biology, The Hospital for Sick Children, Toronto, Ontario, Canada*

AMY J. SEHNERT • *Department of Pediatrics, University of California at San Francisco, Pediatric Heart Center, San Francisco, CA; CardioDX Inc., Palo Alto, CA*

SILKE SPERLING • *Department of Vertebrate Genomics, Max Planck Institute for Molecular Genetics, Berlin, Germany*

NANCY B. SPINNER • *The Division of Human Genetics, The Children's Hospital of Philadelphia, Abramson Research Center, Philadelphia, PA*

MAY TASSABEHJI • *Academic Unit of Medical Genetics, The University of Manchester, St Mary's Hospital, Manchester, United Kingdom*

JEFFREY A. TOWBIN • *Pediatric Cardiology, Texas Children's Hospital, Houston, TX*

ZSOLT URBAN • *Departments of Pediatrics and Genetics, Washington University School of Medicine, St. Louis, MO*

PETRA VAN ACKER • *Department of Medical Genetics, Ghent University Hospital, Ghent, Belgium*

STEPHANIE M. WARE • *Divisions of Molecular Cardiovascular Biology and Human Genetics, Department of Pediatrics, Cincinnati Children's Hospital Medical Center, Cincinnati, OH*

1

Introduction

D. Woodrow Benson

Summary

This chapter introduces the book by providing a summary of the detailed technical information regarding the materials, reagents, and experimental procedures presented in each chapter.

Key Words: Pediatric heart disease; cardiovascular disease in the young; congenital heart disease; cardiovascular genetics; heterotaxy syndrome; vasculopathy.

1. Introduction

The close of the 20th century marked the beginning of the era of molecular medicine, which gave birth to the field of cardiovascular genetics. Insight into the genetic basis of cardiovascular disease is having a transforming effect on this field of medicine, long dominated by biophysical models of disease thought to result largely from environmental effects. Major genetic effects, caused by chromosomal and single-gene defects, have been identified from studies of humans affected with cardiovascular disease at young ages. Identification of disease-causing human gene mutations has provided the means to study the pathogenesis of these conditions in model systems and has supplied new tools for the developmental biologist.

Because of these human genetic discoveries, genetic techniques have become important for scientists, geneticists, and physicians. This book, *Congenital Heart Disease: Molecular Diagnostics*, contributes a compilation of laboratory tools and provides the latest information on the use of molecular genetics for the diagnosis of cardiovascular disease. Each chapter provides detailed technical information regarding the materials, reagents, and experimental procedures necessary to identify genetic alteration associated with specific disease phenotypes. A wide variety of techniques for detecting single-gene defects, analyzing cytogenetic abnormalities, and gene expression studies using microarray techniques are presented. The techniques are applied to diverse

From: *Methods in Molecular Medicine, vol. 126: Congenital Heart Disease: Molecular Diagnostics*
Edited by: M. Kearns-Jonker © Humana Press Inc., Totowa, NJ

phenotypes, including congenital cardiac malformations, cardiomyopathies, cardiac tumors, and cardiac arrhythmias.

2. Genetics of Cardiac Septation Defects and Their Pre-Implantation Diagnosis

Major advances in the understanding of the underlying genetic basis of cardiac septation defects has provided insight into the molecular basis of cardiac development *(1)*. At the same time, advances in ultrasound technology has made possible precise prenatal diagnosis of both syndromic and nonsyndromic forms of these cardiac malformations, which may, in some instances, be amenable to fetal intervention. In addition, improved therapeutic strategies during the last several decades have dramatically increased the number of individuals living to reproductive age, raising the possibility that, as these individuals have their own families, clinicians are likely to see an increase in familial clustering of cardiac malformations.

In Chapter 2, by McDermott et al., an overview of genes whose mutation is known to cause atrial and/or ventricular septal defects is provided. This is a rapidly increasing list, and, at present, genetic testing for most of the genes implicated in septal defects is available only on a research basis. It is to be expected that, as pointed out in many chapters in this book, advances in technology and improved understanding to the genotype–phenotype correlations will ameliorate this problem somewhat.

However, even with advances in technology, it is impractical to screen all septation defect-associated genes in any given patient, and, as the list increases, this will be an increasingly challenging problem. Rather than focusing on the debate about the technology best used to screen for mutations in a particular gene (e.g., denaturing high-performance liquid chromatography [DHPLC], denaturing gel electrophoresis, single-strand conformational polymorphism analysis, or automated sequencing), emphasis in this chapter is on the biological processes underlying different genetically determined septation defects. The idea being that such understanding may appropriately inform the choice of genes to be screened for mutations on a patient-by-patient basis; the methods used to prioritize genes selected for mutation analysis should rely on a thorough understanding of the phenotypes, expression patterns, and functional developmental defects associated with mutations in each gene.

Chapter 2 also includes discussion regarding the use of molecular genetic techniques in concert with in vitro fertilization. Before identification of genes whose mutations cause septation defects, couples interested in prenatal diagnosis for cardiac malformations were limited to genetic counseling and general recurrence risk assessments, ultrasound imagining, or testing for chromosomal causes of cardiac malformations in conjunction with amniocentesis or chorionic villus sampling. With the identification of single genes responsible for cardiac malformations, the ability to offer pre-implantation genetic diagnosis in combination with in vitro fertilization is now a potential option for some couples that prefer earlier diagnosis.

3. Molecular and Genetic Aspects of DiGeorge/Velocardiofacial Syndrome

The deletion 22q11.2 syndrome (del22q11; OMIM 188400, 192430), which includes DiGeorge syndrome, Shprintzen syndrome, velocardiofacial syndrome, conotruncal anomaly face syndrome, and CATCH-22, results from a heterozygous, submicroscopic deletion on chromosome 22q11.2 at the DiGeorge chromosomal region *(2–5)*. Although approx 90% of del22q11 cases are said to occur sporadically, family occurrence has been well-documented since the syndrome was first recognized nearly 40 yr ago *(6–8)*. The associated phenotype is variable, and more than 150 manifestations have been acknowledged by the advocacy group, Velo-Cardio-Facial Syndrome Educational Foundation *(9)*. Common manifestations can be broadly grouped as cardiovascular abnormalities, dysmorphic facial features, speech problems, and learning problems *(10–12)*.

Cardiovascular malformations are common in patients with del22q11. In reviewing the three largest groups of patients reported to date ($N = 810$) in which cardiac phenotypes were analyzed, the most common types were tetralogy of Fallot (TOF; 22–35%), interrupted aortic arch (15–19%), ventricular septal defect (13–18%), truncus arteriosus (7–12%), and vascular ring (5%) *(13–15)*. Overall, cardiovascular malformations have been reported to be present in approx 75% of individuals with del22q11 *(13–15)*, and infant patients frequently come to medical attention because of symptoms caused by heart disease. However, the prevalence is much lower in pediatric patients diagnosed after 6 mo (38%) and in adult patients (~30%), suggesting that the prevalence figure of 75% is likely an overestimation resulting from ascertainment bias caused by selecting sporadic cases presenting with cardiovascular malformations *(8,15–18)*.

As pointed out in Chapter 3, by Driscoll, fluorescence *in situ* hybridization (FISH) with commercially available probes is a sensitive test for detecting the 22q11.2 deletion. The deletion detection rate varies with the type of cardiac defect and the extent of extracardiac anomalies. Identifying individuals with the deletion is important for ascertaining individuals who are at risk for related health and learning problems, so that diagnosis, management, and treatment can be implemented early. Further, diagnosis of the deletion will allow for identification of additional family members who may be at risk for learning disabilities, who also may benefit from appropriate intervention strategies.

Finally, identifying family members with the deletion allows more accurate risk counseling and reproductive decision making. Risk counseling for del22q11 will become more advanced as more is learned about the phenotype; for example, recent investigation suggests that individuals with del22q11 may have poorer outcomes after cardiac surgery *(19)*.

4. Mutation Screening for the Genes Causing Cardiac Arrhythmias

This chapter details our current understanding of the clinical and molecular genetic aspects of cardiac arrhythmias as well as the methodology for mutation analysis of the causative genes. Information regarding the molecular genetic basis of these important clinical problems has accumulated at an explosive pace since the initial report of linkage of long QT syndrome in 1991 *(20)*. Subsequent reports have identified the molecular genetic basis of a number of arrhythmia phenotypes, including atrioventricular block *(21)*, idiopathic ventricular fibrillation or Brugada syndrome *(22)*, atrial fibrillation *(23,24)*, sick sinus syndrome *(25)*, ventricular preexcitation *(26)*, and polymorphic ventricular tachycardia *(27–30)*, using genetic linkage analysis and candidate gene approaches. Mutations in ion channels, referred to as channelopathies, have been identified most often.

Mutation analysis of genes causing arrhythmia disorders has been greatly assisted by the development of rapid, high-technology and high-throughput methods. The methodology presented in Chapter 4, by Towbin, includes DHPLC and DNA sequencing. The methodological approaches are important because not only are a larger number of genes associated with cardiac arrhythmias, but also because most of the mutations are private (i.e., only seen in one family). This creates a challenge for mutation analysis. A test, FAMILION, is available on a fee-for-service basis from Genaissance Pharmaceuticals (http://www.familion.com/). Identification of cardiac arrhythmia-causing mutations will become increasingly important in the future, as therapies become gene specific *(31)*.

5. The Molecular Genetics of Marfan Syndrome

Marfan syndrome (MFS; OMIM 154700) is a disorder of connective tissue, which affects mainly the skeleton, the cardiovascular system, and the eyes. MFS shows autosomal-dominant transmission, with a prevalence of approx 1 in 10,000 people. The phenotype is pleiotropic and characterized by tall stature, arachnodactyly, lens subluxation, mitral valve prolapse, and aortic root dilation with a high risk of aortic aneurysm and dissection, which may result in aortic rupture and sudden death.

Genetic linkage of MFS to chromosome 15, where the fibrillin *(FBN)1* gene is encoded *(32)* was followed by identification of mutations in *FBN1* in individuals with MFS *(33)*. Subsequently, more than 600 mutations in the *FBN1* gene have been identified *(34)*, and the list of known phenotypic effects resulting from these mutations has been extended. *FBN1* is a major component of extracellular matrix structures known as microfibrils, on which elastin (ELN) seems to be deposited. It has been widely thought that the loss of tissue integrity (e.g., lens and aorta) associated with MFS is the consequence of altered microfibril structural integrity, i.e., the presence of a population of abnormal molecules alters the entire fibril structure (a dominant-negative effect; refs. *35* and *36*).

FBN1 has a pattern of structural motifs, also common to *FBN2* and *FBN3*, that includes more than 40 calcium-binding, epidermal growth factor precursor-like units arranged in similarly sized blocks, separated by modules known as eight cysteine-binding or transforming growth factor (TGF)-β-binding domains. Recently, it was proposed that the loss of the FBN1 protein by any of several mechanisms and the subsequent effect on the pool of TGF-β may be more relevant in the development of MFS than mechanisms previously proposed in the dominant-negative disease model *(37)*. The possibility that FBN haploinsufficiency is a significant factor in the pathogenesis of MFS suggests that strategies aimed at boosting protein expression may warrant consideration.

The contribution by Coucke et al. (Chapter 5) provides methods for mutation analysis of *FBN1* by both DHPLC and direct sequencing of genomic DNA and complementary DNA (cDNA) isolated from peripheral blood leukocytes or skin fibroblasts. Identification of *FBN1* mutations can be important for confirming the diagnosis of MFS and for characterizing genetic risk, and may play a key role in management of patients with MFS.

6. Mutation Analysis of *PTPN11* in Noonan Syndrome by WAVE Analysis

Noonan syndrome (NS; MIM 163950) is an autosomal-dominant disorder characterized by dysmorphic facial features, short stature, cardiac defects, and skeletal malformations *(38,39)*. Linkage to chromosome 12q24 *(NS1)* and genetic heterogeneity were established *(40,41)* before *PTPN11*, the gene encoding the src-homology region 2-domain phosphatase-2 (SHP-2), which is a nonreceptor-type protein tyrosine phosphatase, was identified as the *NS1* disease gene *(42)*. Heterozygous *PTPN11* mutations are present in approx 50% of NS cases *(43)*. *PTPN11* mutations are found more often among familial cases than among sporadic cases. Genotype–phenotype analysis revealed that pulmonic stenosis was more prevalent among the patients with NS who had *PTPN11* mutations than it was in the group without *PTPN11* mutations (70.6% vs 46.2%), whereas hypertrophic cardiomyopathy was less prevalent among those with *PTPN11* mutations (5.9 vs 26.2%; $p < 0.001$).

PTPN11 mutations causing NS are heterozygous missense mutations that alter amino acid residues located in or around the N-SH2 and phosphotyrosine phosphatase domains, which interact to switch the protein between its inactive and active conformations. An energetics-based structural analysis of SHP-2 mutants indicated that NS-causing mutations might result in a shift of the equilibrium favoring the active conformation, suggesting that the mutations are gain-of-function changes and that the pathogenesis of NS arises from excessive SHP-2 activity *(42)*. This possibility was confirmed by demonstrating an increase in phosphatase activity of the two most common mutants *(44)*.

Although studies are underway to identify additional NS genes, the identification of *PTPN11* mutations is already exhibiting clinical usefulness. Chapter 6, by Elanko and Jeffrey, details the methodology for polymerase chain reaction amplification and WAVE DHPLC analysis for all coding exons for the gene *PTPN11*, which is mutated in approx 50% of cases of NS. Although DNA sequencing is initially required to determine the mutation(s) detected by WAVE (sequencing methods are not described), each mutation has its own DHPLC signature, and experienced operators can determine known mutations on this basis. The new Navigator™ software has made this process more reliable.

7. Williams–Beuren Syndrome

Williams–Beuren syndrome (WBS; MIM 194050) and autosomal-dominant familial supravalvar aortic stenosis (SVAS; MIM 185500) are related disorders *(45–47)*. The cardiovascular malformations of both conditions are thought to result from haploinsufficiency of ELN. The cardiovascular manifestations of these elastinopathies, often referred to as arteriopathies, typically include SVAS, branch pulmonary artery hypoplasia, coronary artery stenosis, and coarctation of the aorta. Aortic or mitral valve defects have been identified in 10 to 20% of cases *(48,49)*, and isolated pulmonary valve stenosis has been reported *(48)*.

WBS is a developmental disorder affecting approx 1 in 20,000 live births *(50)*. Individuals with this syndrome, which is usually sporadic, exhibit characteristic physical and behavioral features. Affected individuals have a distinctive elfin-like facial appearance and mild-to-moderate mental retardation; however, they typically have relatively good verbal skills and characteristic personality traits. Cardiovascular abnormalities occur in approx 75% of affected individuals *(49)*.

WBS is caused by a hemizygous chromosomal microdeletion (~1.5 Mb) at chromosome 7q11.23; ELN is one of the 24 genes assigned to the deleted WBS critical region, and virtually all (98–99%) people with typical features of WBS have a deletion of the ELN gene *(46)*. This observation, coupled with the coincident distribution of ELN expression and cardiovascular malformations suggest that ELN haploinsufficiency may contribute to the pathogenesis of the characteristic cardiovascular anomalies. Other genomic rearrangements of this region have also been described *(51)*, and a partial deletion of the WBS region also resulting in ELN haploinsufficiency has been identified in a small group of patients with a phenotype intermediate to WBS and SVAS *(52)*.

FISH of either metaphase or interphase nuclei can be used to detect all of these chromosomal rearrangements, providing the ability to test this segment of chromosome 7 in individuals with a suspected diagnosis of WBS. Chapter 7, by Osborne et al., outlines performance of an initial screen using commercially available FISH probes. Karyotyping (performed in parallel or subsequent to the standard diagnostic FISH test) and targeted FISH analyses could then be used to detect macroscopic changes, such as translocations or smaller deletions/inversions, respectively. Each type of analysis varies in the number of probes used and the cell stage analyzed after hybridization.

8. Congenital Heart Disease: Molecular Diagnostics of Supravalvular Aortic Stenosis

Mutation or deletion of the *ELN* gene results in ELN haploinsufficiency, which has been established as the cause of autosomal-dominant SVAS, which, as discussed in Chapter 7, is related to WBS. In addition, *ELN*, whose mutation also results in the connective tissue disorder autosomal-dominant cutis laxa, has been implicated as a susceptibility gene for hypertension and intracranial aneurysms. Chapter 8, by Tassabehji and Urban, describes methodology to identify point mutations, chromosomal deletions and translocation involving the *ELN* gene.

9. "Chip"ping Away at Heart Failure

Cardiomyopathy refers to cardiac dysfunction of unknown cause; the World Health Organization has defined clinical subtypes that include dilated, hypertrophic, restrictive, arrhythmogenic, and unclassified (which includes mitochondrial problems) *(53)*. Through use of genetic linkage analysis, positional cloning, and candidate gene analyses, disease-causing mutations have been identified in nearly 30 genes from diverse functional categories (reviewed in refs. *54–56*). However, in most human cases of cardiomyopathy, the cause is still unknown. Although the cardiomyopathies share common clinical endpoints, e.g., heart failure, the molecular mechanisms contributing to the underlying pathogenesis are quite varied *(57,58)*.

In the past decade, there has been increasing interest in analyzing profile similarities of global gene expressions using microarray technology to identify candidate genes contributing to disease pathogenesis *(59)*. For example, analysis of the expression profiles of colorectal cancers led to identification of a novel gene subsequently identified as playing a role in regulating cell growth *(60)*. Chapter 9, by Barrans and Liew, reviews the technical approaches to microarray studies and describes their experience with a custom-made, cardio-vascular-based cDNA microarray, termed the CardioChip, in characterizing gene expression in end-stage cardiomyopathies relative to gene expression associated with normal heart function *(61)*.

10. Molecular Diagnostics of Catecholaminergic Polymorphic Ventricular Tachycardia

Polymorphic ventricular tachycardia is a term used to describe a beat-to-beat alternating QRS axis and morphology during ventricular tachycardia. The duration is usually nonsustained, with a slower rate than *torsade de pointes*. Catecholaminergic polymorphic ventricular tachycardia (CPVT) has the added feature of being induced by adrenergic stimulation. CPVT is an important clinical problem with a high mortality rate, of up to 50% by the age of 30 yr. Recently, the molecular diagnostics of this disease have become increasingly important because disease-causing mutations have been identified in approx 60% of CPVT patients.

In Chapter 10, by Postma et al., the molecular diagnostics are presented for three genes whose mutations are known to cause polymorphic ventricular tachycardia: the cardiac ryanodine receptor 2 *(27,28)*, the calsequestrin 2 gene *(29)*, and an inward-rectifying potassium channel gene *(62–64)*. Genetic diagnosis of this clinical problem is likely to become increasingly important both in selecting gene-specific therapies and to augment early diagnosis and subsequent preventive strategies.

11. Mutation Detection in Tumor Suppressor Genes Using Archival Tissue Specimens

Tuberous sclerosis complex (TSC; OMIM 191090 and 191100) is a neurocutaneous syndrome characterized by seizures, mental retardation, and benign tumors of many organs, including the heart. Rhabdomyoma, the most common cardiac tumor discovered in the perinatal period, is a signature finding of TSC *(65)*. TSC is caused by mutations in the *TSC1* and *TSC2* tumor suppressor genes (reviewed in **ref.** *66*); TSC is inherited as an autosomal-dominant trait, but 60 to 70% of cases are sporadic and represent new mutations. The absence of obvious mutational hot spots in *TSC1* or *TSC2* and their relatively large size (21 and 41 coding exons, respectively) make the screening for mutations challenging. Because rhabdomyomas often spontaneously regress during early childhood, the usual clinical approach avoids surgical intervention. Consequently, access to tissue (particularly fresh tissue) is very limited, and relatively little is known about the pathogenesis of rhabdomyoma. Importantly, the contribution by Astrinidis and Henske presents methodology for mutation detection using paraffin-embedded tissue.

12. Friedreich Ataxia

Friedreich ataxia (FRDA; OMIM 229300), named for the physician who first described it nearly 150 yr ago, is an autosomal-recessive disease that involves the nervous system and the heart (reviewed in **refs.** **67** and **68**). The disease phenotype is characterized by degenerative neurological disorder (ataxia) and hypertrophic cardiomyopathy; males and females are equally affected *(69)*. Although rare, FRDA is the most prevalent inherited ataxia, affecting approx 1 in 50,000 people in the United States. In most affected individuals, symptom onset occurs in the first two decades of life, and, usually, the neurological symptoms dominate the clinical picture. However, the cardiomyopathy is observed in all patients, and, in 70% of patients, cardiomyopathy develops into a life-threatening condition. Rarely, initial disease manifestations are caused by cardiomyopathy.

The disease gene was mapped to chromosome 9q13, where a 210 amino-acid protein called frataxin is encoded *(70,71)*. The most common mutation, present in 95% of cases, is the expansion of a GAA triplet-repeat polymorphism localized within an Alu sequence (*FRDA*-Alu) in the first intron of the *FRDA* gene *(72)*. Because of a founder effect of the main responsible mutation, the disease usually affects individuals of European, North African, Middle Eastern, and Indian origin. Truncating or missense mutations in FRDA have been identified *(73)*.

The GAA expansion in *FRDA*-Alu impairs transcription and reduces frataxin levels *(72)*. Frataxin is involved in the control of mitochondrial iron metabolism *(74)*, and it is thought to be involved in the iron–sulphur cluster biogenesis *(75)*. Whatever the exact primary role of frataxin might be, its deficiency leads to potentially harmful oxidative injury associated with excessive iron deposits in mitochondria. Current therapeutic attempts use antioxidant strategies, and such efforts are likely to be enhanced by the availability of animal models of the disease *(76)*. The promise of effective therapy is a rationale for genetic diagnosis. As outlined in Chapter 12, by Pandolfo, the diagnostic molecular test for FRDA is aimed at detecting the common mutation, the GAA triplet repeats in the first intron of the *FRDA* gene. Methods are also given for sequence analysis in individuals suspected of having point mutations.

13. The Cardiovascular Manifestations of Alagille Syndrome and *JAG1* Mutations

It has been longer than 30 yr since the original descriptions of Alagille syndrome as an autosomal-dominant disorder characterized by hepatic, cardiac, ocular, skeletal, and facial abnormalities *(77,78)*. The varied cardiovascular malformations with high penetrance were established early on. The recognition of abnormal karyotypes in 5 to 10% of patients resulted in the identification of a locus on chromosome 20, which eventually lead to the identification of *JAG1* as the Alagille syndrome disease gene.

Specific types of cardiovascular malformation are a cardinal feature of Alagille syndrome *(79)*. More than 90% of patients with Alagille syndrome have a cardiovascular anomaly, ranging from mild peripheral pulmonary stenosis to TOF with pulmonary atresia. Although right-sided defects are most common, left-sided cardiac abnormalities and septal defects are also present. A correlation between the type and location of the *JAG1* mutation, cardiac phenotype, and other manifestations has not been identified *(80–83)*. For the investigator pursuing genetic causes of cardiovascular disease in the young, *JAG1* deserves consideration even in the absence of extracardiac manifestations.

As pointed out in Chapter 13, by Goldmuntz et al., identifying *JAG1* mutations is challenging because of the size of *JAG1* (26 exons) and the type of the mutations, which include whole-gene deletions in 3 to 7% of cases. For this reason, methods include mutation detection by conformation-sensitive gel electrophoresis using genomic DNA, direct cDNA sequencing, and FISH to identify whole-gene deletions.

14. Array Analysis Applied to Malformed Hearts: Molecular Dissection of Tetralogy of Fallot

TOF (OMIM 187500) is the most common type of cyanotic congenital heart disease; it is estimated to occur in 3.3 per 10,000 live births and accounts for 6.8% of all congenital heart disease *(84)*. Genetic causes of TOF are being increasingly recognized. For example, approx 15% of patients with TOF have a deletion of chromosome 22q11 *(85)*, and nearly 7% of TOF patients have trisomy 21 (Down syndrome) *(86)*. Heterozygous mutations in the transcription factor, NKX2.5, have been identified in approx 4% of TOF patients *(87,88)*. TOF patients with Alagille syndrome have mutations in *JAG1 (81,89)*. Recently, mutations in the *ZFPM2* gene were identified in sporadic cases of TOF *(90)*. Despite these advances, the genetic cause of TOF is unknown in approx 70% of cases. Identification of specific genetic causes for TOF will allow for improved family counseling and provide insight into the developmental mechanisms that result in the TOF phenotype.

Microarray technology as a method for large-scale gene expression analysis is being increasingly used in the field of cardiovascular research. Chapter 14, by Sperling, summarizes the application of arrays to study gene expression profiles of congenital heart diseases, in particular the molecular portrait of TOF.

The sections of this chapter correspond to the several distinct steps of microarray experiments. A general introduction to the method, information on the selection of arrays, and preparation of labeled cDNA samples are given in Chapter 14. A specific focus of Chapter 14 is experimental design and data analysis.

15. DNA Mutational Analysis in Heterotaxy

Heterotaxy refers to a complex of multiple malformations with various *situs* abnormalities, primarily of the heart, lung, and spleen, as well as midline defects involving the gut and kidney, which, together, suggest a defect in left–right patterning. Heterotaxy is characterized by complex cardiac malformations; in addition to dextrocardia, the cardiac phenotype includes total anomalous pulmonary venous return, atrioventricular septal defect, pulmonary stenosis, double-outlet right ventricle, and systemic vein anomalies. Most cases of heterotaxy seem to occur sporadically; however, pedigree analysis of familial *situs* abnormalities have suggested both autosomal and X-linked transmission, supporting the idea that heterotaxy is genetically heterogeneous *(91)*. Defining the developmental basis of left–right patterning has been daunting because of the large number of genes involved and the different roles that these genes play across species. However, human genetic studies in individuals with heterotaxy syndromes, complemented by mechanistic studies in animal models, are illuminating the molecular basis for this complex phenotype.

Chapter 15, by Ware, provides methods for analysis of four genes whose mutations have been identified in human heterotaxy *(92–97)*. *ZIC3*, a zinc-finger transcription factor, causes X-linked heterotaxy. *Epidermal growth factor-CFC*, *ACVR2B*, and *LEFTYA* are all members of a TGF-β signal transduction pathway that is critical for proper left–right development. Point mutations have been identified in each of these genes using polymerase chain reaction-based mutation analysis strategies.

16. Use of DHPLC to Detect Mutations in Pediatric Cardiomyopathies

Cardiomyopathy, referring to cardiac dysfunction of unknown cause, is an important form of cardiovascular disease in the young. To date, the most common forms of dilated, hypertrophic, and restrictive cardiomyopathy, and of arrhythmogenic right ventricular dysplasia have been caused by heterozygous mutations in sarcomeric or cytoskeletal genes, and, in this way, exhibit overlap with neuromuscular disorders (reviewed in **refs. *54*, *56*,** and ***98–100***). However, recent reports have identified mutations in genes with diverse other functions, such as regulation of cell energy status *(26)* and transcriptional regulation *(101)*. As the list of genes whose mutations cause cardiomyopathy continues to grow, we can expect the diversity of gene functions to expand.

Despite this exciting progress, the genetic basis of many cases of pediatric cardiomyopathy remains unknown (idiopathic). Chapter 16, by Sehnert, is timely because identification of the genetic basis of cardiomyopathy continues to be primarily a research effort. To detect genetic variations (polymorphisms and mutations) in human DNA samples, a variety of methods are needed. Chapter 16 focuses on the use of DHPLC as a high-throughput method for mutation analysis.

Conclusion

This publication, a compilation of laboratory tools, is timely, because the genetic insights into cardiovascular disease, having moved from the bedside to the bench, now move from the bench back to the bedside. Consequently, it can be anticipated that the approaches outlined in this book will continue to move from the research laboratory to the clinical laboratory.

References

1. Hinton, R. B., Yutzey, K. E., and Benson, D. W. (2005) Congenital heart disease: genetic causes and developmental insights. *Prog. Pediatr. Cardiol.* **20,** 101–111.
2. Matsuoka, R., Kimura, M., Scambler, P. J., et al. (1998) Molecular and clinical study of 183 patients with conotruncal anomaly face syndrome. *Hum. Genet.* **103,** 70–80.
3. Driscoll, D. A., Budarf, M. L., and Emanuel, B. S. (1992) A genetic etiology for DiGeorge syndrome: consistent deletions and microdeletions of 22q11. *Am. J. Hum. Genet.* **50,** 924–933.
4. Wilson, D. I., Cross, I. E., Goodship, J. A., et al. (1992) A prospective cytogenetic study of 36 cases of DiGeorge syndrome. *Am. J. Hum. Genet.* **51,** 957–963.
5. Desmaze, C., Scambler, P., Prieur, M., et al. (1993) Routine diagnosis of DiGeorge syndrome by fluorescent *in situ* hybridization. *Hum. Genet.* **90,** 663–665.
6. McDonald-McGinn, D. M., Tonnesen, M. K., Laufer-Cahana, A., et al. (2001) Phenotype of the 22q11.2 deletion in individuals identified through an affected relative: cast a wide FISHing net! *Genet. Med.* **3,** 23–29.
7. Digilio, M. C., Angioni, A., De Santis, M., et al. (2003) Spectrum of clinical variability in familial deletion 22q11.2: from full manifestation to extremely mild clinical anomalies. *Clin. Genet.* **63,** 308–313.
8. Shooner, K. A., Rope, A. F., Hopkin, R. J., Andelfinger, G. U., and Benson, D. W. (2005) Genetic analyses in two extended families with deletion 22q11 syndrome: importance of extracardiac manifestations. *J. Pediatr.* **146,** 382–387.
9. Foundation V-C-FSE. VCFS Educational Foundation specialist fact sheet. Available at: http://www.vcfsef.org/. Last accessed 2004.
10. McDonald-McGinn, D. M., LaRossa, D., Goldmuntz, E., et al. (1997) The 22q11.2 deletion: screening, diagnostic workup, and outcome of results; report on 181 patients. *Genet. Test.* **1,** 99–108.

11. Perez, E. and Sullivan, K. E. (2002) Chromosome 22q11.2 deletion syndrome (DiGeorge and velocardiofacial syndromes). *Curr. Opin. Pediatr.* **14,** 678–683.
12. Cuneo, B. F. (2001) 22q11.2 deletion syndrome: DiGeorge, velocardiofacial, and conotruncal anomaly face syndromes. *Curr. Opin. Pediatr.* **13,** 465–472.
13. McDonald-McGinn, D. M., Kirschner, R., Goldmuntz, E., et al. (1999) The Philadelphia story: the 22q11.2 deletion: report on 250 patients. *Genet. Couns.* **10,** 11–24.
14. Botto, L. D., May, K., Fernhoff, P. M., et al. (2003) A population-based study of the 22q11.2 deletion: phenotype, incidence, and contribution to major birth defects in the population. *Pediatrics* 112, 101–107.
15. Ryan, A. K., Goodship, J. A., Wilson, D. I., et al. (1997) Spectrum of clinical features associated with interstitial chromosome 22q11 deletions: a European collaborative study. *J. Med. Genet.* **34,** 798–804.
16. Swillen, A., Devriendt, K., Vantrappen, G., et al. (1998) Familial deletions of chromosome 22q11: the Leuven experience. *Am. J. Med. Genet.* **80,** 531–532.
17. McElhinney, D. B., McDonald-McGinn, D., Zackai, E. H., and Goldmuntz, E. (2001) Cardiovascular anomalies in patients diagnosed with a chromosome 22q11 deletion beyond 6 months of age. *Pediatrics* 108, E104.
18. Cohen, E., Chow, E. W., Weksberg, R., and Bassett, A. S. (1999) Phenotype of adults with the 22q11 deletion syndrome: a review. *Am. J. Med. Genet.* **86,** 359–365.
19. Mahle, W. T., Crisalli, J., Coleman, K., et al. (2003) Deletion of chromosome 22q11.2 and outcome in patients with pulmonary atresia and ventricular septal defect. *Ann. Thorac. Surg.* **76,** 567–571.
20. Keating, M., Atkinson, D., Dunn, C., Timothy, K., Vincent, G. M., and Leppert, M. (1991) Linkage of a cardiac arrhythmia, the long QT syndrome, and the Harvey ras-1 gene. *Science* **252,** 704–706.
21. Benson, D. W. (2004) Genetics of atrioventricular conduction disease in humans. *Anat. Rec. A. Discov. Mol. Cell. Evol. Biol.* **280,** 934–939.
22. Brugada, P., Brugada, R., Antzelevitch, C., and Brugada, J. (2005) The Brugada syndrome. *Arch. Mal. Coeur. Vaiss.* **98,** 115–122.
23. McNair, W. P., Ku, L., Taylor, M. R., et al. (2004) SCN5A mutation associated with dilated cardiomyopathy, conduction disorder, and arrhythmia. *Circulation* **110,** 2163–2167.
24. Olson, T. M., Michels, V. V., Ballew, J. D., et al. (2005) Sodium channel mutations and susceptibility to heart failure and atrial fibrillation. *JAMA.* **293,** 447–454.
25. Benson, D. W., Wang, D. W., Dyment, M., et al. (2003) Congenital sick sinus syndrome caused by recessive mutations in the cardiac sodium channel gene (SCN5A). *J. Clin. Invest.* **112,** 1019–1028.
26. Arad, M., Benson, D. W., Perez-Atayde, A. R., et al. (2002) Constitutively active AMP kinase mutations cause glycogen storage disease mimicking hypertrophic cardiomyopathy. *J. Clin. Invest.* 109, 357–362.
27. Laitinen, P. J., Brown, K. M., Piippo, K., et al. (2001) Mutations of the cardiac ryanodine receptor (RyR2) gene in familial polymorphic ventricular tachycardia. *Circulation* **103,** 485–490.

28. Priori, S. G., Napolitano, C., Tiso, N., et al. (2001) Mutations in the cardiac ryanodine receptor gene (hRyR2) underlie catecholaminergic polymorphic ventricular tachycardia. *Circulation* **103**, 196–200.

29. Lahat H, Pras E, Olender T, et al. (2001) A missense mutation in a highly conserved region of CASQ2 is associated with autosomal recessive catecholamine-induced polymorphic ventricular tachycardia in Bedouin families from Israel. *Am. J. Hum. Genet.* **69**, 1378–1384.

30. Laohakunakorn, P., Benson, D. W., Yang, P., Yang, T., Roden, D. M., and Kugler, J. D. (2003) Bidirectional ventricular tachycardia and channelopathy. *Am. J. Cardiol.* **92**, 991–995.

31. Bloise, R., Napolitano, C., and Priori, S. G. (2002) Romano-Ward and other congenital long QT syndromes. *Cardiovasc. Drugs Ther.* **16**, 19–23.

32. Kainulainen, K., Pulkkinen, L., Savolainen, A., Kaitila, I., and Peltonen, L. (1990) Location on chromosome 15 of the gene defect causing Marfan syndrome. *N. Engl. J. Med.* **323**, 935–939.

33. Dietz, H. C., Cutting, G. R., Pyeritz, R. E., et al. (1991) Marfan syndrome caused by a recurrent de novo missense mutation in the fibrillin gene. *Nature* **352**, 337–339.

34. The FBN1 mutations database. 2004. Available from: www.umd.be:2030.

35. Robinson, P. N. and Godfrey, M. (2000) The molecular genetics of Marfan syndrome and related microfibrillopathies. *J. Med. Genet.* **37**, 9–25.

36. Byers, P. H. (2004) Determination of the molecular basis of Marfan syndrome: a growth industry. *J. Clin. Invest.* **114**, 161–163.

37. Judge DP, Biery NJ, Keene DR, et al. (2004) Evidence for a critical contribution of haploinsufficiency in the complex pathogenesis of Marfan syndrome. *J. Clin. Invest.* **114**, 172–181.

38. Allanson, J. E. (1987) Noonan syndrome. *J. Med. Genet.* **24**, 9–13.

39. Noonan, J. A. (1968) Hypertelorism with Turner phenotype. A new syndrome with associated congenital heart disease. *Am. J. Dis. Child.* **116**, 373–380.

40. Jamieson, C. R., van der Burgt, I., Brady, A. F., et al. (1994) Mapping a gene for Noonan syndrome to the long arm of chromosome 12. *Nat. Genet.* 8, 357–360.

41. Brady, A. F., Jamieson, C. R., van der Burgt, I., et al. (1997) Further delineation of the critical region for noonan syndrome on the long arm of chromosome 12. *Eur. J. Hum. Genet.* 5, 336–337.

42. Tartaglia, M., Mehler, E. L., Goldberg, R., et al. (2001) Mutations in PTPN11, encoding the protein tyrosine phosphatase SHP-2, cause Noonan syndrome. *Nat. Genet.* **29**, 465–468.

43. Tartaglia, M., Kalidas, K., Shaw, A., et al. (2002) PTPN11 mutations in Noonan syndrome: molecular spectrum, genotype-phenotype correlation, and phenotypic heterogeneity. *Am. J. Hum. Genet.* **70**, 1555–1563.

44. Tartaglia, M., Niemeyer, C. M., Fragale, A., et al. (2003) Somatic mutations in PTPN11 in juvenile myelomonocytic leukemia, myelodysplastic syndromes and acute myeloid leukemia. *Nat. Genet.* **34**, 148–150.

45. Curran, M. E., Atkinson, D. L., Ewart, A. K., Morris, C. A., Leppert, M. F., and Keating, M. T. (1993) The elastin gene is disrupted by a translocation associated with supravalvular aortic stenosis. *Cell* **73**, 159–168.

46. Ewart, A. K., Morris, C. A., Atkinson, D., et al. (1993) Hemizygosity at the elastin locus in a developmental disorder, Williams syndrome. *Nat. Genet.* **5,** 11–16.

47. Li, D. Y., Toland, A. E., Boak, B. B., et al. (1997) Elastin point mutations cause an obstructive vascular disease, supravalvular aortic stenosis. *Hum. Mol. Genet.* **6,** 1021–1028.

48. Hallidie-Smith, K. A. and Karas, S. (1988) Cardiac anomalies in Williams-Beuren syndrome. *Arch. Dis. Child.* **63,** 809–813.

49. Eronen, M., Peippo, M., Hiippala, A., et al. (2002) Cardiovascular manifestations in 75 patients with Williams syndrome. *J. Med. Genet.* **39,** 554–558.

50. Stromme, P., Bjornstad, P. G., and Ramstad, K. (2002) Prevalence estimation of Williams syndrome. *J. Child. Neurol.* **17,** 269–271.

51. Osborne, L. R., Li, M., Pober, B., et al. (2001) A 1.5 million-base pair inversion polymorphism in families with Williams-Beuren syndrome. *Nat. Genet.* **29,** 321–325.

52. Morris, C. A., Mervis, C. B., Hobart, H. H., et al. (2003) GTF2I hemizygosity implicated in mental retardation in Williams syndrome: genotype-phenotype analysis of five families with deletions in the Williams syndrome region. *Am. J. Med. Genet. A.* **123,** 45–59.

53. Richardson, P., McKenna, W., Bristow, M., et al. (1996) Report of the 1995 World Health Organization/International Society and Federation of Cardiology Task Force on the definition and classification of cardiomyopathies. *Circulation* **93,** 841–842.

54. Seidman, J. G. and Seidman, C. (2001) The genetic basis for cardiomyopathy: from mutation identification to mechanistic paradigms. *Cell* **104,** 557–567.

55. Ahmad, F. (2003) The molecular genetics of arrhythmogenic right ventricular dysplasia-cardiomyopathy. *Clin. Invest. Med.* **26,** 167–178.

56. Chien, K. R. (2003) Genotype, phenotype: upstairs, downstairs in the family of cardiomyopathies. *J. Clin. Invest.* **111,** 175–178.

57. Hwang, J. J., Dzau, V. J., and Liew, C. C. (2001) Genomics and the pathophysiology of heart failure. *Curr. Cardiol. Rep.* **3,** 198–207.

58. Hwang, J. J., Allen, P. D., Tseng, G. C., et al. (2002) Microarray gene expression profiles in dilated and hypertrophic cardiomyopathic end-stage heart failure. *Physiol. Genomics* **10,** 31–44.

59. Li, K. C., Liu, C. T., Sun, W., Yuan, S., and Yu, T. (2004) A system for enhancing genome-wide coexpression dynamics study. *Proc. Natl. Acad. Sci. USA* **101,** 15,561–15,566.

60. Takahashi, M., Lin, Y. M., Nakamura, Y., and Furukawa, Y. (2004) Isolation and characterization of a novel gene CLUAP1 whose expression is frequently upregulated in colon cancer. *Oncogene* **23,** 9289–9294.

61. Barrans, J. D., Allen, P. D., Stamatiou, D., Dzau, V. J., and Liew, C. C. (2002) Global gene expression profiling of end-stage dilated cardiomyopathy using a human cardiovascular-based cDNA microarray. *Am. J. Pathol.* **160,** 2035–2043.

62. Plaster, N. M., Tawil, R., Tristani-Firouzi, M., et al. (2001) Mutations in Kir2.1 cause the developmental and episodic electrical phenotypes of Andersen's syndrome. *Cell* **105,** 511–519.

63. Andelfinger, G., Tapper, A. R., Welch, R. C., Vanoye, C. G., George, A. L., Jr., and Benson, D. W. (2002) KCNJ2 mutation results in Andersen syndrome with sex-specific cardiac and skeletal muscle phenotypes. *Am. J. Hum. Genet.* **71,** 663–668.

64. Tristani-Firouzi, M., Jensen, J. L., Donaldson, M. R., et al. (2002) Functional and clinical characterization of KCNJ2 mutations associated with LQT7 (Andersen syndrome). *J. Clin. Invest.* **110,** 381–388.

65. Isaacs, H., Jr. (2004) Fetal and neonatal cardiac tumors. *Pediatr. Cardiol.* **25,** 252–273.

66. Jones, A. C., Shyamsundar, M. M., Thomas, M. W., et al. (1999) Comprehensive mutation analysis of TSC1 and TSC2-and phenotypic correlations in 150 families with tuberous sclerosis. *Am. J. Hum. Genet.* **64,** 1305–1315.

67. Pandolfo, M. (2001) Molecular basis of Friedreich ataxia. *Mov. Disord.* **16,** 815–821.

68. Palau, F. (2001) Friedreich's ataxia and frataxin: molecular genetics, evolution and pathogenesis (Review). *Int. J. Mol. Med.* **7,** 581–589.

69. Harding, A. E. (1981) Friedreich's ataxia: a clinical and genetic study of 90 families with an analysis of early diagnostic criteria and intrafamilial clustering of clinical features. *Brain* **104,** 589–620.

70. Chamberlain, S., Shaw, J., Rowland, A., et al. (1988) Mapping of mutation causing Friedreich's ataxia to human chromosome 9. *Nature* **334,** 248–250.

71. Campuzano, V., Montermini, L., Molto, M. D., et al. (1996) Friedreich's ataxia: autosomal recessive disease caused by an intronic GAA triplet repeat expansion. *Science* **271,** 1423–1427.

72. Campuzano, V., Montermini, L., Lutz, Y., et al. (1997) Frataxin is reduced in Friedreich ataxia patients and is associated with mitochondrial membranes. *Hum. Mol. Genet.* **6,** 1771–1780.

73. Cossee, M., Durr, A., Schmitt, M., et al. (1999) Friedreich's ataxia: point mutations and clinical presentation of compound heterozygotes. *Ann. Neurol.* **45,** 200–206.

74. Cavadini, P., Gellera, C., Patel, P. I., and Isaya, G. (2000) Human frataxin maintains mitochondrial iron homeostasis in Saccharomyces cerevisiae. *Hum. Mol. Genet.* **9,** 2523–2530.

75. Yoon, T. and Cowan, J. A. (2004) Frataxin-mediated iron delivery to ferrochelatase in the final step of heme biosynthesis. *J. Biol. Chem.* **279,** 25,943–25,946.

76. Voncken, M., Ioannou, P., and Delatycki, M. B. (2004) Friedreich ataxia-update on pathogenesis and possible therapies. *Neurogenetics* **5,** 1–8.

77. Watson, G. H. and Miller, V. (1973) Arteriohepatic dysplasia: familial pulmonary arterial stenosis with neonatal liver disease. *Arch. Dis. Child.* **48,** 459–466.

78. Alagille, D., Odievre, M., Gautier, M. and Dommergues, J. P. (1975) Hepatic ductular hypoplasia associated with characteristic facies, vertebral malformations, retarded physical, mental, and sexual development, and cardiac murmur. *J. Pediatr.* **86,** 63–71.

79. McElhinney, D. B., Krantz, I. D., Bason, L., et al. (2002) Analysis of cardiovascular phenotype and genotype-phenotype correlation in individuals with a JAG1 mutation and/or Alagille syndrome. *Circulation* **106**, 2567–2574.
80. Krantz, I. D., Smith, R., Colliton, R. P., et al. (1999) Jagged1 mutations in patients ascertained with isolated congenital heart defects. *Am. J. Med. Genet.* **84,** 56–60.
81. Eldadah, Z. A., Hamosh, A., Biery, N. J., et al. (2001) Familial tetralogy of Fallot caused by mutation in the jagged1 gene. *Hum. Mol. Genet.* **10,** 163–169.
82. Le Caignec, C., Lefevre, M., Schott, J. J., et al. (2002) Familial deafness, congenital heart defects, and posterior embryotoxon caused by cysteine substitution in the first epidermal-growth-factor-like domain of jagged 1. *Am. J. Hum. Genet.* **71,** 180–186.
83. Kamath, B. M., Spinner, N. B., Emerick, K. M., et al. (2004) Vascular anomalies in Alagille syndrome: a significant cause of morbidity and mortality. *Circulation* **109**, 1354–1358.
84. Ferencz, C., Rubin, J. D., McCarter, R. J. et al. (1985) Congenital heart disease: prevalence at livebirth. The Baltimore-Washington Infant Study. *Am. J. Epidemiol.* **121,** 31–36.
85. Goldmuntz, E., Clark, B. J., Mitchell, L. E., et al. (1998) Frequency of 22q11 deletions in patients with conotruncal defects. *J. Am. Coll. Cardiol.* **32,** 492–498.
86. Ferenz, C., Correa-Villasenor, A., Loffredo, C. A. and Wilson, P. D. (1997) Malformations of the cardiac outflow tract. Genetic and environmental risk factors of major cardiovascular malformations: the Baltimore-Washington Infant Study: 1081–1989. Futura Publishing, Armonk, NY.
87. Benson, D. W., Silberbach, G. M., Kavanaugh-McHugh, A., et al. (1999) Mutations in the cardiac transcription factor NKX2.5 affect diverse cardiac developmental pathways. *J. Clin. Invest.* **104,** 1567–1573.
88. Goldmuntz, E., Geiger, E. and Benson, D. W. (2001) NKX2.5 mutations in patients with tetralogy of fallot. *Circulation* **104,** 2565–2568.
89. Kamath, B. M., Bason, L., Piccoli, D. A., Krantz, I. D. and Spinner, N. B. (2003) Consequences of JAG1 mutations. *J. Med. Genet.* **40,** 891–895.
90. Pizzuti, A., Sarkozy, A., Newton, A. L., et al. (2003) Mutations of ZFPM2/FOG2 gene in sporadic cases of tetralogy of Fallot. *Hum. Mutat.* **22,** 372–377.
91. Carmi, R., Boughman, J. A. and Rosenbaum, K. R. (1992) Human situs determination is probably controlled by several different genes. *Am. J. Med. Genet.* **44,** 246–249.
92. Gebbia, M., Ferrero, G. B., Pilia, G., et al. (1997) X-linked situs abnormalities result from mutations in ZIC3. *Nat. Genet.* **17,** 305–308.
93. Kosaki, K., Bassi, M. T., Kosaki, R., et al. (1999) Characterization and mutation analysis of human LEFTY A and LEFTY B, homologues of murine genes implicated in left-right axis development. *Am. J. Hum. Genet.* **64,** 712–721.
94. Kosaki, R., Gebbia, M., Kosaki, K., et al. (1999) Left-right axis malformations associated with mutations in ACVR2B, the gene for human activin receptor type IIB. *Am. J. Med. Genet.* **82,** 70–76.

95. Megarbane, A., Salem, N., Stephan, E., et al. (2000) X-linked transposition of the great arteries and incomplete penetrance among males with a nonsense mutation in ZIC3. *Eur. J. Hum. Genet.* **8,** 704–708.

96. Ware, S. M., Peng, J., Zhu, L., et al. (2004) Identification and functional analysis of ZIC3 mutations in heterotaxy and related congenital heart defects. *Am. J. Hum. Genet.* **74,** 93–105.

97. Bamford, R. N., Roessler, E., Burdine, R. D., et al. (2000) Loss-of-function mutations in the EGF-CFC gene CFC1 are associated with human left-right laterality defects. *Nat. Genet.* **26,** 365–369.

98. Fatkin, D. and Graham, R. M. (2002) Molecular mechanisms of inherited cardiomyopathies. *Physiol. Rev.* **82,** 945–980.

99. Gerull, B., Heuser, A., Wichter, T., et al. (2004) Mutations in the desmosomal protein plakophilin-2 are common in arrhythmogenic right ventricular cardiomyopathy. *Nat. Genet.* **36,** 1162–1164.

100. Burkett E. L. and Hershberger R. E. (2005) Clinical and genetic issues in familial dilated cardiomyopathy. *J. Am. Coll. Cardiol.* **45,** 969–981.

101. Schonberger, J., Wang, L., Shin, J. T., et al. (2005) Mutation in the transcriptional coactivator EYA4 causes dilated cardiomyopathy and sensorineural hearing loss. *Nat. Genet.* **37,** 418–422.

2

Genetics of Cardiac Septation Defects and Their Pre-Implantation Diagnosis

Deborah A. McDermott, Craig T. Basson, and Cathy J. Hatcher

Summary

Cardiac septation defects are among the most common birth defects in humans. The frequency of these defects reflects the complexity of cardiogenesis, which involves such processes as cell proliferation, migration, differentiation, and morphogenetic interactions.

Major advances in the understanding of the underlying genetic etiologies of cardiac septation defects have provided insight into the genetic pathways involved. These genetic factors are most often transcription factors involved in the early stages of cardiogenesis. The ability to modify these genes in animal models is providing a better understanding of the role of these genes in common pathways leading to diverse forms of cardiac defects. Ultimately, our understanding of these basic processes should lead to molecular-based treatment and prevention options for those individuals most at risk for such birth defects.

Key Words: Heart; congenital; genetics; septation defect; transcription factor.

1. Introduction

Congenital heart malformations (CHMs) occur in more than 0.5 to 1% of live births *(1)* and are among the most common birth defects in newborns. Atrial septal defects (ASDs) and ventricular septal defects (VSDs) account for the greatest proportion of CHMs *(2)*. Serial echocardiography of large newborn populations has revealed that VSDs are present at birth in approx 5% of all newborns *(3)*, but most VSDs close spontaneously before adolescence *(4)*. In recent years, our understanding of the etiology of certain CHMs has increased significantly. Great strides have been made in the identification of genes responsible for both syndromic and nonsyndromic forms of CHM, and their role in cardiogenesis. By identifying human gene mutations associated with syndromes affecting cardiac chamber septation, in vitro and in vivo mod-

From: *Methods in Molecular Medicine, vol. 126: Congenital Heart Disease: Molecular Diagnostics*
Edited by: M. Kearns-Jonker © Humana Press Inc., Totowa, NJ

els of abnormal cardiogenesis can be created, and investigators can define genetic interactions that regulate cardiogenesis.

To understand how gene mutations cause syndromic and nonsyndromic forms of septal defects, one must delineate the process of septal formation during cardiogenesis. Cardiogenesis requires a complex series of events, including proliferation, migration, differentiation, and morphogenetic interactions involving cells from several embryonic origins. The susceptibility of the heart to developmental anomalies reflects the complexity of these embryonic processes. Among the most sensitive cardiac structures are the atrial and ventricular septa. Separation of the four cardiac chambers involves more than mere formation of simple partitions between the chambers. After formation of the primary heart tube, this linear tube loops to the right, creating inflow and outflow limbs. The primitive chambers become recognizable by the constrictions that demarcate the sinus venosus, common atrial chamber, atrioventricular (AV) canal, ventricular chamber, and conotruncus. Initially, endocardial cushions form within the common AV junction. Simultaneously, the myocardium of the atrial and ventricular chambers develop trabeculations of endocardium-covered myocardium that extend into the lumen of the heart tube. Ultimately, all of the septa fuse with the AV cushions, and these cushions divide the AV canal into left and right canals. Although many genes that regulate septogenesis remain to be identified, several genes have been shown to play key roles in septation.

Historically, recurrence risk assessment for CHM in individuals and their relatives was based on epidemiological data *(5,6)*. As the genetic bases for many types of CHMs are elucidated, genetic counseling for such families is increasingly refined and effective. The ability to offer genetic testing will aid in identifying those at-risk individuals who may present with normal cardiac evaluations but who may be susceptible to complications later in life, or for having children with more severe presentations of disease. A detailed three-generation family history is useful in the evaluation of the individual with a CHM. Additionally, a peripheral blood karyotype is warranted in those individuals with multiple congenital anomalies.

CHMs can be detected and diagnosed prenatally, and, in some instances, may be amenable to fetal intervention *(7)*. Furthermore, vast improvements in the surgical and medical management of individuals with CHMs during the last several decades has dramatically increased the number of adults living with CHMs *(4)*. ASDs, which occur more commonly in women than men, are among the most common CHMs to be identified in the adult CHM patient *(4)*. Because these individuals have their own families, clinicians are likely to see an increase in clusters of familial CHMs.

At present, genetic testing for the majority of the genes implicated in CHMs is available only on a research basis *(8)*. Continued research to better understand the incidence, penetrance, and expressivity of mutations in these and other genes involved in CHMs is critical before such tests warrant widespread clinical application. In this chapter, we discuss syndromes that are characterized by the presence of ASDs and/or VSDs and their causative genes. We provide an overview of some of the better understood genes investigated to date, but this overview is not a comprehensive list. Mendelian syndromes and chromosomal etiologies with associated CHMs that can include septation defects are listed in **Table 1** *(9–11)*. The number of genes associated with ASDs and VSDs in patients is rapidly increasing.

Although the technology best used to screen for mutations (e.g., denaturing high-performance liquid chromatography, denaturing gel electrophoresis, single-strand conformational polymorphism analysis, and automated sequencing) can be legitimately debated, and largely reflects institutional and laboratory biases, we do not focus on this technical aspect. Instead, we focus on the biological processes underlying different genetically determined septation defects so that such understanding may appropriately inform the choice of genes to be screened for mutations in any given patient. From the perspective of routine clinical testing, it is already impractical to screen all septation defect-associated genes in any given patient, and the selection of genes to be screened by the clinician evaluating the patient to undergo testing will be an increasingly challenging problem. Thus, the methods used to make this selection should rely on a thorough understanding of the phenotypes, expression patterns, and functional developmental defects associated with mutations in each gene.

1.1. Holt–Oram Syndrome: TBX5

Holt–Oram syndrome (HOS) is an autosomal-dominant disorder characterized by structural and/or conductive heart deformities in the setting of upper-limb radial ray anomalies *(12)*. HOS is estimated to occur in approx 1 in 100,000 live births, and most individuals represent sporadic cases, i.e., new mutations. There is significant phenotypic variability observed between affected individuals even in a single family, suggesting a role for modifying genetic factors. The limb findings associated with HOS are fully penetrant and may be unilateral, bilateral/symmetric, or bilateral/asymmetric. A range of upper-limb deformities (ULDs) with varying severity may be observed, such as triphalangeal or absent thumb(s), severe limb hypoplasia, phocomelia, abnormal forearm pronation and supination, possible sloping shoulders, and restriction of shoulder joint movement. Polydactyly is not a feature of HOS. Left-sided ULDs are often more severe than right-sided ULDs. In some affected

Table 1
Mendelian and Chromosomal Forms of ASD, VSD, and AVSD

Disease	Gene (chromosomal location)	OMIM or reference no.	Clinical features, including CHMs
Autosomal-dominant conditions			
Alagille syndrome	JAG1 (20p12)	118450	Peripheral PS, ASD, TOF, deafness, decreased number of intrahepatic bile ducts, posterior embryotoxon, triangular facies
ASD with AV conduction defects	NKX2.5 (5q34)	108900	ASD progressive AV block, TOF, VSD, tricuspid valve anomalies
ASD2	GATA4 (8p23.1–p22)	607941	ASD, VSD, AVSD, PS, mitral and aortic valve regurgitation
Autosomal-dominant ASD	(5p)	10	Incomplete penetrance, aortic stenosis, atrial septal aneurysm, persistent left superior vena cava
ASD1	(6p21.3)	108800	Autosomal-dominant ASD
AVSD	(1p31–p21)	600309	Autosomal-dominant AVSD, incomplete penetrance, and variable expressivity
AVSD2	CRELD1/CIRRIN	607170	Partial AVSD with heterotaxy
DiGeorge syndrome	TBX1 (del22q11)	188400	VSD, right sided aortic arch, TOF, learning disabilities, secondary palate clefts
Holt–Oram syndrome	TBX5 (12q24.1)	142900	Ostium secundum ASD, VSD, progressive heart block, upper-limb deformity
Duane–Radial Ray syndrome (Okihiro syndrome)	SALL4 (20q13.13–q13.2)	607323	Radial ray abnormalities, Duane anomaly, sensorineural and/or conductive deafness, ASD (infrequent), Hirschsprung disease, anal stenosis, imperforate anus, renal abnormalities, fused cervical vertebrae, hypoplasia of pectoral and upper-limb musculature

	Gene (location)	OMIM	Clinical features
Noonan syndrome	PTPN11 (12q24.1)	163950	PS, left ventricular hypertrophy, cardiac septal defects, webbed neck, postnatal short stature, characteristic facial features, cryptorchidism, bleeding diathesis, vertebral anomalies
Autosomal-recessive conditions			
Ellis–van Creveld syndrome	EVC (4p16), EVC2 (4p16)	225500	Common atrium, ASD, AVSD, short limbs, short ribs, postaxial polydactyly, dysplastic teeth and nails
Ivemark syndrome	Not identified	208530	Asplenia or polysplenia, abnormal lobation of lungs, malposition and maldevelopment of abdominal organs, ASD, VSD, AVSD, PS
McKusick–Kaufmann syndrome	MKKS (20p12)	236700	Hydrometrocolpos, postaxial polydactyly, ASD, VSD, AVSD, common atrium
Smith–Lemli–Opitz	DHCR7 (11q12–q13)	270400	ASD, VSD, AVSD, PDA, aortic coarctation, short stature, failure to thrive, low cholesterol levels, facial dysmorphism, abnormal male external genitalia
TARP syndrome	Xp11.23–q13.3	300442	Club foot, ASD, Robin sequence, persistent left superior vena cava, lethal in infancy

Chromosomal etiologies			
Chromosomal anomaly			Clinical features
Down syndrome/trisomy 21			AVSD, common neonatal findings include hypotonia, flat facial profile, poor motor reflex, slanted palpebral fissures, joint hyperflexibility, excess skin on posterior neck, transpalmar crease
Trisomy 13			AVSD, holoprosencephaly-type defects, severe mental defect, minor motor seizures, polydactyly, rocker-bottom feet, mild microcephaly, single umbilical artery

(continued)

Table 1 (continued)

Disease	Clinical features
Trisomy 18	AVSD, clenched hand and overlapping fingers, polyhydramnios, single umbilical artery, hypertonic, mental deficiency, short sternum, small nipples, inguinal or umbilical hernia, hypoplastic nails
3pdel	AVSD, mental and growth retardation (prenatal onset), hypotonia, microcephaly, bilateral ptosis, upper limb postaxial polydactyly
Turner syndrome (45,X)	Bicuspid aortic valve, aortic coarctation, MVP, AVSD, short stature (female), congenital lymphedema, broad chest with widely spaced nipples, ovarian dysgenesis, narrow convex nails
Interstitial dupl 19p	VSD, urinary tract anomalies, renal anomalies, rocker-bottom feet, small thorax, mild hydrops fetalis, nuchal edema

ASD, atrial septal defect; AV, atrioventricular; AVSD, AV septal defect; MVP, mitral valve prolapse; PDA, patent ductus arteriosis; PS, pulmonic stenosis; TOF, Tetrology of Fallot; VSD, ventricular septal defect.

individuals, the ULD may involve only the carpal bones and be visible only on X-ray. Initial clinical evaluation should, therefore, include posterior–anterior hand X-rays of the affected individual's parents to rule out any carpal bone anomalies. This information, in the absence of mutational analysis, is critical for offering accurate recurrence risk estimates for the family.

Heart defects in HOS are incompletely penetrant, occurring in approx 75% of affected individuals *(13)*. When they do occur, expressivity is highly variable. The most typical CHMs associated with HOS are ostium secundum ASDs, which may be associated with isomerism and can present as a common atrium. Similarly, VSDs, particularly of the muscular trabeculated septum are frequent manifestations *(13,14)*. Such defects are often associated with abnormal ventricular trabeculation. Numerous other complex CHMs have been associated with HOS, but conotruncal anomalies and ostium primum ASDs are not cardinal features of this syndrome. All individuals with HOS, regardless of the presence of a CHM, are at risk for cardiac conduction disease. Such conduction disease can be progressive, resulting in complete heart block with or without atrial fibrillation, and mandates routine electrocardiographic evaluation for all individuals with HOS.

Mutations in *TBX5,* a member of the T-box transcription factor gene family, cause HOS. This gene is located at chromosome 12q24.1 *(14,15)*. The T-box gene family is characterized by a highly conserved T-box DNA-binding domain. Of the many *TBX5* mutations identified to date, most are nonsense or frameshift mutations, splice mutations, or chromosomal rearrangements that are predicted to produce HOS through *TBX5* haploinsufficiency. *TBX5* missense mutations do occur, and, unlike *TBX5* haploinsufficiency mutations, they have been associated in large family studies with more significant organ bias in their manifestations *(13)*. Because such genotype–phenotype correlations are only evident as statistically significant findings in population studies, they are not useful in predicting the individual patient's phenotype *(13,16)*. Only a single family potentially affected by HOS *(17)* has been shown not to be linked to chromosome 12q24.1, and, thus, if any intergenic genetic heterogeneity exists in HOS, it is very small.

The specific role of TBX5 in heart development is slowly being elucidated. TBX5 has been shown to play a role in chamber specification *(18)* as well as in inhibition of cardiomyocyte proliferation *(19)*. Therefore, TBX5 may participate in cardiogenesis by regulating cell proliferation in specific cardiac domains, resulting in the regional morphological features of the heart. Creation of a *Tbx5* knockout mouse *(20)* has provided an in vivo method for identifying downstream targets of Tbx5. Although these embryos died early in development, before cardiac looping, several observations were made before their death. Failed development of posterior sinoatrial structures resulted in a common atrium and a distorted right ventricle, thus, adding credence to the hypothesis that Tbx5 plays a role in cardiac septation. In addition, expression of several cardiac-specific genes, such as *Mlc2v*, *Irx4*, *Hey2*, *ANF*, *Nkx2.5*, and *Gata-4* were noted to be either decreased or absent in the *Tbx5*-null mice. However, only expressions of *ANF* and *Cx40* were altered in heterozygous *Tbx5* mice, which were also observed to have enlarged hearts with ASDs. Bruneau et al. *(20)* further demonstrated that Tbx5 acts synergistically with Nkx2.5 to transactivate expression of *Cx40*. Other biochemical studies have confirmed this finding and have demonstrated a synergy between Tbx5 and Nkx2.5 to transactivate expression of *ANF* *(21,22)*. Recent data from Garg et al. *(23)* suggests that Tbx5 also interacts with Gata-4. Identification of the downstream targets and cofactors of TBX5 is helpful in understanding the role of this transcription factor in cardiogenesis.

1.2. Familial ASDs With Progressive AV Block: NKX2.5

Schott et al. *(24)* identified mutations in *NKX2.5* (a member of the highly conserved NK homeobox transcription factor gene family) as the underlying cause for an autosomal-dominant cardiac disorder characterized by ostium secundum ASDs and postnatal progressive AV conduction defects. Unlike individuals with HOS, these patients did not exhibit limb deformity *(25)*. The families in this cohort had members with various other CHMs, including VSD, tetralogy of Fallot (TOF), subvalvular aortic stenosis, ventricular hypertrophy, pulmonary atresia, and mitral valve malformations. In another case, Pauli et al. *(26)* reported a patient with a distal 5q deletion, including the *NKX2.5* locus and who presented with an ASD, AV block, and ventricular myocardial noncompaction.

Benson and colleagues *(27)* provided further evidence for a diverse role for *NKX2.5* mutations in a variety of forms of congenital heart disease, including ASD, muscular VSD, VSD associated with TOF or double-outlet right ventricle (DORV), tricuspid valve abnormalities, and familial cardiomyopathy. Goldmuntz et al. *(28)* identified *NKX2.5* mutations in nonsyndromic TOF and estimated that *NKX2.5* mutations account for at least 4% of such cases. In a series of 114 prospectively enrolled individuals with TOF (in whom 22q11 deletions were excluded), they identified six individuals with *NKX2.5* mutations. The combination of right-sided aortic arch and pulmonary atresia were more common in the mutation-positive group. The authors demonstrated that reduced penetrance and variable expressivity were associated with these mutations, and that AV conduction disease was not associated with mutations located outside of the gene's DNA-binding homeodomain.

NKX2.5 mutations are proposed to contribute to a small but significant proportion of sporadic cases of ASD and hypoplastic left-heart syndrome (HLHS)

(29). One hundred forty-six individuals with a diagnosis of secundum ASD (n = 102), patent foramen ovale complicated by paradoxical embolism (n = 25), or HLHS (n = 19) were analyzed. Ten percent of the patients with ASD or patent foramen ovale reported a family history of heart defects, and 4% of the patients had AV block. A missense mutation, T178M, was identified in an ASD family without AV block, and in one child in the family with HLHS. A second previously reported disease-causing mutation, E21Q, was also identified, but did not segregate with disease in a family with ASD, leading one to question the significance of this variant. These findings also highlight the difficulty in establishing whether unique sequence variants found in isolated individuals with CHMs are truly responsible for disease pathogenesis.

McElhinney et al. *(30)* reported *NKX2.5* mutations in 3% of a population of prospectively enrolled patients afflicted with the following CHMs: TOF, secundum ASD (with and without AV block), truncus arteriosus, DORV, left transposition of the great arteries, interrupted aortic arch, HLHS, and aortic coarctation. Almost 90% of patients with *NKX2.5* mutations in this group reportedly had no family history of CHMs. Heterozygote status was confirmed in some available parents, suggesting decreased penetrance of these mutations. Interestingly, none of the 18 mutations, which consisted of missense mutations, an in-frame deletion, and an insertion resulting in premature translation termination, were localized to the homeodomain region. Thus, these studies highlighted the importance of mutational analysis, suggesting *NKX2.5* in nonhomeodomain NKX2.5 regions.

Given the various cardiac phenotypes observed in the previously mentioned families, the role of *NKX2.5* in other forms of CHMs as well as cardiac morphogenesis seems diverse. Although genotype–phenotype correlations have not borne out, the variable expressivity among affected individuals may reflect various interactions between *NKX2.5* and other modifier genes. Located on chromosome 5q35 *(31)*, the *NKX2.5* gene, the human homolog of *Drosophila* gene, *tinman,* is a marker of the cardiac lineage and is expressed in atrial and ventricular myocardium during development *(32)*. Mutations in the *Drosophila* gene, *tinman*, result in absence of the dorsal vessel, a relative of the vertebrate heart *(33)*. In vertebrates, *NKX2.5* is an important regulator of cardiac-restricted gene activity required during cardiogenesis; as demonstrated in mice deficient in *Nkx2.5*, which died before looping of the linear heart tube *(32)*. Biochemical analysis of mutant proteins demonstrated NKX2.5 haploinsufficiency as a cause of these cardiac defects *(34)*. The wide range of *NKX2.5* mutational cardiac phenotypes suggests a primary involvement of this transcription factor with other modifier genes at various stages of cardiogenesis. Ongoing efforts to uncover the downstream targets and synergistic partners of NKX2.5 have revealed a number of myocardial genes, including *ANF*, *MLC-2v*, *N-Myc*, *Msx2*, *eHAND*, *MEF2C (32)*, *TBX5 (21)*, and *GATA-4 (35)*.

1.3. Familial ASDs and VSDs: GATA4

A subset of familial, nonsyndromic cardiac septal defects has recently been linked to mutations in *GATA-4 (23)*, a member of the conserved GATA zinc-finger transcription factor family. Before this, Pehlivan demonstrated that individuals with a chromosomal deletion of 8p23.1, where *GATA-4* localizes, characteristically had a variety of cardiac septal defects *(36)*. Taken together, these data suggest that *GATA-4* and, potentially, other 8p genes, regulate septogenesis during cardiac development.

Initially, linkage of these CHMs to a single locus on chromosome 8p22–23 in a large, multigenerational family with an autosomal-dominant inheritance of ASDs revealed the presence of *GATA-4* within this region. Through sequence analysis of *GATA-4* in two large kindreds, Garg et al. *(23)* were able to associate two *GATA-4* mutations with these congenital heart defects. Besides the characteristic ASDs found in all affected members, individuals also presented with a variety of other congenital heart defects, including VSDs, AV septal defects (AVSDs), and pulmonic valvular stenosis. The association with AVSD and conotruncal anomalies distinguishes this syndrome from HOS. Nevertheless, missense mutation of *GATA-4* diminished DNA-binding activity and transcriptional activity of the transcription factor, and it abrogated a physical interaction between GATA-4 and TBX5.

GATA-4 mutations were not demonstrated in some ASD and VSD kindreds that were analyzed *(23)*. This observation, in addition to the finding that *GATA-4* is not consistently deleted in all individuals with CHMs who have 8p mutations *(36)*, suggests a role for other genes in close proximity to *GATA-4* as causative for the familial clusters. It is also conceivable that such genes may mediate the effects of *GATA-4* on cardiogenesis.

During mouse cardiogenesis, *Gata-4* is expressed in the atrial and ventricular myocardium, endocardium, endocardial cushions, and outflow tract *(37)*. Disruption of *Gata-4* in the mouse has revealed a phenotype that is consistent with its expression pattern. Deletion of *Gata-4* in mice causes arrested development between embryonic days 7.0 and 9.5, caused by defects in cardiac morphogenesis, specifically cardia bifida *(38)*. However, Pu et al. *(39)* showed that a conditional deletion of mouse *Gata-4* leads to DORV, common AV canal, and marked hypoplasia of both the trabecular and compact myocardium. In vitro experiments using embryonic stem cells showed that GATA-4 is essential for survival of cardioblasts and for terminal cardiomyocyte differentiation *(40,41)*. Several genes, such as α- and β-*MHC*, *ANF*, and cardiac *TnC*, are transcriptionally regulated by *Gata-4* *(42)* when studied by in vitro assays.

Data also show that *Gata-4* acts synergistically with *Nkx2.5* to activate *ANF* *(43)* as well as cardiac α-*actin* via the serum response factors *(44)*, and is influenced by interactions with FOG-2 to modulate GATA-dependent transcriptional activation, thus, acting as either an activator or repressor *(45,46)*. A potentially cooperative relationship between TBX5 and GATA-4 *(23)* is appealing, given the overlap in cardiac phenotypes associated with the mutations in these genes.

1.4. Ellis–van Creveld Syndrome: EVC and EVC2

Unlike other Mendelian forms of CHMs, Ellis van–Creveld syndrome (EvC) is inherited in an autosomal-recessive manner *(47)*. The hallmark features of EvC are congenital heart defects, which occur in at least 50% of affected individuals, as well as chondroectodermal dysplasia and bilateral postaxial polydactyly *(48,49)*. Such findings have not been reported in syndromes with septation defects caused by mutations in *TBX5*, *NKX2.5*, or *GATA-4*. Cardinal cardiac features include ostium secundum or ostium primum ASDs, as well as a common atrium. Complex CHMs have also been observed *(48–52)*. Occasional findings include polydactyly of the feet, and genitourinary anomalies *(49,51)*. EvC has been reported in a number of ethnic groups, but is particularly common in the Lancaster County, PA Amish population, where more than 12% of individuals are carriers for the disease, and approx 1 in 5000 people are affected *(50)*.

By studying affected families of Amish, Mexican, Ecuadorian, and Brazilian descent, Polymeropoulos et al. *(52)* initially mapped the genetic locus for EvC to chromosome 4p16.1. Subsequent positional cloning studies of affected Amish individuals enabled investigators to identify the novel *EVC* gene at this locus as a disease gene. The EVC protein is predicted to contain a leucine zipper, as well as putative nuclear localization signals and a transmembrane domain *(53)*, but its function remains unknown. Galdzicka et al. *(54)* also identified the *EVC2* gene. This gene is mutated in individuals affected by EvC, and also localizes to chromosome 4p16. Ruiz-Perez et al. *(55)* reported mutations in *EVC2* in a number of other affected individuals of varying ethnicities, but not in Amish families. *EVC* and *EVC2* are arranged in the genome in a "head-to-head" configuration, with transcription start sites separated by 2624 bp in humans. Expression of *EVC* and *EVC2* could be coordinated by the same promoter or by shared elements of overlapping promoters *(55)*. The EVC2 protein is predicted to encode a transmembrane domain, three coil-coiled regions, and a RhoGEF domain, and shares sequence homology to class IX nonmuscle myosin tail domains, but is not homologous to *EVC*. Northern blot analysis of *EVC2* revealed expression in the heart, placenta, lung, liver, skeletal muscle, kidney, and pancreas *(54)*. *In situ* hybridization of human embryonic tissue for *EVC* revealed low levels of mRNA in the developing bone, heart, kidney, and lung. Specifically, *EVC* expression was observed in the atrial and ventricular myocardium, as well as the atrial and interventricular septa *(53)*.

The availability of genetic testing, particularly in the setting of ultrasound diagnosis *(56)*, is an important advance in the management of at-risk pregnancies and newborns with EvC. By identifying new mutations in the *EVC* and *EVC2* genes, more information can be gained to understand how these two genes participate in cardiac and skeletal development. Further studies to elucidate the downstream targets may explain not only the mechanism by which mutations in *EVC* and *EVC2* lead to the manifestations of disease observed in affected individuals, but also may explain the mechanism by which these mutations produce either a skeletal or cardiac phenotype, or both.

1.5. VSD: 22q11.2 Genes and Other Candidates

VSDs are the most common form of CHM observed. They may occur as isolated defects, or in conjunction with other CHMs, such as those discussed in **Subheading 1.3**. VSDs are a common occurrence in individuals with 22q11-deletion syndrome, also referred to as DiGeorge syndrome and velocardiofacial syndrome *(57,58)*. Individuals with 22q11 chromosomal deletions often have characteristic facial features, palatal anomalies, mental/learning deficiencies, and endocrine and immunological findings, in addition to the cardiovascular defects. These characteristics aid in the diagnosis. McElhinney et al. *(59)* sought to determine the contribution of 22q11 deletion to VSDs in a group of 125 prospectively enrolled individuals with conoventricular, posterior malalignment, or conoseptal hypoplasia VSD. Although the authors identified 22q11 deletion in 10% of those individuals enrolled, the strongest predictors for chromosomal deletion were anomalies of aortic arch branching or sidedness, anomalies of the cervical aortic arch, or discontinuous pulmonary arteries in conjunction with VSD. In general, the contribution of 22q11 deletion to certain isolated VSDs is predicted to be minimal.

Recent evidence suggests that many features associated with DiGeorge syndrome are caused by haploinsufficiency of the *TBX1* gene, a member of the T-box gene family *(60–62)*. Mice with a hemizygous deletion of the 1.5-Mb region corresponding to human chromosome 22q11 exhibited conotruncal and parathyroid defects. After insertion of a human bacterial artificial chromosome containing the *TBX1* gene, however, only the conotruncal defects could be partially rescued *(62)*. Individuals who have the phenotypical features of 22q11.2-deletion syndrome, but have intact 22q11.2 chromosomes, have been shown to have mutations in *TBX1*, which localizes to this chromosomal region. Thus, *TBX1* may be a major determinant of the 22q11.2-deletion syndrome *(63)*.

Membranous VSD, with variable muscular septal involvement, has been observed in association with biventricular cardiomyopathy in transgenic mice lacking *Hey-2/CHF1 (64)*. Based on its expression pattern, *Hey-2/CHF1* has been implicated in the development of the ventricle, vasculature, somites, and retina *(65,66)*. The *Drosophila* gene, *gridlock*, a member of the hairy/enhancer of split-related family of genes, is expressed in a pattern similar to the mouse *Hey* genes, and functions downstream of Notch *(67)*. Although these genes have yet to be implicated in human CHMs, other Notch ligands have been implicated. Mutations in the *JAG1* gene, a Notch-receptor ligand, result in the autosomal dominantly inherited Alagille syndrome *(68,69)*, a multisystemic disorder with frequent cardiac involvement. Primarily, peripheral pulmonic stenosis occurs, although ASD, VSD, and TOF can also occur.

1.6. AV Septal Defects

AVSDs, also referred to as endocardial cushion defects or AV canal defects, result from developmental anomalies of the AV canal. The resulting AVSDs can range in severity and complexity, and may be partial (atrial or ventricular form) or complete (involve atrial and ventricular septa), which could reflect a polygenic basis for the various clinical presentations.

Epidemiological data on AVSDs from the Baltimore–Washington infant study have supported the idea of genetic heterogeneity and have provided other useful information regarding the various subtypes of AVSD *(70)*. Family history of CHMs is more commonly observed in individuals with the complete form of AVSD and with the partial atrial form. Also of note, complete AVSD and the partial ventricular form are more likely to occur in association with extracardiac anomalies, whereas nearly 55% of the partial atrial form occur as an isolated finding *(70)*. Preconceptual maternal diabetes is a risk factor for the complete form of AVSD, as well as other cardiac and noncardiac complications in newborns, thus, highlighting the importance of eliciting a detailed pregnancy history in the evaluation of such cases *(71)*.

In humans, AVSDs are most commonly associated with Down syndrome (trisomy 21). Down syndrome cell adhesion molecule has been proposed as a candidate gene for CHMs associated with Down syndrome *(70)*. AVSDs are also commonly associated with other chromosomal anomalies, including 3p25 deletion, 8p2 deletion, trisomy 13, and trisomy 18, often presenting as ventricular AVSDs *(70,72)*. Such chromosomal etiologies are generally characterized by additional clinical manifestations, including mental and growth retardation, as well other multiple congenital anomalies. AVSD is occasionally detected in Turner syndrome (chromosomal complement 45,X) and 22q11.2-deletion syndrome *(72)*. Autosomal-dominant AVSD, exhibiting incomplete penetrance and variable expressivity, has also been reported, with linkage to chromosomes 1p31–p21 and 3p25 *(73,74)*.

The *CRELD1*, or *cirrin*, gene was proposed as an AVSD candidate gene on 3p25. CRELD1 is a cell adhesion molecule that is expressed during heart development *(75)*. Robinson and colleagues *(76)* analyzed the *CRELD1* gene in individuals with both the complete and partial forms of AVSD. They reported distinct missense mutations in three patients, two patients with isolated partial AVSD (ostium primum ASD) and one patient with AVSD and heterotaxy. There were no mutations identified in 13 individuals with complete AVSD, suggesting genetic heterogeneity among the various subtypes. Each of the detected mutations occurred at highly conserved amino acid residues. Paternal inheritance was confirmed in one of the individuals with isolated partial AVSD, and the mutation was also detected in two of the subject's siblings. Neither the father nor the siblings had any identifiable CHM on echocardiogram, suggesting incomplete penetrance. These findings prompted Robinson et al. *(76)* to conclude that *CRELD1* is an AVSD susceptibility gene and that mutations in *CRELD1* are associated with an increased risk of developing partial AVSDs.

In some cases, Noonan syndrome, an autosomal-dominant, genetically heterogeneous syndrome that occurs in approximately every 1 in 1000 to 2500 live births, has been shown to result from mutations in the *PTPN11*, or *SHP-2*, gene on chromosome 12q24.1 *(77)*. This gene has been demonstrated to have a role in cardiac semilunar valvulogenesis, among other developmental activities. The CHMs typically associated with Noonan syndrome are pulmonic stenosis and hypertrophic cardiomyopathy, although AVSD has been reported in approx 15% of cases *(78)*. Individuals with Noonan syndrome also commonly have other diagnostic features, including webbed neck, dysmorphic facial features, proportionate short stature, chest deformity, cryptorchidism, mental retardation, and bleeding diatheses. Mutations in *PTPN11* have also been identified in individuals with multiple lentigines, electrocardiographic-conduction abnormalities, ocular hypertelorism, pulmonary stenosis, abnormal genitalia, retardation of growth, and sensorineural deafness syndrome *(79)*.

AVSD has been reported, although very rarely, in individuals suggested to have other Mendelian syndromes (e.g., EvC and HOS), but genetic analyses of genes associated with these syndromes have not been reported to confirm these clinical diagnoses. Similar to EvC, many autosomal-recessive syndromes in which AVSD and other CHMs have been observed involve skeletal abnormalities. McKusick–Kaufman syndrome, similar to EvC, is common in the Amish population and is caused by mutations in the *MKKS* gene on chromosome 20p12 *(80)*. This gene encodes a protein similar to the chaperonin proteins.

Clinical features include hydrometrocolpos in females, postaxial polydactyly, and CHMs. The autosomal-recessive oral–facial–digital syndromes, including short-rib polydactyly, have also been reported to have a risk for AVSD.

In addition to the syndromes discussed in **Subheading 1.6.**, AVSD is also commonly seen in association with developmental defects involving left–right axis formation. One example is Ivemark syndrome, characterized by asplenia, CHMs (mostly ASDs, AVSDs, and conotruncal malformations) *(81)*, malposition and maldevelopment of the abdominal organs, and abnormal lobation of the lungs. Ivemark syndrome is a recessive condition, but is most often sporadic.

Individuals with Smith–Lemli–Opitz syndrome, a recessive condition caused by mutations in the sterol δ-7-reductase on chromosome 11q12–q13 *(82)*, are also afflicted with AVSDs. In one report, approx 21% affected individuals had a diagnosis of AVSD *(83)*. Other common features of Smith–Lemli–Opitz include failure to thrive, low birth weight, dysmorphic facies, renal anomalies, genital anomalies in males, postaxial polydactyly, mental retardation, and low cholesterol levels.

1.7. Pre-Implantation Genetic Diagnosis for Congenital Heart Defects

The ability to offer genetic testing for CHM has been limited until recent years. Now that several causative gene defects, as discussed in **Subheadings 1.1.–1.7.**, have been identified for some cases of familial CHMs, increasing numbers of options are available. Before identification of these genes, couples interested in prenatal diagnosis for CHMs were limited to genetic counseling and general recurrence risk assessments, and to imaging modalities (such as ultrasound) or testing for chromosomal causes of CHMs in conjunction with amniocentesis or chorionic villus sampling. With the identification of single genes responsible for Mendelian forms of CHMs, the ability to offer pre-implantation genetic diagnosis (PGD) in combination with in vitro fertilization (IVF) is now a potential option for some couples who prefer earlier diagnosis than afforded by amniocentesis or chorionic villus sampling.

Successful PGD for CHM has been achieved for a pregnancy at 50% risk for HOS *(84)* in a couple pursuing IVF for premature ovarian failure. The proband had a previously reported mutation in exon 3 of *TBX5*, predicting a truncated protein(Glu69ter) *(14)*. The proband and his spouse wished to achieve a pregnancy unaffected by HOS, if possible.

2. Materials
1. *TBX5* oligonucleotide primers.
2. Polymerase chain reaction (PCR) reagents and equipment.

3. DNA-sequencing equipment.
4. DNA from single blastomeres and genomic DNA from parents and controls.
5. DNA restriction enzymes.
6. Lymphocyte separation gradient.
7. Single-cell separation methods.

3. Methods

3.1. IVF and Blastomere Biopsy

IVF procedures, intracytoplasmic sperm injection (ICSI), and blastomere biopsies were performed by the Cornell Center for Reproductive Medicine and Infertility using standard techniques *(85,86)*. This particular case required synchronization of an oocyte donor and the proband's spouse. Sperm from the proband, who has a personal history of HOS, was used for ICSI. Informed consent was obtained for all clinical procedures, blastomere biopsies, and genetic testing, in accordance with Weill Medical College of Cornell University Committee on Human Rights in Research.

3.2. Sequence Analysis for TBX5 Glu69ter Mutation

DNA was isolated from single blastomere biopsies. Biopsies were performed at 3 d after fertilization on five blastocysts obtained from fertilization (by ICSI) of five donor oocytes, using methods previously described *(85)*. DNA was isolated from peripheral blood samples from the proband (positive control heterozygous for Glu69ter), as well as the oocyte donor (negative control), who was previously determined not to carry a *TBX5* mutation by bidirectional sequence analysis of protein-coding exons 2 to 9.

Exon 3 of *TBX5*, as well as its flanking introns, was amplified from the blastomeres using a nested PCR approach. This approach was used because of the limited template DNA able to be isolated from these single cells. The validity of this method was confirmed by analyses of single lymphocytes isolated from whole-blood samples from the proband, the oocyte donor, and controls, in anticipation of testing the blastomeres.

Lymphocytes were separated from whole-blood samples by Ficoll–Paque density gradient, using previously described techniques *(14)*. Single lymphocytes were selected by direct micropipetting. Single lymphocytes and blastomeres were prepared using techniques described by Xu et al. *(86)*. Single cells and blastomeres were placed into 500-μL microcentrifuge tubes, stored at –30°C with 25 μL of lysis buffer. These samples were heated at 65°C for 10 min and placed immediately on ice, and 5 μL of neutralization buffer was added.

PCR was performed using standard techniques previously described for amplification of exon 2 and exons 4 to 9 of *TBX5*. A nested PCR approach was used to amplify exon 3. First-round PCR for exon 3 and its flanking introns was performed using primers 3GRN2 (5'-GGAAGGAGGAGCAGTCTC TGTGTT-3') and 3GFN (5'-GTGTCTTTTCTCCTCGTCCCTCTCTCTAC ACA-3') *(84)*. Standard PCR reagents and AmpliTaqGold polymerase (Applied Biosystems [ABI], Foster City, CA) were used with PCR conditions of 40 cycles of (95°C for 20 s; 67°C for 30 s; and 72°C for 45 s). The resultant PCR product was 242 bp.

Second-round PCR (final volume, 50 µL) was performed using 6 µL of first-round PCR product (1:100 dilution) as a template. Nested primers for the second-round PCR amplification of exon 3 were: 3GRN (5'-AGTTTGGGG AAGGAATGCCCACTAC-3') and 3GF1 (5'-GTGTCTTCTACACAACAA ACCATCTCACCTT-3') *(84)*. PCR was again performed with standard reagents and AmpliTaq Gold polymerase with PCR conditions of 35 cycles of (95°C for 20 s; 65°C for 30 s; and 72°C for 45 s). The product of the second-round amplification was 182 bp. Negative controls were included in both rounds of PCR. Two second-round PCR reactions were performed in parallel. One reaction used a NED fluorescent dye (ABI)-labeled 3GRN *(84)* primer to allow for visualization of restriction fragment length polymorphism (RFLP) products. After PCR amplification, sequence and RFLP analysis of the PCR products were performed.

Bidirectional sequence analysis was performed on an ABI 377 automated sequencer, using BigDye Terminator sequencing (ABI) reagents, according to the manufacturer's recommended techniques.

3.3. RFLP Analysis

Twenty-five microliters of amplified PCR product were digested with *Dde*I [4U] (Promega, Madison, WI) for 90 min at 37°C and analyzed by gel electrophoresis, as previously described *(14)*. The presence of the Glu69ter mutation resulted in a 123-bp product that could be visualized because of the use of the fluorescent 3GRN primer (*see* **Notes 1** and **2**).

Four of the five blastocysts were determined to be homozygous normal for *TBX5*. One blastocyst was determined to carry the Glu69ter mutation. The four normal blastocysts continued to grow well in culture after the blastomere biopsies. Two of the four blastocysts were transferred to the recipient. The two remaining blastocysts that were *TBX5* homozygous normal were cryopreserved through the clinical IVF program at Cornell for future transfer (*see* **Note 3**).

3.4. Clinical Follow-Up

Confirmation of pregnancy was confirmed by serum Γ-human chorionic gonadotropin. High-resolution ultrasound and amniocentesis were performed in the second trimester. There were no ultrasound anomalies suggestive of HOS. Sequence and RFLP analysis of DNA extracted from waste amniocytes confirmed the homozygous normal *TBX5* genotype. Clinical karyotype was normal. At delivery, cord blood was obtained for *TBX5* genotyping, which again was normal.

3.5. Conclusion

We have discussed several human genetic disorders that have primary malformations of the atrial and/or ventricular septa. Although great strides have been made in our understanding of the molecular basis of cardiac development, specifically septation of the heart, many modulatory genes and signaling pathways remain unknown or poorly characterized. Gene mutations may cause a spectrum of cardiac defects. Not yet available on a routine clinical basis, molecular genetic testing is performed via scientific research protocols. Mutational screening of genomic DNA derived from patient blood samples is routinely performed using DNA confirmation-sensitive techniques and automated sequencing. Although these standard genetic testing methods have allowed basic scientists to rapidly screen numerous kilobases of genomic DNA, they remain costly and are often not reimbursable by the patient's health insurance coverage. In the future, molecular genetic testing will become more readily available as a standard clinical diagnostic test, allowing clarification of risks for an individual's family members, for reproductive options, and for possible progression of their own cardiac disease. Choosing which specific genes to be analyzed based on specific clinical presentation of probands will remain a critical challenge.

4. Notes

1. RFLP analysis has been successfully used for identification of gene mutations in individuals *(14)*. The presence of an RFLP is detected in DNA products obtained from PCR amplification. Although RFLP analysis could be performed on primary PCR products, the yield of DNA obtained after PCR amplification from single-cell biopsies is rather low in many cases. Therefore, it may be necessary to perform a nested PCR reaction by using the product from the primary PCR as a template and to perform the RFLP analysis on the DNA generated from this secondary PCR reaction *(84,86)*.
2. The presence of a mutation should be confirmed by both sequence and RFLP analyses of two distinct nested PCR reactions. It is necessary to examine two distinct nested PCR reactions to exclude the likelihood that PCR-induced errors have been introduced in the DNA *(84,86)*.
3. After we successfully performed PGD for HOS using the assay design presented in **Subheading 3.2.**, the usefulness of coamplifying flanking single tandem repeats to address preferential allelic amplification has been suggested, and such a strategy should be taken into consideration when designing PGD assays *(87)*.

Acknowledgments

The authors are grateful to the patients and their physicians. Dr. Basson is an Established Investigator of the American Heart Association and an Irma T. Hirschl Scholar. Dr. Hatcher is supported by National Institutes of Health grant K01HL080948. This work wasw also supported by the Smart Cardiovascular Fund.

References

1. D'Alton, M. E. and DeCherney, A. H. (1993) Prenatal diagnosis. *N. Engl. J. Med.* **328**, 114–120.
2. Hoffman, J. I. (1995) Incidence of congenital heart disease: I. postnatal incidence. *Pediatr. Cardiol.* **16**, 103–113.
3. Roguin, N., Du, Z. D., Barak, M., Nasser, N., Hershkowitz, S. and Milgram, E. (1995) High prevalence of muscular ventricular septal defect in neonates. *J. Am. Coll. Cardiol.* **26**, 1545–1548.
4. Brickner, M. E., Hillis, L. D., and Lange, R. A. (2000) Congenital heart disease in adults. First of two parts. *N. Engl. J. Med.* **342**, 256–263.
5. Nora, J. J. and Nora, A. H. (1988) Update on counseling the family with a first-degree relative with a congenital heart defect. *Am. J. Med. Genet.* **29**, 137–142.
6. Nora, J. J. and Nora, A. H. (1976) Recurrence risks in children having one parent with a congenital heart disease. *Circulation* **53**, 701–702.
7. Sklansky, M. (2003) New dimensions and directions in fetal cardiology. *Curr. Opin. Pediatr.* **15**, 463–471.
8. University of Washington and Children's Health System (March 24, 2004). *GeneTests: Medical Genetics Information Resource.* Available at http://www.genetests.org.
9. McKusick-Nathans Institute for Genetic Medicine, Johns Hopkins University (Baltimore, MD) and National Center for Biotechnology Information, National Library of Medicine (April 13, 2004). *Online Mendelian Inheritance in Man,* OMIM (TM). Available at http://www.ncbi.nlm.nih.gov/omim.
10. Benson, D. W., Sharkey, A., Fatkin, D., et al. (1998) Reduced penetrance, variable expressivity, and genetic heterogeneity of familial atrial septal defects. *Circulation* **97**, 2043–2048.
11. Jones, K. L., ed. (1997) *Smith's Recognizable Patterns of Human Malformation,* 5th ed, W. B. Saunders, Philadelphia.
12. Holt, M. and Oram S. (1960) Familial heart disease with skeletal malformations. *Br. Heart. J.* **22**, 236–242.
13. Basson, C. T., Huang, T., Lin, R. C., et al. (1999) Different TBX5 interactions in heart and limb defined by Holt–Oram syndrome mutations. *Proc. Natl. Acad. Sci. USA* **96**, 2919–2924.
14. Basson, C. T., Bachinsky, D. R., Lin, R. C., et al. (1997) Mutations in human TBX5 cause limb and cardiac malformation in Holt–Oram syndrome. *Nat. Genet.* **15**, 30–35.

15. Li, Q. Y., Newbury-Ecob, R. A., Terrett, J. A., et al. (1997) Holt–Oram syndrome is caused by mutations in TBX5, a member of the Brachyury (T) gene family. *Nat. Genet.* **15**, 21–29.
16. Brassington, A. M., Sung, S. S., Toydemir, R. M., et al. (2003) Expressivity of Holt–Oram syndrome is not predicted by TBX5 genotype. *Am. J. Hum. Genet.* **73**, 74–85.
17. Terrett, J. A., Newbury-Ecob, R., Cross, G. S., et al. (1994) Holt–Oram syndrome is a genetically heterogeneous disease with one locus mapping to human chromosome 12q. *Nat. Genet.* **6**, 401–404.
18. Bruneau, B. G., Logan, M., Davis, N., et al. (1999) Chamber-specific cardiac expression of Tbx5 and heart defects in Holt–Oram syndrome. *Dev. Biol.* **211**, 100–108.
19. Hatcher, C. J., Kim, M. S., Mah, C. S., et al. (2001) TBX5 transcription factor regulates cell proliferation during cardiogenesis. *Dev. Biol.* **230**, 177–188.
20. Bruneau, B. G., Nemer, G., Schmitt, J. P., et al. (2001) A murine model of Holt–Oram syndrome defines roles of the T-box transcription factor Tbx5 in cardiogenesis and disease. *Cell* **106**, 709–721.
21. Ghosh, T. K., Packham, E. A., Bonser, A. J., Robinson, T. E., Cross, S. J., and Brook, J. D. (2001) Characterization of the TBX5 binding site and analysis of mutations that cause Holt–Oram syndrome. *Hum. Mol. Genet.* **10**, 1983–1994.
22. Hiroi, Y., Kudoh, S., Monzen, K., et al. (2001) Tbx5 associates with Nkx2-5 and synergistically promotes cardiomyocyte differentiation. *Nat. Genet.* **28**, 276–280.
23. Garg, V., Kathiriya, I. S., Barnes, R., et al. (2003) GATA4 mutations cause human congenital heart defects and reveal an interaction with TBX5. *Nature* **424**, 443–447.
24. Schott, J. J., Benson, D. W., Basson, C. T., et al. (1998) Congenital heart disease caused by mutations in the transcription factor NKX2-5. *Science* **281**, 108–111.
25. Basson, C. T., Solomon, S. D., Weissman, B., et al. (1995) Genetic heterogeneity of heart-hand syndromes. *Circulation* **91**, 1326–1329.
26. Pauli, R. M., Scheib-Wixted, S., Cripe, L., Izumo, S., and Sekhon, G.S. (1999) Ventricular noncompaction and distal chromosome 5q deletion. *Am. J. Med. Genet.* **85**, 419–423.
27. Benson, D. W., Silberbach, G. M., Kavanaugh-McHugh, A., et al. (1999) Mutations in the cardiac transcription factor NKX2.5 affect diverse cardiac developmental pathways. *J. Clin. Invest.* **104**, 1567–1573.
28. Goldmuntz, E., Geiger, E., and Benson, D. W. (2001) NKX2.5 mutations in patients with Tetralogy of Fallot. *Circulation* **104**, 2565–2568.
29. Elliott, D. A., Kirk, E. P., Yeoh, T., et al. (2003) Cardiac homeobox gene NKX2-5 mutations and congenital heart disease: associations with atrial septal defect and hypoplastic left heart syndrome. *J. Am. Coll. Cardiol.* **41**, 2072–2076.
30. McElhinney, D. B., Geiger, E., Blinder, J., Benson, D. W., and Goldmuntz, E. (2003) NKX2.5 mutations in patients with congenital heart disease. *J. Am. Coll. Cardiol.* **42**, 1650–1655.

31. Turbay, D., Wechsler, S. B., Blanchard, K. M. and Izumo, S. (1996) Molecular cloning, chromosomal mapping, and characterization of the human cardiac-specific homeobox gene hCsx. *Mol. Med.* **2**, 86–96.

32. Tanaka, M., Chen, Z., Bartunkova, S., Yamasaki, N., and Izumo, S. (1999) The cardiac homeobox gene Csx/Nkx2.5 lies genetically upstream of multiple genes essential for heart development. *Development* **126**, 1269–1280.

33. Bodmer, R. (1993) The gene tinman is required for specification of the heart and visceral muscles in Drosophila. *Development* **118**, 719–729.

34. Kasahara, H., Lee, B., Schott, J. J., et al. (2000) Loss of function and inhibitory effects of human CSX/NKX2.5 homeoprotein mutations associated with congenital heart disease. *J. Clin. Invest.* **106**, 299–308.

35. Jamali, M., Rogerson, P. J., Wilton, S., and Skerjanc, I. S. (2001) Nkx2-5 activity is essential for cardiomyogenesis. *J. Biol. Chem.* **276**, 42,252–42,258.

36. Pehlivan, T., Pober, B. R., Brueckner, M., et al. (1999) GATA4 haploinsufficiency in patients with interstitial deletion of chromosome region 8p23.1 and congenital heart disease. *Am. J. Med. Genet.* **83**, 201–206.

37. Nemer, G. and Nemer, M. (2003) Transcriptional activation of BMP-4 and regulation of mammalian organogenesis by GATA-4 and -6. *Dev. Biol.* **254**, 131–148.

38. Molkentin, J. D., Lin, Q., Duncan, S. A., and Olson, E. N. (1997) Requirement of the transcription factor GATA4 for heart tube formation and ventral morphogenesis. *Genes Dev.* **11**, 1061–1072.

39. Pu, W. T., Ishiwata, T., Juraszek, A. L., Ma, Q., and Izumo, S. (2004) GATA4 is a dosage-sensitive regulator of cardiac morphogenesis. *Dev. Biol.* **275,** 235–244.

40. Grepin, C., Robitaille, L., Antakly, T. and Nemer, M. (1995) Inhibition of transcription factor GATA-4 expression blocks in vitro cardiac muscle differentiation. *Mol. Cell. Biol.* **15**, 4095–4102.

41. Grepin, C., Nemer, G., and Nemer, M. (1997) Enhanced cardiogenesis in embryonic stem cells overexpressing the GATA-4 transcription factor. *Development* **124**, 2387–2395.

42. Charron, F., Paradis, P., Bronchain, O., Nemer, G., and Nemer, M. (1999) Cooperative interaction between GATA-4 and GATA-6 regulates myocardial gene expression. *Mol. Cell. Biol.* **19**, 4355–4365.

43. Durocher, D., Charron, F., Warren, R., Schwartz, R. J., and Nemer, M. (1997) The cardiac transcription factors Nkx2-5 and GATA-4 are mutual cofactors. *Embo. J.* **16**, 5687–5696.

44. Sepulveda, J. L., Vlahopoulos, S., Iyer, D., Belaguli, N., and Schwartz, R.J. (2002) Combinatorial expression of GATA4, Nkx2-5, and serum response factor directs early cardiac gene activity. *J. Biol. Chem.* **277**, 25,775–25,782.

45. Lu, J. R., McKinsey, T. A., Xu, H., Wang, D. Z., Richardson, J. A., and Olson, E. N. (1999) FOG-2, a heart- and brain-enriched cofactor for GATA transcription factors. *Mol. Cell. Biol.* **19**, 4495–4502.

46. Svensson, E. C., Tufts, R. L., Polk, C. E., and Leiden, J. M. (1999) Molecular cloning of FOG-2: a modulator of transcription factor GATA-4 in cardiomyocytes. *Proc. Natl. Acad. Sci. USA* **96**, 956–961.

47. Ellis, R. W. B. and van Creveld, S. (1940) A syndrome characterized by ectodermal dysplasia, polydactyly, chondrodysplasia, and congenital *morbus cordis*: report of three cases. *Arch. Dis. Child.* **15**, 65.
48. McKusick, V. A., Egeland, J. A., Eldridge, R., and Krusen, D. E. (1964) Dwarfism in the Amish I. The Ellis-van Creveld Syndrome. *Bull. Johns Hopkins Hosp.* **115**, 306–336.
49. da Silva, E. O., Janovitz, D., and de Albuquerque, S. C. (1980) Ellis-van Creveld syndrome: report of 15 cases in an inbred kindred. *J. Med. Genet.* **17**, 349–356.
50. McKusick, V. A. (2000) Ellis-van Creveld syndrome and the Amish. *Nat. Genet.* **24**, 203–204.
51. Kunze, P. (1980) [Ellis-van-Creveld syndrome]. *Kinderarztl. Prax.* **48**, 193–198.
52. Polymeropoulos, M. H., Ide, S. E., Wright, M., et al. (1996) The gene for the Ellis-van Creveld syndrome is located on chromosome 4p16. *Genomics* **35**, 1–5.
53. Ruiz-Perez, V. L., Ide, S. E., Strom, T. M., et al. (2000) Mutations in a new gene in Ellis-van Creveld syndrome and Weyers acrodental dysostosis. *Nat. Genet.* **24**, 283–286.
54. Galdzicka, M., Patnala, S., Hirshman, M. G., et al. (2002) A new gene, EVC2, is mutated in Ellis-van Creveld syndrome. *Mol. Genet. Metab.* **77**, 291–295.
55. Ruiz-Perez, V. L., Tompson, S. W., Blair, H. J., et al. (2003) Mutations in two nonhomologous genes in a head-to-head configuration cause Ellis-van Creveld syndrome. *Am. J. Hum. Genet.* **72**, 728–732.
56. Dugoff, L., Thieme, G., and Hobbins, J. C. (2001) First trimester prenatal diagnosis of chondroectodermal dysplasia (Ellis-van Creveld syndrome) with ultrasound. *Ultrasound. Obstet. Gynecol.* **17**, 86–88.
57. Vincent, M. C., Heitz, F., Tricoire, J., et al. (1999) 22q11 deletion in DGS/VCFS monozygotic twins with discordant phenotypes. *Genet. Couns.* **10**, 43–49.
58. Wilson, D. I., Cross, I. E., Goodship, J. A., et al. (1991) DiGeorge syndrome with isolated aortic coarctation and isolated ventricular septal defect in three sibs with a 22q11 deletion of maternal origin. *Br. Heart. J.* **66**, 308–312.
59. McElhinney, D. B., Driscoll, D. A., Levin, E. R., Jawad, A. F., Emanuel, B. S., and Goldmuntz, E. (2003) Chromosome 22q11 deletion in patients with ventricular septal defect: frequency and associated cardiovascular anomalies. *Pediatrics* **112**, e472.
60. Jerome, L. A. and Papaioannou, V. E. (2001) DiGeorge syndrome phenotype in mice mutant for the T-box gene, Tbx1. *Nat. Genet.* **27**, 286–291.
61. Lindsay, E. A., Vitelli, F., Su, H., et al. (2001) Tbx1 haploinsufficieny in the DiGeorge syndrome region causes aortic arch defects in mice. *Nature* **410**, 97–101.
62. Merscher, S., Funke, B., Epstein, J. A., et al. (2001) TBX1 is responsible for cardiovascular defects in velo-cardio-facial/DiGeorge syndrome. *Cell* **104**, 619–629.
63. Yagi, H., Furutani, Y., Hamada, H., et al. (2003) Role of TBX1 in human del22q11.2 syndrome. *Lancet* **362**, 1366–1373.
64. Sakata, Y., Kamei, C. N., Nakagami, H., Bronson, R., Liao, J. K., and Chin, M. T. (2002) Ventricular septal defect and cardiomyopathy in mice lacking the transcription factor CHF1/Hey2. *Proc. Natl. Acad. Sci. USA* **99**, 16,197–16,202.

65. Chin, M. T., Maemura, K., Fukumoto, S., et al. (2000) Cardiovascular basic helix loop helix factor 1, a novel transcriptional repressor expressed preferentially in the developing and adult cardiovascular system. *J. Biol. Chem.* **275**, 6381–6387.
66. Leimeister, C., Externbrink, A., Klamt, B., and Gessler, M. (1999) Hey genes: a novel subfamily of hairy- and Enhancer of split related genes specifically expressed during mouse embryogenesis. *Mech. Dev.* **85**, 173–177.
67. Zhong, T. P., Childs, S., Leu, J. P. and Fishman, M. C. (2001) Gridlock signalling pathway fashions the first embryonic artery. *Nature* **414**, 216–220.
68. Oda, T., Elkahloun, A. G., Pike, B. L., et al. (1997) Mutations in the human Jagged1 gene are responsible for Alagille syndrome. *Nat. Genet.* **16**, 235–242.
69. Li, L., Krantz, I. D., Deng, Y., et al. (1997) Alagille syndrome is caused by mutations in human Jagged1, which encodes a ligand for Notch1. *Nat. Genet.* **16**, 243–251.
70. Loffredo, C. A., Hirata, J., Wilson, P. D., Ferencz, C. and Lurie, I. W. (2001) Atrioventricular septal defects: possible etiologic differences between complete and partial defects. *Teratology* **63**, 87–93.
71. Loffredo, C. A., Wilson, P. D., and Ferencz, C. (2001) Maternal diabetes: an independent risk factor for major cardiovascular malformations with increased mortality of affected infants. *Teratology* **64**, 98–106.
72. Pierpont, M. E., Markwald, R. R., and Lin, A. E. (2000) Genetic aspects of atrioventricular septal defects. *Am. J. Med. Genet.* **97**, 289–296.
73. Green, E. K., Priestley, M. D., Waters, J., Maliszewska, C., Latif, F., and Maher, E. R. (2000) Detailed mapping of a congenital heart disease gene in chromosome 3p25. *J. Med. Genet.* **37**, 581–587.
74. Sheffield, V. C., Pierpont, M. E., Nishimura, D., et al. (1997) Identification of a complex congenital heart defect susceptibility locus by using DNA pooling and shared segment analysis. *Hum. Mol. Genet.* **6**, 117–121.
75. Rupp, P. A., Fouad, G. T., Egelston, C. A., et al. (2002) Identification, genomic organization and mRNA expression of CRELD1, the founding member of a unique family of matricellular proteins. *Gene* **293**, 47–57.
76. Robinson, S. W., Morris, C. D., Goldmuntz, E., et al. (2003) Missense mutations in CRELD1 are associated with cardiac atrioventricular septal defects. *Am. J. Hum. Genet.* **72**, 1047–1052.
77. Tartaglia, M., Mehler, E. L., Goldberg, R., et al. (2001) Mutations in PTPN11, encoding the protein tyrosine phosphatase SHP-2, cause Noonan syndrome. *Nat. Genet.* **29**, 465–468.
78. Marino, B., Gagliardi, M. G., Digilio, M. C., et al. (1995) Noonan syndrome: structural abnormalities of the mitral valve causing subaortic obstruction. *Eur. J. Pediatr.* **154**, 949–952.
79. Digilio, M. C., Conti, E., Sarkozy, A., et al. (2002) Grouping of multiple-lentigines/LEOPARD and Noonan syndromes on the PTPN11 gene. *Am. J. Hum. Genet.* **71**, 389–394.
80. Stone, D. L., Slavotinek, A., Bouffard, G. G., et al. (2000) Mutation of a gene encoding a putative chaperonin causes McKusick-Kaufman syndrome. *Nat. Genet.* **25**, 79–82.

81. Phoon, C. K. and Neill, C. A. (1994) Asplenia syndrome: insight into embryology through an analysis of cardiac and extracardiac anomalies. *Am. J. Cardiol.* **73**, 581–587.

82. Wassif, C. A., Maslen, C., Kachilele-Linjewile, S., et al. (1998) Mutations in the human sterol delta7-reductase gene at 11q12-13 cause Smith-Lemli-Opitz syndrome. *Am. J. Hum. Genet.* **63**, 55–62.

83. Lin, A. E., Ardinger, H. H., Ardinger, R. H., Jr., Cunniff, C., and Kelley, R. I. (1997) Cardiovascular malformations in Smith-Lemli-Opitz syndrome. *Am. J. Med. Genet.* **68**, 270–278.

84. He, J., McDermott, D. A., Song, Y., Gilbert, F., Kligman, I., and Basson, C. T. (2004) Preimplantation genetic diagnosis of human congenital heart malformation and Holt–Oram syndrome. *Am. J. Med. Genet.* **126A**, 93–98.

85. Davis, O. and Rosenwaks, Z. (1996) In vitro fertilization, in *Reproductive Endocrinology, Surgery, and Technology* (Adashi, E. Y., Rock, J. A., and Rosenwaks, Z., eds.), Lippincott-Raven, Philadelphia, pp. 2319–2334.

86. Xu, K., Shi, Z. M., Veeck, L. L., Hughes, M. R., and Rosenwaks, Z. (1999). First unaffected pregnancy using preimplantation genetic diagnosis for sickle cell anemia. *JAMA* **281**, 1701–1706.

87. Verlinsky, Y., Rechitsky, S., Verlinsky, O., et al. (2003) Preimplantation diagnosis for sonic hedgehog mutation causing familial holoprosencephaly. *N. Engl. J. Med.* **348**, 1449–1454.

3

Molecular and Genetic Aspects of DiGeorge/Velocardiofacial Syndrome

Deborah A. Driscoll

Summary

Cytogenetic, molecular, and clinical genetic studies have contributed to our understanding of the etiology, pathogenesis, and natural history of DiGeorge syndrome (DGS) and velocardiofacial syndrome (VCFS). Submicroscopic deletions of chromosome 22q11.2 are the leading cause of both of these disorders. The 22q11.2 deletion syndrome is recognized as one of the most common microdeletion syndromes. The clinical features are highly variable and include a variety of congenital anomalies, medical problems, and cognitive and neuropsychological difficulties.

Infrequently, other chromosomal rearrangements are found in patients with DGS/VCFS, and, rarely, point mutations in the gene *TBX1*, a transcription factor, that maps to the deleted region. The most sensitive and widely used diagnostic test for detecting the 22q11.2 deletion is fluorescence *in situ* hybridization using probes from the commonly deleted region. Alternatively, polymerase chain reaction can be performed to confirm failure to inherit a parental allele in the region or to determine copy number. Prenatal diagnosis is also available, particularly when a conotruncal cardiac defect is identified during a pregnancy or when a parent carries a deletion. Genetic counseling is recommended before testing to review the natural history of the disorder, testing options, and test sensitivity and limitations.

Key Words: 22q11.2 deletion; DiGeorge syndrome; velocardiofacial syndrome; fluorescence *in situ* hybridization.

1. Introduction

DiGeorge syndrome (DGS) was initially recognized in 1965, in a group of children with congenital absence of the thymus and parathyroid glands *(1)*. Later, congenital heart defects and facial dysmorphia were also considered classic features *(2)*. Until the mid-1990s, DGS was considered a relatively rare sporadic developmental defect of the third and fourth pharyngeal arches *(3)*. During the past decade, numerous cytogenetic, molecular, and clinical genetic

From: *Methods in Molecular Medicine, vol. 126: Congenital Heart Disease: Molecular Diagnostics*
Edited by: M. Kearns-Jonker © Humana Press Inc., Totowa, NJ

studies of patients with DGS have contributed to our current understanding of this disorder. Not long after the discovery that deletions of chromosome 22q11.2 are the leading cause of DGS, studies identified deletions in individuals with velocardiofacial syndrome (VCFS) and conotruncal anomaly face syndrome (CTAFS) *(4–7)*. Shortly thereafter, it became apparent that deletions of 22q11.2 were a frequent cause of conotruncal cardiac malformations *(8)*. Today, diagnostic testing for the 22q11.2 deletion is widely available and DGS/VCFS is recognized as one of the most common microdeletion syndromes, and a frequent cause of congenital heart disease.

1.1. Clinical Features

The classic features of DGS/VCFS include congenital heart defects, immune deficiencies secondary to aplasia or hypoplasia of the thymus, hypocalcemia caused by small or absent parathyroid glands, palatal anomalies, and speech and learning difficulties. In addition to case reports and smaller series, there are several recent large, prospective studies that have contributed to our knowledge of the types and frequency of congenital anomalies, medical problems, and cognitive and neuropsychological difficulties that these patients are likely to develop *(9–11)*. Cardiovascular malformations found in 70 to 80% of DGS/VCFS patients, typically involve the conotruncus and outflow tract including interrupted aortic arch type B, truncus arteriosus (TA), tetralogy of Fallot (TOF), and aortic arch anomalies. Although some patients can have a profound immunodeficiency, requiring thymic transplantation, many maintain reasonable lymphocyte counts. Characteristic facial features have been described, which include a long face, a prominent nose with a bulbous nasal tip and narrow alar base, almond-shaped or narrow palpebral fissures, malar flattening, recessed chin, hooded eyelids, and low-set prominent ears. Palatal abnormalities, including cleft palate, submucous cleft palate, and velopharyngeal insufficiency, occur in approx 70% of DGS/VCFS patients. Other features include feeding difficulties, renal anomalies, inguinal and umbilical hernias, skeletal abnormalities, short stature, juvenile rheumatoid arthritis, hematological abnormalities, neural tube defects, craniosynostosis, diaphragmatic hernia, and hypospadias.

Neuropsychological evaluations indicate that these children are at risk for cognitive impairment and neurological and psychiatric problems *(9–13)*. Seizures, asymmetric crying facies, ataxia, polymicrogyria, and cerebellar hypoplasia have been reported. A wide range of developmental outcomes has been documented in children with the 22q11.2 deletion. Approximately 80% of these children demonstrate significant motor delay. Expressive and receptive language is delayed in more than three-fourths of these children. Cognitive development ranges from normal intelligence to moderate retardation. Studies have found that verbal IQ scores are significantly higher than performance IQ scores and suggest that these children are at risk for nonverbal learning disabilities. Attention deficit disorder, with or without hyperactivity, emotional difficulties, anxiety, and shyness, has been observed. There also seems to be a higher than expected rate of psychiatric disorders, including depression, schizophrenia, and bipolar disorder, in adolescents and adults with the 22q11.2 deletion.

A wide range of phenotypic variability is associated with the 22q11.2 deletion. Although some individuals present with classic findings of DGS/VCFS, others have relatively subtle features, such as minor dysmorphic facial features and mild cognitive impairment. Other disorders associated with the 22q11.2 deletion include CTAFS, Opitz/GBBB syndrome, and Cayler cardiofacial syndrome (asymmetric crying facies) *(14–16)*.

1.2. Etiology

Deletions of chromosomal region 22q11.2 are the leading cause of DGS/VCFS. Interstitial and submicroscopic deletions have been detected in approx 90% of patients with the diagnosis of DGS *(17)*. The frequency of 22q11.2 deletions reported in VCFS patients is 76 to 81% *(17,18)*. Chromosome 22q11.2 deletions were found in 84% of patients diagnosed with CTAFS *(14)*. Deletions of 22q11.2 are estimated to occur in as many as 1 in 4000 live births. The estimated annual incidence in the Flemish region of Belgium in 1992–1996 was 1 in 6395 newborns *(19)*. A similar incidence of 1 in 5950 births (95% confidence interval, 1 in 4417 to 1 in 8224) was reported in a large population-based study in the United States. It has been estimated that 700 children are born with the 22q11.2 deletion each year in the United States alone *(20)*.

Less frequently, haploinsufficiency for this region of 22q11 occurs because of an unbalanced translocation with monosomy 22pter→q11.2 *(21)*. In rare instances, DGS has been associated with other chromosomal abnormalities, in particular, deletions of the short arm of chromosome 10 (del[10][p13]). Other chromosomal rearrangements reported in association with DGS include monosomy and trisomy 18q, monosomy 18p, monosomy 12p with trisomy 1q, monosomy 5p, partial trisomy 1q, and duplication 9q *(22)*. DGS may also occur because of *in utero* retinoic acid and alcohol exposure, and poorly controlled maternal insulin-dependent diabetes *(3)*.

The 22q11.2 deletion is a common cause of conotruncal cardiac malformations. The reported frequency of the 22q11.2 deletion among individuals with conotruncal cardiac defects is highly variable because of differences in ascertainment and inclusion criteria. A large, prospective study of infants and children with conotruncal cardiac defects, ascertained by cardiologists, reported an overall deletion rate of 18% *(23)*. However, the probands in this study were not evaluated for the presence of extracardiac malformations, phenotypic features of DGS/VCFS, or dysmorphia. Studies report lower detection rates when only individuals with isolated, nonsyndromic cardiac defects are included. Fokstuen et al. identified a 22q11.2 deletion in 8% of 110 cardiac patients, but all of the patients with the deletion had additional anomalies or dysmorphisms, whereas none of the isolated cases had the deletion *(24)*. Voight et al. identified 22q11.2 deletions in only 2 of 81 patients with isolated TOF *(25)*. The majority of cardiac patients with the 22q11.2 deletion will have multiple minor anomalies and dysmorphic features *(20,24)*. In some cases, the dysmorphic features can be very subtle, and features such as speech delay and learning difficulties cannot be evaluated in a newborn or infant child *(10)*.

The deletion frequency varies with the primary cardiac diagnosis and is higher in patients with associated aortic arch abnormalities. Deletions of 22q11.2 occur in 50 to 82% of patients with an interrupted aortic arch, in particular, type B *(23,26,27)*. Deletions of 22q11.2 have been identified in 30 to 40% of patients with TA *(28,29)*. Patients with TA were more likely to have a 22q11.2 deletion in the presence of a right aortic arch and/or abnormal aortic arch branching patterns *(29)*. This also held true for ventricular septal defects (VSD). In a prospective study of 125 patients with a conoventricular, posterior malalignment, or conoseptal hypoplasia VSD, 10% had a 22q11.2 deletion. Of these patients, 45% had an abnormal aortic arch laterality, abnormal aortic arch branching patterns, or discontinuous pulmonary arteries had a deletion; whereas only 3% of VSD patients with a normal aortic arch and normal branch pulmonary arteries had a deletion *(30)*. Approximately 16% of patients with TOF have a 22q11.2 deletion *(23,31)*. Deletions of 22q11.2 are rarely seen in patients with transposition of the great arteries and double-outlet right ventricle, but, when they occur, they are usually associated with anomalies of the pulmonary artery, aortic arch, or ductus arteriosus *(23,32)*.

1.3. Diagnostic Testing for DGS/VCFS

As part of the evaluation of an infant or child with suspected DGS/VCFS, a karyotype and testing for the 22q11.2 deletion is recommended. When a chromosomal abnormality is identified (translocation or deletion), then parental testing is indicated. The value of testing patients with conotruncal defects has been debated *(33,34)*. There is no doubt that the 22q11.2 deletion is a significant cause of some types of outflow tract defects; the presence of this deletion should prompt a more thorough evaluation of the patient to look for extracardiac manifestations. However, some of these features are subtle or may not be apparent until childhood. Early identification of the deletion can lead to increased awareness of possible medical problems and speech and learning difficulties, and, thus, to earlier intervention *(34,35)*. Further, early identification will assure that familial cases are identified and that families receive accurate counseling of their risk and reproductive options in subsequent pregnancies. Therefore, diagnostic testing for the 22q11.2 deletion is recommended in patients with features of DGS/VCFS or a conotruncal cardiac defect, particularly in the presence of aortic arch and pulmonary artery anomalies.

Indications for prenatal testing include the following:

1. Previous child with DGS/VCFS or the 22q11.2 deletion.
2. Parent with 22q11.2 deletion or mosaicism for the deletion.
3. Conotruncal cardiac defect is identified *in utero (36,37)*.

Pre-implantation genetic diagnosis has been reported in a mildly affected parent with a 22q11.2 deletion *(38)*. The risk of an affected child in this case is 50%. Unaffected parents, without a deletion, who have had a previous child with DGS/VCFS may consider prenatal testing because of the small possibility of germline mosaicism *(39,40)*.

Although there are several types of tests available, fluorescence *in situ* hybridization (FISH) has become the standard method of choice for clinical diagnosis and prenatal testing for the 22q11.2 deletion *(17,36,41)*. In some circumstances, polymerase chain reaction (PCR)-based studies may be helpful. Mutation analysis has been performed in a research setting but has not been particularly useful clinically.

1.3.1. Cytogenetic Analysis

High-resolution cytogenetic analysis detects up to 25% of interstitial deletions in the chromosome 22q11.2 region *(6,42)*. The majority of deletions are submicroscopic and are only detected by FISH. However, a karyotype is still valuable for identifying other chromosomal rearrangements that have been reported in patients with DGS, including translocations. Correct identification of a cytogenetic abnormality in these patients has important implications for their recurrence risk.

1.3.2. Fluorescence In Situ Hybridization

FISH is a sensitive and efficient test to detect submicroscopic deletions (*see* **Subheadings 2.** and **3.**). It is routinely used in commercial and hospital-based cytogenetic laboratories as an adjunct to a routine karyotype. FISH can be performed on metaphase spreads or interphase nuclei from peripheral blood lymphocytes, cultured amniocytes, or chorionic villi. FISH has also been used on blastomeres obtained from a 6- to 10-cell embryo *(38)*. In addition to testing for the 22q11.2 deletion, FISH has also been used to simultaneously detect chromosome 10p13p14 deletions in patients with features of DGS/VCFS *(43)*.

2. Materials

1. Slides with chromosome preparations.
2. LSI DiGeorge/VCFS region/ARSA dual-color DNA probe (Vysis, Downers Grove, IL).
3. 70, 80, and 100% ethanol.
4. LSI hybridization buffer (Vysis).
5. 50 and 70% formamide.
6. 2X standard sodium citrate (SSC).
7. 0.1% NP-40.
8. DAPI solution.
9. Cover slips.
10. Rubber cement.
11. Coplin jars.
12. Water baths.
13. Incubator.
14. Humidified box.
15. Slide warmer.
16. Fluorescence microscope equipped with a triple-band filter.

3. Methods

A detailed protocol and reagents, including labeled probes, are available from Vysis (Downers Grove, IL). The test probes from the DiGeorge minimal critical region are cosmid clones for loci D22S75 (N25) and TUPLE1. The control probe, arylsulfatase A (ARSA), maps to 22q13.3 and is used to ensure proper hybridization (*see* **Note 1**). If commercial probes are not available, cosmids from the commonly deleted region can be labeled with Spectrum–Orange–dUTP (Vysis) by nick translation. An internal control probe for the distal long arm of chromosome 22 is always recommended. FISH is performed on glass slides with metaphase chromosomes or interphase nuclei. The slides are denatured in 70% formamide/2X SSC, dehydrated in a series of ethanol washes (70, 85, and 100%), and air-dried. The probes are denatured in hybridization buffer at 73 to 74°C. The probe is applied to the slides and allowed to hybridize in a moist chamber overnight (12–16 h) at 37°C. A series of washes with formamide, SSC, and NP-40 are performed at 46°C to remove the excess probe. Slides are air dried and counterstained with DAPI to permit identification of the chromosomes. The slides are viewed with a fluorescence microscope. The test probe from the DGS critical region appears orange; a single hybridization signal is consistent with a deletion. The control probe that maps to the distal long arm, 22q13.3, appears green, and two signals should be present. Rarely, absence of a signal from the control probe occurs and indicates a deletion of 22q13.3 (*see* **Note 1**). At least 15 metaphases should be analyzed.

3.1. Characteristics of the 22q11.2 Deletion

The vast majority of DGS/VCFS patients have a common 3-Mb deletion of 22q11.2. The majority of these deletions arise *de novo*. The deletion endpoints are identical and have been shown to contain large (250–500 kb) blocks of highly homologous chromosome low-copy repeats that predispose to aberrant interchromosomal exchange events in proximal chromosome 22 during meiosis I *(44,45)*. Crossover frequency is not related to proband gender, parental age, or the presence of chromosome inversions *(45)*. Further, no bias in parental origin of the deletion was found. The extent and size of the deletion can be determined with FISH, using pairs of probes labeled with different colors. However, because the size and location of the deletion within this region does not seem to correlate with the phenotype, it is not recommended for clinical use. Smaller deletions (1.5 Mb) within the commonly deleted region occur in approx 15% of patients. The smaller deletions seem to be mediated by smaller duplicated blocks of repeats *(44)*.

3.2. Conclusion

In summary, genetic counseling is highly recommended when testing an affected child or an at-risk pregnancy and should include a discussion of the clinical features, the variability, the etiology, and the diagnostic tests, including the test sensitivity and limitations. In general, FISH is a reliable and accurate test for detecting the 22q11.2 deletion and is usually used as an adjunct to a routine karyotype. Occasionally, the FISH assay can be difficult to interpret and require additional studies (*see* **Notes 1–3**). In some laboratories or situations, PCR-based testing may be preferable to FISH. PCR is an efficient and cost-effective method of screening patients for a deletion, and requires only a small amount of DNA. It also eliminates the need to culture and harvest peripheral blood lymphocytes, and to prepare metaphase chromosome spreads. Further, a variety of sources of DNA can be used, including cheek swabs and postmortem and paraffin-embedded tissue. Two types of PCR-based assays have been developed as an alternative to FISH for the detection of the 22q11.2 deletion. These alternatives to FISH are described in **Notes 4** and **5**.

4. Notes

1. Control probe absent. Infrequently, one of the control probes may fail to hybridize. This hybridization failure is highly suggestive of a distal deletion of chromosome 22q13.3 and should be confirmed using a chromosome 22-specific subtelomeric probe. This may occur because of a terminal deletion or a malsegregation of a subtle balanced translocation. In these cases, it is helpful to analyze the parental chromosomes and to perform FISH with the chromosome 22-specific probes.

2. No evidence of 22q11.2 deletion in a patient with DGS/VCFS. Although the 22q11.2 deletion is the most common cause of DGS/VCFS, 10 to 15% of individuals with DGS/VCFS do not have a deletion in this region. A small number of DGS/VCFS cases will result from another chromosomal abnormality, therefore, a karyotype is recommended. Rarely, a point mutation may be implicated (*see* **Note 3**). In some cases, a definitive etiology may not be identified. This is particularly true in a prenatal setting, in which most cases are suspected because of an abnormal fetal echocardiogram. Because the detection rate for 22q11.2 deletions varies with the type of cardiac defect, unless there are extracardiac anomalies suggestive of DGS/VCFS, the detection rate will be much lower. Clinicians are often perplexed when a patient with clinical features highly suggestive of DGS or VCFS has a negative 22q11.2 deletion result (i.e., no evidence of a 22q11.2 deletion) and an apparently normal karyotype. The probes that are commercially available (D22S75 [N25] and TUPLE1) are from the DGS/VCFS critical region and are deleted in the overwhelming majority of DGS/VCFS patients. However, there have been a few reports of rare deletions outside of this region *(46,47)*. In research laboratories, it has been possible to characterize these deletions using FISH with cosmid clones from region 22q11.2. Mutation studies of patients with no evidence of a 22q11.2 deletion have also been performed (*see* **Note 3**).

3. Mutation analysis. Approximately 25 genes reside within the commonly deleted region of 22q11.2. Many of these genes have been considered as candidates for DGS/VCFS, however, there is now compelling evidence that *TBX1* is the causative gene *(48–50)*. Heterozygous mice for a null mutation in *Tbx1* develop the outflow tract anomalies seen in DGS. Furthermore, the homozygous mutants have other characteristic features, including abnormalities of the thymus, parathyroid gland, facial structures, and cleft palate. Until recently, most studies had failed to find mutations in several genes in the deleted region, including *TBX1*, in patients without the 22q11.2 deletion who were diagnosed with DGS/VCFS, nonsyndromic conotruncal malformations, or aortic arch anomalies *(49,51,52)*. Yagi et al. sequenced the *TBX1* coding regions and identified three mutations in two unrelated individuals and in three affected family members *(53)*. These patients all had features of either CTAFS or DGS, yet there was no evidence of cognitive impairment that is common in the 22q11.2-deletion syndrome. These studies suggest that *TBX1* mutations are a rare cause of the physical manifestations in DGS/VCFS.

4. PCR-based analysis of microsatellite markers. Short tandem repeat polymorphisms or microsatellite markers within the commonly deleted region on chromosome 22q11.2 can be used to detect a deletion by demonstrating failure to inherit a parental allele *(54,55)*. Using microsatellite markers from within the commonly deleted region in infants with conotruncal cardiac malformations, Bonnet et al. have confirmed or rejected a diagnosis of 22q11.2 deletion in 94% of cases within 24 h *(55)*. These markers are also useful for looking for loss of heterozygosity in patients at risk for the deletion. The assay has a 100% sensitiv-

ity and high specificity (85% or higher) when three or more markers in the region proximal to locus D22S264 were used *(54)*. Because the PCR-based assay is cost efficient and rapid, it lends itself to population-based or newborn screening. The assay requires a sample of DNA from blood, a cheek swab, dried blood spots, or pathological specimens. A positive screen should be followed either by FISH to confirm the presence of a 22q11.2 deletion or by parental studies to document failure to inherit a parental allele. A negative screen in a patient suspected of having DGS/VCFS does not exclude the possibility of a smaller deletion. Haplotype analysis using these markers has also been used to confirm or exclude germline mosaicism in families with two or more affected relatives *(39,40,56)*. This has important implications for counseling families regarding the possibility of a recurrence.

5. Quantitative PCR. Quantitiative PCR has also been developed for rapid detection of the 22q11 deletion *(57)*. Karyiazono et al. selected *UFD1L* as the test gene from 22q11.2 and a control gene on chromosome 21, *S100 b*. The TaqMan^{tm} PCR assay was capable of detecting a deletion of *UFD1L* with a 99.7% statistical confidence. It can be performed rapidly on small quantities of DNA. However, quantitiative PCR does require expensive equipment, including an ABI PRISM 7700 Sequence Detection System and software (PE Biosystems) for quantitative analysis, and it cannot detect mosaicism or structural abnormalities, such as translocations.

Acknowledgment

This work was supported in part by grants DC02027 and HL074731 from the National Institutes of Health.

References

1. DiGeorge, A. M. (1965) Discussion on a new concept of the cellular basis of immunology. *J. Pediatr.* **67**, 907.
2. Conley, M. E., Beckwith, J. B., Mancer, J. F. K., and Tenckhoff, L. (1979) The spectrum of the DiGeorge syndrome. *J. Pediatr.* **94**, 883–890.
3. Lammer, E. J. and Opitz, J. M. (1986) The DiGeorge anomaly as a developmental field defect. *Am. J. Med. Genet.* **29**, 113–127.
4. Scambler, P. J., Carey, A. H., Wyse, R. K. H., et al. (1991) Microdeletions within 22q11 associated with sporadic and familial DiGeorge syndrome. *Genomics* **20**, 201–206.
5. Driscoll, D. A., Budarf, M. L., and Emanuel, B. S. (1992a) A genetic etiology for DiGeorge syndrome: consistent deletions and microdeletions of 22q11. *Am. J. Hum. Genet.* **50**, 924–933.
6. Driscoll, D. A., Spinner, N. B., Budarf, M. L., et al. (1992b) Deletions and microdeletions of 22q11.2 in velo–cardio–facial syndrome. *Am. J. Med. Genet.* **44**, 261–268.
7. Burn, J., Takao, A., Wilson, D., et al. (1993) Conotruncal anomaly face syndrome is associated with a deletion within chromosome 22. *J. Med. Genet.* **30**, 822–824.

8. Goldmuntz, E., Driscoll, D., Budarf, M. L., et al. (1993) Microdeletions of chromosomal region 22q11 in patients with congenital conotruncal cardiac defects. *J. Med. Genet.* **30**, 807–812.

9. Ryan, A. K., Goodship, J. A., Wilson, D. I., et al. (1997) Spectrum of clinical features associated with interstitial chromosome 22q11 deletions: a European collaborative study. *J. Med. Genet.* **34**(10), 798–804.

10. McDonald-McGinn, D. M., Kirschner, R., Goldmuntz, E., et al. (1999) The Philadelphia Story: The 22q11.2 Deletion: Report on 250 Patients. *Genetic. Counseling* **10**(1), 11–24.

11. Swillen, A., Vogels, A., Devriendt, K., Fryns, J. P. (2000) Chromosome 22q11 deletion syndrome: Update and review of the clinical features, cognitive-behavioral spectrum, and psychiatric complications. *Am. J. Med. Genet.* **97**, 128–135.

12. Moss, E., Batshaw, M. L., Solot, C. B., et al. (1999) Psychoeducational profile of the 22q11.2 microdeletion: a comples pattern. *J. Pediatr.* **134**, 193–198.

13. Woodin, M., Wang, P. P., Aleman, D., McDonald-McGinn, D., Zackai, E., Moss, E. (2001) Neuropsychological profile of children and adolescents with the 22q11.2 microdeletion. *Genet. Med.* **3**, 34–44.

14. Matsuoka, R., Takao, A., Kimura, M., et al. (1994) Confirmation that the conotruncal anomaly face syndrome is associated with a deletion within 22q11.2. *Am. J. Med. Genet.* **53**, 285–289.

15. McDonald-McGinn, D. M., Driscoll, D. A., Bason, L., et al. (1995) Autosomal dominant "Optiz" GBBB syndrome due to a 22q11.2 deletion. *Am. J. Med. Genet.* **59**, 103–113.

16. Giannotti, A., Digilio, M. C., Marino, B., Mingarelli, R., and Dallapiccola, B. (1994) Cayler cardiofacial syndrome and del 22q11: Part of the CATCH22 phenotype. *Am. J. Med. Genet.* **53**, 303–304.

17. Driscoll D. A., Salvin J., Sellinger B., et al. (1993): Prevalence of 22q11 microdeletions in DiGeorge and velocardiofacial syndromes: implications for genetic counselling and prenatal diagnosis. *J. Med. Genet.* 30:813–817.

18. Lindsay, E. A., Greenberg, F., Shaffer, L. G., Shapira, S. K., Scambler, P. J., and Baldini, A. (1995) Submicroscopic deletions at 22q11.2: variability of the clinical picture and delineation of a commonly deleted region. *Am. J. Med. Genet.* **56**, 191–197.

19. Devriendt, K., Fryns, J.-P., Van Thienen, M.-N., and Keymolen, K. (1998) The annual incidence of DiGeorge/velocardiofacial syndrome. *J. Med. Genet.* **35**, 789–790.

20. Botto, L. D., May, K., Fernhoff, P. M., et al. (2003) A population-based study of the 22q11.2 deletion: phenotype, incidence, and contribution to major birth defects in the population. *Pediatrics* **112**, 101–107.

21. Kelley, R. I., Zackai, E. H., Emanuel, B. S., Kistenmacher, M., Greenberg, F., and Punnett, H. H. (1982) The association of the DiGeorge anomalad with partial monosomy of chromosome 22. *J. Pediatr.* **101**:197–200.

22. Greenberg, F. (1993) DiGeorge syndrome: an historical review of clinical and cytogenetic features. *J. Med. Genet.* **30**, 803–806.

23. Goldmuntz, E., Clark, B. J., Mitchell, L. E., et al. (1998) Frequency of 22q11 deletions in patients with conotruncal defects. *J. Am. Coll. Cardiol.* **32**, 492–298.

24. Fokstuen, S., Arbenz, U., Artan, S., et al. (1998) 22q11.2 deletions in a series of patients with non-selective congenital heart defects: incidence, type of defects and parental origin. *Clin. Genet.* **53**, 64–69.

25. Voigt, R., Maier-Weidmann, M., Lange, P. E., and Haaf, T. (2002) Chromosome 10p13-14 and 22q11 deletion screening in 100 patients with isolated and syndromic conotruncal heart defects. *J. Med. Genet.* **39**, e16.

26. Lewin, M. B., Lindsay, E. A., Jurecic, V., Goytia, V., Towbin, J. A., and Baldini, A. (1997) A genetic etiology for interruption of the aortic arch type B. *Am. J. Cardiol.* **80**, 493–497.

27. Rauch, A., Hofbeck, M., Leipold, G., et al. (1998) Incidence and significance of 22q11.2 hemizygosity in patients with interrupted aortic arch. *Am. J. Med. Genet.* **78**, 322–331.

28. Momma, K., Ando, M., Matsuoka, R. (1997) Truncus arteriosus communis associated with chromosome 22q11 deletion. *J. Am. Coll. Cardiol.* **30**, 1067–1071.

29. McElhinney, D. B., Driscoll, D. A., Emanuel, B. S., and Goldmuntz, E. (2003) Chromosome 22q11 deletion in patients with truncus arteriosus. *Pediatr. Cardiol.* **24**, 569–573.

30. McElhinney, D. B., Driscoll, D. A., Levin, E., Jawad, A. F., Emanuel, B. S., and Goldmuntz, E. (2003) Chromosome 22q11 deletion in patients with ventricular septal defect: frequency and associated cardiovascular anomalies. *Pediatrics* **112**(6 Pt 1), e472–e476.

31. Lu, J.-H., Chung, M.-Y., Hwang, B., and Chien, H.-P. (1999) Prevalence and parental origin in Tetralogy of Fallot associated with chromosome 22q11 microdeletion. *Pediatrics* **104**, 87–90.

32. Derbent, M., Yilmaz, Z., Baltaci, V., Saygih, A., Varan, B., and Tokel, K. (2003) Chromosome 22q11.2 deletion and phenotypic features in 30 patients with conotruncal heart defects. *Am. J. Med. Genet.* **116A**, 129–135.

33. Digilio, M.C., Marino, B., Giannotti, A., Mingarelli, R., and Dallapiccola, B. (1999) Guidelines for 22q11 deletion screening of patients with conotruncal defects. *J. Am. Col. Cardiol.* **33**, 1746–1747.

34. Goldmuntz, E., Clark, B. J., Mitchell, L. E., et al. (1999) Guidelines for 22q11.2 deletion screening of patients with conotruncal defects. *J. Am. Col. Cardiol.* Letter to the Editor. Reply. **33**, 1747–1748.

35. Gerdes, M., Solot, S., Wang, P. P., McDonald-McGinn, D. M., and Zackai, E. Z. (2001) Taking advantage of early diagnosis: preschool children with the 22q11.2 deletion. *Genet. Med.* **3**, 40–44.

36. Driscoll, D. A. (2001) Prenatal diagnosis of the 22q11.2 deletion syndrome. *Genet. Med.* **3**, 14–18.

37. Manji, S., Roberson, J. R., Wiktor, A., et al. (2001) Prenatal diagnosis of 22q11.2 deletion when ultrasound examination reveals a heart defects. *Genet. Med.* **3**, 65–66.

38. Iwarsson, E., Ahrlund-Richter, L., Inzunza, J., et al. (1998) Preimplantation genetic diagnosis of DiGeorge syndrome. *Molec. Hum. Reprod.* **4**, 871–875.

39. Hatchwell, E., Long, F., Wilde, J., Crolla, J., and Temple, K. (1998) Molecular confirmation of germ line mosaicism for a submicroscopic deletion of chromosome 22q11. *Am. J. Med. Genet.* **78**, 103–106.
40. Sandrin-Gardia, P., Macedo, C., Martelli, L. R., et al. (2002) Short report: recurrent 22q11.2 deletion in a sibship suggestive of parental germline mosaicism in velocardiofacial syndrome. *Clin. Genet.* **61**, 380–383.
41. Desmaze C., Scambler P., Prieur M., et al. (1993) Routine diagnosis of DiGeorge syndrome by fluorescent in situ hybridization. *Hum. Genet.* **90**, 663–665.
42. Wilson, D. I., Cross, I. E., Goodship, J. A., et al. (1992) A prospective cytogenetic study of 36 cases of DiGeorge syndrome. *Am. J. Hum. Genet.* **51**, 957–963.
43. Berend, S. A., Spikes, A. S., Kashork, C. D., et al. (2000) Dual-probe fluorescence in situ hybridization assay for detecting deletions associated with VCFS/DiGeorge syndrome I and DiGeorge syndrome II loci. *Am. J. Med. Genet.* **91**, 313–317.
44. Shaikh, T. S., Kurahashi, H., Saitta, S. C., et al. (2000) Chromosome 22-specific low copy repeats and the 22q11.2 deletion syndrome: genomic organization and deletion endpoint analysis. *Hum. Molec. Genet.* **9**, 489–501.
45. Saitta, S. C., Harris, S. E., Gaeth, A. P., et al. (2004) Aberrant interchromosomal exchanges are the predominant cause of the 22q11.2 deletion. *Hum. Mol. Genet.* **13**, 417–428.
46. Rauch, A., Pfeiffer, R. A., Leipold, G., Singer, H., Tigges, M., and Hofbeck, M. (1999) A novel 22q11.2 microdeletion in DiGeorge syndrome. *Am. J. Hum. Genet.* **64**, 659–666.
47. Saitta, S. C., McGrath, J. M., Mensch, H., Shaikh, T. H., Zackai, E. H., and Emanuel, B. S. (1999) A 22q11.2 deletion that excludes UFD1L and CDC45L in a patient with conotruncal and craniofacial defects. *Am. J. Hum. Genet.* **65**, 562–566.
48. Merscher, S., Funke, B., Epstein, J.A., et al. (2001) TBX1 is responsible for cardiovascular defects in velo–cardio–facial/DiGeorge syndrome. *Cell* **104**, 619–629.
49. Lindsay, E. A., Vitelli, F., Su, H., et al. (2002) tbx1 haploinsufficiency in the DiGeorge syndrome region causes aortic arch defects in mice. *Nature* **410**, 97–101.
50. Jerome, L. A. and Papaioannou, V. E. (2001) DiGeorge syndrome phenotype in mice mutant for the T-box gene, TBX1. *Nat. Genet.* **27**, 286–291.
51. Gong, W., Gottlieb, S., Collins, J., et al. (2001) Mutation analysis of TBX1 in non-deleted patients with features of DGS/VCFS or isolated cardiovascular defects. *J. Med. Genet.* **38**, E45.
52. Conti, E., Grifone, N., Sarkozy, A., et al. (2003) DiGeorge subtypes of nonsyndromic conotruncal defects: evidence against a major role of TBX1 gene. *Eur. J. Hum. Genet.* **11**, 349–351.
53. Yagi, H., Furutani, Y., Hamada, H., et al. (2003) Role of TBX1 in human del22q11.2 syndrome. *Lancet* **362**, 1366–1373.
54. Driscoll, D. A., Emanuel, B. S., Mitchell, L. E., and Budarf, M. L. (1997) PCR assay for screening patients at risk for 22q11.2 deletion. *Genet. Test.* **1**, 109–113.

55. Bonnet, D., Cormier-Daire, V., Kachaner, J., et al. (1997) Microsatellite DNA markers detects 95% of chromosome 22q11 deletions. *Am. J. Med. Genet.* **68**, 182–184.
56. Saitta, S. C., Harris, S. E., McDonald-McGinn, D. M., et al. (2004) Independent de novo 22q11.2 deletions in first cousins with DiGeorge/velocardiofacial syndrome. *Am. J. Med. Genet.* **124A**, 313–317.
57. Kariyazono, J., Ohno, T., Ihara, K., et al. (2001) Rapid detection of the 22q11.2 deletion with quantitative real-time PCR. *Molec. Cell. Probes* **25**, 71–73.

4

Mutation Screening for the Genes Causing Cardiac Arrhythmias

Jeffrey A. Towbin

Summary

In this chapter, the up-to-date understanding of the molecular basis of disorders causing arrhythmias are outlined. Several arrhythmic disorders have been well described at the molecular level, including the long QT syndromes (LQTS), Brugada syndrome, and polymorphic ventricular tachycardia. The genes identified have been determined using genetic linkage analysis, cloning, and mutation analyses. In the past, cloning was common, but with completion of the Human Genome Project, cloning is now rarely needed. In this chapter, current mutation screening methods, including denaturing high-performance liquid chromatography (DHPLC) and DNA sequencing are described, and the current knowledge gained using these studies is discussed.

Key Words: Mutation screening; DHPLC; DNA sequencing; long QT syndrome; Brugada syndrome; idiopathic ventricular fibrillation; ion channels; polymorphic ventricular tachycardia; pre-excitation; Wolff–Parkinson–White syndrome.

1. Introduction

Sudden cardiac death in the United States occurs with a reported incidence of more than 300,000 persons per year *(1)*. Although coronary heart disease is a major cause of death, other etiologies contribute to this problem, including arrhythmia disorders, myocardial disorders, and disorders in which both arrhythmias and structural heart disease coexist. In cases in which no structural heart disease can be identified, cardiac arrhythmias are usually suspected, in particular, these disorders include the long QT syndromes (LQTS) *(1,2)*, characterized by electrocardiographic evidence of the measured interval between the Q wave and T wave and T wave morphology abnormalities; ventricular preexcitation *(3)*; idiopathic ventricular fibrillation or Brugada syndrome *(4)*, characterized by electrocardiographic evidence of ST-segment elevation in the

From: *Methods in Molecular Medicine, vol. 126: Congenital Heart Disease: Molecular Diagnostics*
Edited by: M. Kearns-Jonker © Humana Press Inc., Totowa, NJ

right precordial leads with or without right bundle branch block; and catecholaminergic polymorphic ventricular tachycardia *(5)*. In this chapter, the current understandings of the clinical and molecular genetic aspects of inherited arrhythmia diseases are discussed, and the methods used to identify the genes causing these disorders are outlined. These methods include denaturing high-performance liquid chromotography (DHPLC) and DNA sequencing.

2. Materials

2.1. Denaturing High-Performance Liquid Chromatography

1. Polymerase chain reaction (PCR)-quality deionized water.
2. GeneAMP 10X PCR buffer II (Applied Biosystems [ABI]) or equivalent (500 mM KCl; 100 mM Tris-HCl, pH 8.3).
3. 25 mM MgCl$_2$.
4. 5 mM solutions of each dNTP (dCTP, dATP, dTTP, and dGTP).
5. 1 pmol/µL of each of the forward and reverse amplification primers (standard 20- to 25-mers) designed to amplify single-copy loci (recommended size, ≤500 bp).
6. 5 U/µL AmpliTaq Gold polymerase (ABI) or standard *Taq* DNA polymerase in conjunction with alternative "hot-start" schemes *(6)*.
7. 25 to 50 ng/µL human genomic DNA: samples known to contain polymorphism or mutation; and homozygous positive controls.
8. High-performance liquid chromatography (HPLC) buffers A and B (*see* **Subheadings 2.2.1.** and **2.2.2.**).
9. *Hae*III restriction digest of pUC18 DNA (Sigma-Aldrich, St. Louis, MO) or other commercially available plasmid digest.
10. Thermal cycler (e.g., ABI Model 9600 or equivalent).
11. Appropriately configured HPLC instrumentation (WAVE DNA Fragment Analysis System; Transgenomic; or similar systems from Varian or Hewlett-Packard).
12. Heat exchanger (HEX-440.010; Timberline Instruments).
13. DNASep column (Transgenomic) or Prototype dsDNA Column (Hewlett-Packard).
14. Precolumn filter with 0–5-µm frit (Upchurch Scientific).

2.2. DHPLC *(see Notes 1–3)*

1. Buffer A: 100 mM triethylamine acetate (TEAA), pH 7.0., 0.1 mM EDTA. Store up to 1 wk at room temperature.
2. Buffer B: 100 mM TEAA, pH 7.0., 0.1 mM EDTA, 25% (v/v) acetonitrile. Store up to 1 wk at room temperature.

2.3. Cycle Sequencing With a 5'-End-Labeled Primer

1. Blood or other DNA source from individual(s) to be tested.
2. 5 M sodium acetate, pH 4.8.
3. Isopropanol (pure).
4. 10 mM Tris-HCl, 1 mM EDTA (TE) buffer, pH 7.4.

5. Molecular weight markers: e.g., φX-174 plasmid digested with *Hae*III (Hoefer Pharmacia Biotech or Invitrogen).
6. 12.5 pmol oligonucleotide.
7. 10X T4 polynucleotide kinase reaction buffer.
8. 10 μCi/μL [γ-^{32}P]ATP (3000 Ci/mmol), 10 μCi/μL [γ-^{33}P]ATP (3000 Ci/mmol), or 10 μCi/μL [γ-^{35}S]ATP (1000 Ci/mmol).
9. 5 U/μL T4 polynucleotide kinase.
10. Dideoxynucleotides: 100 μ*M* ddGTP (*or* 7-deaza-dGTP for GC-rich templates), 600 μ*M* ddATP, 1000 μ*M* ddTTP, and 600 μ*M* ddCTP.
11. 5 U/μL *Taq* DNA polymerase.
12. 10X cycle-sequencing reaction buffer (*see* **Subheading 2.4.1.**).
13. Mineral oil (if needed, depending on thermal cycler).
14. Stop solution (*see* **Subheading 2.4.2.**).
15. Thermal cycler and thermal cycler tubes.

2.4. Reagents and Solutions for Cycle Sequencing

1. 10X cycle-sequencing reaction buffer (*see* **Note 4**): 100 m*M* Tris-HCl, pH 9.0., 500 m*M* KCl, 40 m*M* MgCl$_2$, 20 μ*M* dATP, 20 μ*M* dGTP or 7-deaza-dGTP, 20 μ*M* dCTP, 20 μ*M* dTTP.
2. Stop solution (*see* **Note 5**): 90% (v/v) formamide, 0.1% (w/v) bromphenol blue, 0.1% (w/v) xylene cyanol.
3. 10X T4 polynucleotide kinase reaction buffer (*see* **Note 6**): 500 m*M* Tris-HCl, pH 7.5., 80 m*M* MgCl$_2$, 20 m*M* dithiothreitol.

3. Methods

Genetic mutations may be identified using a number of approaches. In 2005, the most common approaches include DHPLC and/or DNA sequencing.

3.1. Denaturing High-Performance Liquid Chromatography

Single base substitutions, small insertions, or deletions can be detected in 100- to 1500-bp DNA fragments by fractionation of heteroduplexes on reverse-phase columns by DHPLC *(7)*. All single-copy regions of genomic DNA that can be amplified by PCR can be rapidly evaluated using automated machines. Heteroduplexes formed during PCR amplification of DNA from a heterozygous individual will have different melting properties than exactly matched homoduplexes amplified from the DNA of homozygous individuals *(8)*. DNA mutation detection by DHPLC analysis exploits the differential retention of double-stranded homoduplex and heteroduplex species under conditions of partial thermal denaturation, and involves a two-step process. DNA fragments are:

1. Amplified by PCR from genomic template DNA of hetero- or homozygous individuals.
2. Subsequently fractionated under partially denaturing conditions by HPLC.

Because the primary sequence is often known for candidate regions subjected to mutational analysis, the optimal temperature for DHPLC analysis for each fragment (e.g., exon) can be determined by computer software analysis (http://hardy-weinberg.stanford.edu/dhplc/melt.html). When more than one significant melting domain is present in a fragment, additional analysis temperatures are automatically provided. In cases in which the primary sequence between the primer sequence regions is unknown, the optimal temperature required for successful resolution of heteroduplex molecules has to be determined empirically by injecting PCR products at increasing mobile-phase temperatures until a significant decrease in retention time is observed, indicating that the duplexes are almost completely denatured *(9)*. Subsequent analysis at a temperature 1YC lower than the temperature that was determined is generally recommended. The analysis of each sample by DHPLC is very rapid, and nearly 100% of sequence alterations (polymorphisms or mutations) can be detected *(7–9)* (**Fig. 1**).

3.1.1. Amplify Target Sequences (see **Notes 7–10**)

1. Prepare sufficient PCR mix for 100 reactions (i.e., 2.5 mL total), according to **Table 1**.
2. Mix well and dispense 24 µL into each PCR tube.
3. Add 1 µL genomic DNA (25 to 50 ng/µL).
4. Set up tubes containing negative (1 µL of water or some DNA not represented in the genome of interest) controls, and, if possible, positive controls, of known homozygous and heterozygous samples that carry a polymorphism or mutation.
5. Amplify using an ABI 9600 thermal cycler or equivalent, according settings given in **Table 2**.
6. Denature for a final 3 min at 95°C, then allow to gradually reanneal during 30 min from 95°C to 65°C. Store PCR products at 4°C until DHPLC analysis.
7. Analyze 5 µL of PCR product by electrophoresis on a 1- to 1.5%-agarose gel and stain with ethidium bromide to confirm amplification of desired target sequence.

3.1.2. Analyze PCR Products by DHPLC (see **Notes 11–14**)

1. Condition newly packed columns with 50% buffer A and 50% buffer B, using a flow rate of 0.5 mL/min for at least 60 min at 50°C.
2. Test column performance at 50°C by injecting approx 0.5 µg of commercially available *Hae*III restriction digest of pUC18. Use a flow rate of 0.9 mL/min and the following gradient conditions:
   a. From 43% buffer B to 56% buffer B in 3 min.
   b. From 56% buffer B to 68% buffer B in 7 min.
   c. From 68% buffer B to 95% buffer B in 0.1 min.
   d. 95% buffer B for 0.5 min.
   e. From 95% buffer B to 43% buffer B in 0.1 min.

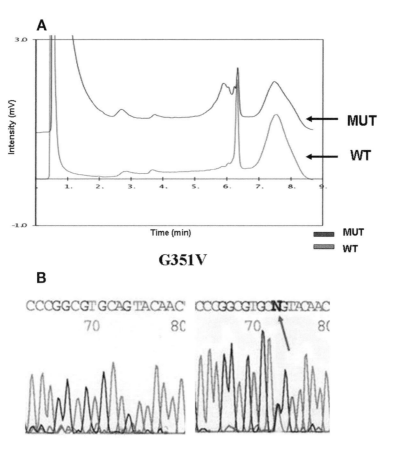

Fig. 1. Analysis of a gene by DHPLC and direct sequencing. (**A**) DHPLC analysis of an exon of this gene identifies an abnormal DHPLC pattern in the affected subject (top arrow) compared with the normal pattern present in controls (bottom arrow). (**B**) DNA sequence analysis of genomic DNA identifies a A-to-G base substitution leading to an amino acid change in the affected subject.

Successful separation of the restriction fragments is monitored at the column outlet by on-line UV absorbance at 254 nm.
3. Equilibrate column to analysis temperature predicted by the computation algorithm at http://hardy-weinberg.stanford.edu/dhplc/melt.html. Alternatively, determine optimum temperature conditions empirically by increasing column temperature with 2 to 3°C increments, until a shift of approx 1 min in retention is observed.
4. Equilibrate column to starting buffer conditions (usually 50% buffer B) at a flow rate of 0.9 mL/min.
5. Adjust gradient startpoints and endpoints according to the size of the PCR products (*2*) based on the retention times of the DNA restriction fragments of the digest used to test the column performance (**Subheading 3.1.2., step 2**).

Table 1
PCR Mix

	Volume per 25-mL reaction (μL)	Final concentration
Deionized water	16.4	—
10X PCR buffer	2.5	1X
25 mM MgCl$_2$	2.0	2 mM
DNTPs (5 mM each)	0.5 each	0.1 mM each
Forward primer (10 μM)	0.5	0.2 μM
Reverse primer (10 μM)	0.5	0.2 μM
5 U/μL AmpliTaq Gold polymerase	0.1	0.5 U

Table 2
PCR Amplification Cycles

1 cycle	10 min	95°C (denaturation)
14 cycles	20 s	94°C (denaturation)
	45 s	72°C (extension)
	20 s	63°C decreased by 0.5°C increments (annealing)
16 cycles	20 s	94°C (denaturation)
	45 s	72°C (extension)
	20 s	56°C (annealing)

6. Set autosampler to inject between 5 and 10 μL of sample, and begin DHPLC analysis.
7. When not in use, continue to perfuse column at a very low flow rate (0.05 mL/ min) with 50% buffer A and 50% buffer B.

3.1.3. Sequence Polymorphic PCR Products (see **Note 15**)

Determine the exact chemical nature and the position of the mutation(s) by sequencing the PCR product.

3.2. Cycle Sequencing (see **Notes 16–18**)

Candidate genes are screened for mutations by a DNA sequencing procedure known as cycle sequencing *(10)*. First, using PCR, a segment of the candidate gene is amplified from the genomic DNA of an affected individual *(11)*. The PCR product is then subjected to multiple rounds of further amplification in a thermal cycler using a heat-stable DNA polymerase in the presence of different dideoxynucleotides and a radiolabeled primer. The resulting ^{32}P-labeled sequence reaction products are fractionated on a denaturing polyacrylamide gel and visualized by autoradiography. DNA segments on the order of 200 bp from 10 to 30 individuals can be screened on each gel. Cycle sequencing eliminates the need to subclone genomic fragments or PCR products, which makes it a much simpler method than conventional sequencing for identifying mutations. Clearly, automated DNA sequencing is a highly used modality. However, this will not be described because it is an automated process.

3.2.1. Prepare Template DNA

1. Isolate and purify human genomic DNA using standard methods, resuspending the DNA in water or TE buffer (pH 7.4 at the end of the procedure).
2. Using PCR, amplify the segment of interest from genomic DNA.
3. Add 50 μL of 5 N sodium acetate, pH 4.8, and 100 μL pure isopropanol to the 50-μL PCR reaction. Incubate for 10 min at room temperature.
4. Microcentrifuge for 10 min at maximum speed (~16,000g), at room temperature. Discard supernatant, and air-dry.
5. Resuspend the pellet in 50 μL water or TE buffer (pH 7.4). Quantify the amount of resuspended DNA by analyzing a 5-μL aliquot on an agarose gel and comparing the resulting band to a known amount of a size marker (e.g., 1 μg of φX-174 plasmid digested with *Hae*III).

3.2.2. 5'-End-Label the Sequencing Primer

1. Prepare a 25-μL reaction mixture containing:
   a. 12.5 pmol oligonucleotide sequencing primer.
   b. 2.5 μL 1X T4 polynucleotide kinase reaction buffer.
   c. 1.0 μL 5 U/μL T4 polynucleotide kinase (5 U total).
   d. 3.0 μL 10 μCi/μL [γ-^{32}P]ATP or [γ-^{33}P]ATP (3000 Ci/mmol; 30 μCi total) or 2.0 μL 10 μCi/μL [γ-^{35}S]ATP (1000 Ci/mol; 20 μCi total).
   e. H$_2$O to total volume of 25 μL.
2. Incubate 30 min at 37°C.

3.2.3. Perform Cycle-Sequencing Reaction

1. For each DNA template, prepare four thermal cycler tubes and add 3 μL of one of the following to each tube: 100 μM ddGTP, 600 μM ddATP, 1000 μM ddTTP, or 600 μM ddCTP. Store tubes on ice.
2. Prepare sequencing cocktail by placing in a fresh tube:
   a. 10 to 20 fmol sequencing template (DNA solution from **Subheading 3.2.1., step 5**).
   b. 1 μL 5'-end-labeled sequencing primer (from **Subheading 3.2.2., step 1**).
   c. 4 μL 10X cycle-sequencing reaction buffer.
   d. 1 μL 2 U/μL Taq DNA polymerase (2 U total).
   e. H$_2$O to total volume of 30 μL.
3. Place 7-μL aliquots of cocktail into each of the four cycle sequencing reaction tubes.

4. Add mineral oil (if necessary), close caps, and start thermal cycling. Cycling conditions will vary for different templates, sequencing primers, thermal cycler designs, and so on. It is advisable to begin with standard PCR conditions and
   optimize the sequencing reaction by varying reaction temperatures, cycling times,
   and/or number of cycling rounds.
5. After completion of thermal cycling, add 5 µL stop solution to each reaction, heat
   denature for 5 min at 95°C, and cool rapidly to less than 4°C.
6. Analyze sequencing reaction products on a 6 or 8% denaturing polyacrylamide
   sequencing gel by loading 5 µL of the denatured reaction and running the gel as
   far as required. If screening the DNA of multiple individuals simultaneously, the
   G reactions, A reactions, T reactions, and C reactions should each be loaded
   together on the gel.
7. Store sequencing reaction at –20°C, and load repeatedly, if necessary.
8. Dry gel and autoradiograph overnight.

3.3. Anticipated Results

3.3.1. DHPLC

In any mutational analysis scheme, it is important to distinguish between
common polymorphisms and clinically relevant mutations. This is achieved by
assessing the background polymorphic variation associated with normal control individuals (unaffected individuals of similar ethnicity or population composition). Estimates of the frequency of common sequence variation associated
with the human genome are approx 1 per kilobase in noncoding sequences and
lower in coding sequences. Therefore, most samples can be expected to be
monomorphic and, thus, display homoduplex signatures. However, the frequency of a mutation or polymorphism may be high relative to the normal
control sample. Although DHPLC typically generates heteroduplex profiles
clearly distinct from homoduplexes (often of similar height), certain fragments
may display only subtle differences in profile topography. If additional resolution is not achieved by using a different analysis temperature, then the size of
the homoduplex peak becomes more significant than usual. Any significant
decrease in height with concomitant appearance of an earlier-eluting peak or a
pronounced shoulder is suggestive of sequence variation. In cases in which
multiple mismatches exist, it is possible that, very rarely, the heteroduplex may
completely denature and coelute with primers, dNTPs, and so on. The only
indication of such a situation would be a significant decrease in the homoduplex
peak height. Whenever possible, positive controls of known heteroduplex composition should be run at least once during the analysis process.

3.3.2. Anticipated Results: Cycle Sequencing

Cycle sequencing is best used to screen relatively short sequences (e.g., those
≤300 bp) for mutations. If the samples are loaded with all of the G reactions

next to one another, all of the A reactions next to one another, and so on, mutations can be rapidly identified from the autoradiogram. That is, a single nucleotide difference in a probands will be reflected by the presence of a unique band (and absence of another band normally seen) in one lane of the sequencing gel. If the proband is heterozygous, there should also be a band at that normal position, but its intensity should be diminished compared with the products derived from other individuals.

3.4. Clinical Diseases

3.4.1. The Long QT Syndromes

3.4.1.1. CLINICAL DESCRIPTION

The LQTS are inherited or acquired disorders of repolarization, identified by the electrocardiographic (ECG) abnormalities of prolongation of the QT interval corrected for heart rate (QTc) higher than 460 to 480 ms, relative bradycardia, T-wave abnormalities, and episodic ventricular tachyarrhythmias *(1,2)*, particularly *torsade de pointes*. The inherited form of LQTS is transmitted as an autosomal-dominant or autosomal-recessive trait. Acquired LQTS may be seen as a complication of various drug therapies or electrolyte abnormalities *(1,2)*. Whether the abnormality is genetic based or acquired, the clinical presentation is similar. In many cases, the initial presentation is syncope, whereas, in others, an ECG leads to the diagnosis. Tragically, some individuals have sudden death as their initial presenting feature, and this has been reported to occur in families in some cases. Typically, autopsy evaluation identifies a normal structural heart with no apparent cardiac cause of death.

3.4.1.2. CLINICAL GENETICS

Two differently inherited forms of familial LQTS have been reported. The Romano–Ward Syndrome is the most common of the inherited forms of LQTS and seems to be transmitted as an autosomal-dominant trait *(1,2)*. In this disorder, the disease gene is transmitted to 50% of the offspring of an affected individual. However, low penetrance has been described and, therefore, gene carriers may, in fact, have no clinical features of disease *(12)*. Individuals with Romano–Ward syndrome have the pure syndrome of prolonged QT interval on ECG, with the associated symptom complex of syncope, sudden death, and, in some patients, seizures *(1)*.

The Jervell and Lange-Nielsen Syndrome (JLNS) is a relatively uncommon inherited form of LQTS *(1,2)*. Classically, this disease has been described as having apparent autosomal-recessive transmission *(1,2)*. These patients have the identical clinical presentation as those with Romano–Ward syndrome but also have associated sensorineural deafness. Clinically, patients with JLNS usually have longer QT intervals as compared with individuals with Romano–Ward syndrome, and also have a more malignant course. Priori and colleagues reported autosomal-recessive cases of Romano–Ward syndrome *(13)*, thus, changing one of the *sina qua nons* of JLNS.

To date, six genes for LQTS have been identified *(1,2,14–20)*, and a seventh gene, causing a more complex disorder known as Andersen syndrome (LQTS, ventricular arrhythmias, and hypokalemic periodic paralysis associated with dysmorphisms in some individuals) *(21,22)*, has been discovered *(22–24)*.

3.4.1.3. Gene Identification in Romano–Ward Syndrome

3.4.1.3.1. KVLQT1 or KCNQ1: The *LQT1* Gene. The first of the genes mapped for LQTS, initially termed *LQT1*, required 5 yr from the time that mapping to chromosome 11p15.5 was first reported *(14)* to gene cloning. This gene, originally named *KVLQT1*, but more recently called *KCNQ1*, is a potassium channel gene that consists of 16 exons, spans approx 400 kb, and is widely expressed in human tissues, including heart, inner ear, kidney, lung, placenta, and pancreas, but not in skeletal muscle, liver, or brain *(25)*. This gene is the most commonly mutated of the LQTS genes. Although most of the mutations are private (i.e., only seen in one family), there is at least one frequently mutated region (called a hot spot) *(25)*.

Analysis of the predicted amino acid sequence of KCNQ1 suggested that it encodes a potassium channel subunit *(15)* (**Fig. 2**). Biophysical characterization of the KCNQ1 protein confirmed that this is a voltage-gated potassium channel protein subunit that requires coassembly with a β-subunit (called *minK* or *KCNE1*) to function properly *(26,27)*. Expression of either *KCNQ1* or *minK* (*KCNE1*) alone results in either inefficient or no current development. When *KCNE1* and *KCNQ1* are coexpressed in either mammalian cell lines or *Xenopus* oocytes, however, the slowly activating potassium current (I_{Ks}) is developed in cardiac myocytes *(26,27)*. Combination of normal and mutant KCNQ1 subunits forms abnormal I_{Ks} channels, and these mutations are believed to act through a dominant-negative mechanism (the mutant form of KCNQ1 interferes with the function of the normal wild-type form through a poison pill-type mechanism) or a loss-of-function mechanism (only the mutant form loses activity) *(28)*.

Because KCNQ1 and KCNE1 form a unit, mutations in *KCNE1* could also be expected to cause LQTS, as was subsequently demonstrated *(16)*.

3.4.1.3.2. HERG or KCNH2: The *LQT2* Gene. After the initial localization of *LQT2* to chromosome 7q35–36 by Jiang et al. *(17)*, candidate genes (i.e., genes encoding proteins that could cause repolarization abnormalities if mutated, such as ion channels, modulators of ion channels, members of the

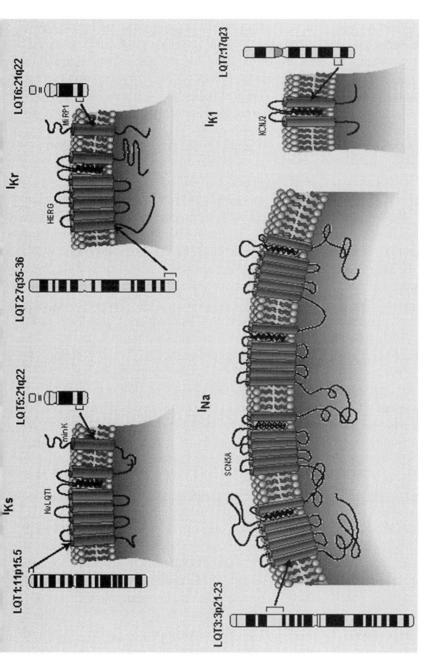

Fig. 2. Topology of ion channels in the heart. (**Top left**) KvLQT1 and minK, which constitute the I_{Ks} potassium channel. (**Top right**) HERG and MiRP1, which constitute the I_{Kr} potassium channel. (**Bottom left**) The cardiac I_{Na} sodium channel encoded by SCN5A. In addition, the *LQT7* gene (**Bottom right**) encoding for Andersen syndrome, known as *KCNJ2*, encodes for the I_{K1} potassium channel.

sympathetic nervous system, and so on) in this region were analyzed. *HERG* (human ether-a-go-go-related gene), now known as *KCNH2*, a cardiac potassium-channel gene, was one of the candidates evaluated and found to be mutated in patients with clinical evidence of LQTS *(18)*. This gene is the second most common gene mutated in LQTS (second to *KCNQ1*). As with *KCNQ1*, private mutations, which are scattered throughout the entire gene without clustering preferentially, are seen.

KCNH2 consists of 16 exons and spans 55 kb of genomic sequence *(18)*, and its predicted topology (**Fig. 2**) is similar to *KCNQ1*. Electrophysiological and biophysical characterization of expressed KCNH2 in *Xenopus* oocytes established that it encodes the rapidly activating, delayed-rectifier potassium current (I_{Kr}) *(29,30)*. Electrophysiological studies of LQTS-associated mutations showed that they act through either a loss-of-function or a dominant-negative mechanism *(31)*. In addition, protein trafficking abnormalities have been shown to occur *(32,33)*. This channel has also been shown to coassemble with β-subunits for normal function, similar to that seen in I_{Ks}. McDonald et al. *(34)* initially suggested that the complexing of KCNH2 with KCNE1 is needed to regulate the I_{Kr} potassium current. Bianchi et al. subsequently provided confirmatory evidence that KCNE1 is involved in regulation of both I_{Ks} and I_{Kr} *(35)*. In addition, Abbott et al. *(36)* identified MiRP1 (or KCNE2) as a β-subunit for KCNH2.

Mutations in the pore region of HERG have been shown to result in an increased risk of syncope and sudden death *(37)*. This, in addition to the newly created fee-for-service mutation analysis laboratory, capable of providing direct sequencing results within weeks (Genaissance Pharmaceuticals), potentially enables the use of genotype to phenotype correlation to effectively prevent episodes of sudden death.

3.4.1.3.3. *SCN5A:* The *LQT3* Gene. The positional candidate gene approach was also used to establish that the gene responsible for the chromosome 3p21–25-linked LQTS *(LQT3)* is the cardiac sodium channel gene, *SCN5A* *(19)*. *SCN5A* is highly expressed in human myocardium and brain, but not in skeletal muscle, liver, or uterus. It consists of 28 exons that span 80 kb and encodes a protein of 2016 amino acids whose structure consists of four homologous domains, each of which contains six membrane-spanning segments, similar to the structure of the potassium channel α-subunits (**Fig. 2**) *(38)*. Expression in *Xenopus* oocytes demonstrated that *SCN5A* mutations act through a gain-of-function mechanism (the mutant channel functions normally, but with altered properties, such as delayed inactivation) and that the mechanism of chromosome 3-linked LQTS is persistent noninactivated sodium current in the plateau phase of the action potential *(38–40)*. Later, An et al. *(41)* showed that not all mutations in *SCN5A* are associated with persistent current, and demonstrated that *SCN5A* interacted with β-subunits.

Polymorphisms in *SCN5A* have been shown to elevate the risk of arrhythmias. Splawski et al. *(42)* showed this to occur in individuals of African descent, whereas Viswanathan and colleagues *(43)* demonstrated modulation of conduction system disease by the H558R polymorphism in a child with a nearby mutation (T512I). These findings have fueled speculation about the potential importance of polymorphisms in clinical features of subjects with ion-channel dysfunction.

3.4.1.3.4. *ankyrin-B*: The *LQT4* Gene. This gene was first localized to chromosome 4q25–27 in a large French kindred in which the clinical syndrome was characterized by sinus node dysfunction, QTc prolongation, episodes of atrial fibrillation, as well as odd T-wave morphology *(44)*. The identity of this gene was uncovered by Mohler et al. using a candidate gene approach *(20)*. The gene, *ankyrin-B* (also known as *ANKB* or *ANK2*), plays a fundamental role in the recognition of important interacting proteins that ensure appropriate localization in cell membranes *(20,45)*. Several of these proteins are involved in ion transport, including the pore-forming subunits of voltage-gated sodium channels, the transmembrane Na^+–K^+ ATPase and Na^+–Ca^{2+} exchanger, and studies of mouse models have demonstrated calcium-handling abnormalities. It was also speculated that ankyrin-B affects sodium channels, leading to this broad, complex phenotype *(20,45)*.

3.4.1.3.5. *minK* or *KCNE1*: The *LQT5* Gene. *minK* (also known as *lsK* or *KCNE1*), was initially localized to chromosome 21 (21q22.1) and found to consist of three exons that span approx 40 kb *(46)*. It encodes a short protein consisting of 130 amino acids and has only one transmembrane-spanning segment, with small extracellular and intercellular regions *(46)*. When expressed in *Xenopus* oocytes, it produces a potassium current that closely resembles the slowly activating, delayed-rectifier potassium current, I_{Ks}, in cardiac cells *(46,47)*. KCNE1 interacts with KCNQ1 to form the cardiac slowly activating, delayed-rectifier I_{Ks} current *(26,27)*; KCNE1 alone cannot form a functional channel, but induces the I_{Ks} current by interacting with the endogenous *KCNQ1* protein in *Xenopus* oocytes and mammalian cells. Bianchi et al. also showed that mutant *minK* results in abnormalities of I_{Ks}, I_{Kr}, and protein trafficking *(35)*. McDonald et al. *(34)* showed that KCNE1 also complexes with HERG to regulate the I_{Kr} potassium current. Splawski et al. *(16)* demonstrated that *KCNE1* mutations cause LQTS when they identified mutations in two families with LQTS. In both cases, missense mutations (S74L, D76N) were identified, which reduced I_{Ks} by shifting the voltage dependence of activation and accelerating channel deactivation. The functional consequences of these mutations includes delayed cardiac repolarization and, hence, an increased risk of arrhythmias.

3.4.1.3.6. *MiRP1* or *KCNE2*: The *LQT6* Gene. *MiRP1*, the *minK*-related peptide 1, also known as *KCNE2*, is a potassium-channel gene similar to KCNE1 *(36)*. This small integral membrane subunit protein assembles with *HERG (LQT2),* to alter its function and enables full development of the I_{Kr} current. It encodes a 123-amino acid channel protein with a single predicted transmembrane segment, and the gene is mapped to chromosome 21q22.1, near *KCNE1* (*minK*) *(36)*.

Three missense mutations associated with LQTS and ventricular fibrillation were initially identified in *KCNE2* by Abbott et al. *(36)*, and biophysical analysis demonstrated that these mutants form channels that open slowly and close rapidly, thus, diminishing potassium currents. In one case, the missense mutation led to the development of *torsade de pointes* and ventricular fibrillation after intravenous clarithromycin infusion (i.e., drug induced).

Therefore, similar to KCNE1, this channel protein acts as a β-subunit but, by itself, leads to ventricular arrhythmia risk when mutated. These similar channel proteins (i.e., KCNE1 and KCNE2*)* suggest that a family of channels exist that regulate ion channel α-subunits.

3.4.1.4. THERAPY FOR *LQTS*

The standard of care for LQTS for many years has been the use of β-blockers *(1,2)*. A large study published by the Long QT Registry Investigators demonstrated significant reduction in syncope, but sudden death still resulted in some patients *(48)*. Gene-specific approaches were originally reported by Schwartz et al. *(49)*, who used the sodium-channel blocking agent, mexiletine, for patients with LQTS, and demonstrated shortening of the QTc. Compton et al. *(50,51)* reported the use of potassium infusion (serum potassium > 4.8) in LQT1 patients, with similar results. However, only the potassium therapy studies have been followed up to show improved outcome *(51)*. Recently, the use of an internal cardioverter defibrillator has become a mainstay of therapy *(52)*. The use of genotype to phenotype correlations to predict those at risk for sudden death may be useful in choosing the proper therapeutic strategy *(53,54)*.

3.4.1.5. GENETICS AND PHYSIOLOGY OF AUTOSOMAL-RECESSIVE LQTS (JLNS)

Neyroud et al. *(55)* reported the first molecular abnormality in patients with JLNS when they reported on two families in which three children were affected by JLNS and in whom a novel homozygous deletion–insertion mutation of *KCNQ1* in three patients was found. At the same time, Splawski et al. *(56)* identified a homozygous insertion of a single nucleotide, which caused a frameshift in the coding sequence after the second putative transmembrane domain of *KCNQ1*. Together, these data strongly suggested that at least one form of JLNS is caused by homozygous mutations in *KCNQ1* (*55–57*).

Generally, heterozygous mutations in *KCNQ1* cause Romano–Ward syndrome (LQTS only), whereas homozygous (or compound heterozygous) mutations in *KCNQ1* cause JLNS (LQTS and deafness). The hypothetical explanation suggests that although heterozygous *KCNQ1* mutations act by a dominant-negative mechanism, some functional KCNQ1 potassium channels still exist in the stria vascularis of the inner ear. Therefore, congenital deafness is averted in patients with heterozygous mutations. For patients with homozygous mutations, no functional KCNQ1 potassium channels can be formed. It has been shown that KCNQ1 is expressed in the inner ear (*55*), suggesting that homozygous mutations can cause the dysfunction of potassium secretion in the inner ear and lead to deafness. However, it should be noted that incomplete penetrance exists, and not all heterozygous or homozygous mutations follow this rule (*13*).

As with Romano–Ward syndrome, if *KCNQ1* mutations can cause the phenotype, it could be expected that *KCNE1* mutations could also be causative of the phenotype (JLNS). Schulze-Bahr et al. (*58*), in fact, showed that mutations in *KCNE1* also result in JLNS syndrome. Hence, abnormal $I_{K}s$ current, whether it occurs because of homozygous or compound heterozygous mutations in *KCNQ1* or *minK*, result in LQTS and deafness.

3.4.1.6. ANDERSEN SYNDROME

This complex phenotype includes hypokalemic periodic paralysis, dysmorphic features, QTc prolongation, and ventricular arrhythmias (*21*). In some patients, polymorphic ventricular tachycardia has been identified. The dysmorphic features include syndactyly, hypertelorism, low-set ears, broad forehead, micrognathia, cleft palate, clinodactyly, and scoliosis (*22*). In some patients, renal anomalies and congenital heart disease, including bicuspid aortic valve, coarctation of the aorta, and valvular pulmonary stenosis, have been identified as well.

Andersen syndrome is inherited as an autosomal-dominant trait. The genetic basis of this complex phenotype was identified as mutations in the chromosome 17q23 *KCNJ2* gene encoding the inward-rectifying potassium current, Kir2.1 (*23*). Mutations expressed in *Xenopus* oocytes demonstrated a strong dominant-negative effect and loss of function (*23*).

In many cell types, particularly cardiomyocytes and neurons, Kir2 channels play an important role in setting the membrane potential and modulating excitability. When inward rectifier current is reduced, the propensity for arrhythmias increases. Hence, in Andersen syndrome, mutations result in reduced current and the development of cardiac arrhythmias *(24)*.

3.4.2. Brugada Syndrome

3.4.2.1. CLINICAL ASPECTS OF BRUGADA SYNDROME

The first identification of the ECG pattern of right bundle branch block (RBBB) with ST-elevation in leads V1–V3 was reported by Osher and Wolff *(59)*. Shortly thereafter, Edeiken *(60)* identified persistent ST-elevation without RBBB in 10 asymptomatic males and Levine et al. *(61)* described ST-elevation in the right chest leads and conduction block in the right ventricle in patients with severe hyperkalemia. The first association of this ECG pattern with sudden death was described by Martini et al. *(62)* and later by Aihara et al. *(63)*. This association was further confirmed in 1991 by Pedro and Josep Brugada *(4)*, who described four patients with sudden and aborted sudden death with ECGs demonstrating RBBB and persistent ST-elevation in leads V1–V3.

3.4.2.2. CLINICAL GENETICS OF BRUGADA SYNDROME

Most of the families thus far identified with Brugada syndrome have apparent autosomal-dominant inheritance *(64)*. In these families, approx 50% of offspring of affected patients develop the disease. Although the number of families reported has been small, it is likely that this is because of underrecognition as well as premature and unexpected death.

3.4.2.3. MOLECULAR GENETICS OF BRUGADA SYNDROME

In 1998, our laboratory reported the findings on six families and several sporadic cases of Brugada syndrome *(65)*. Candidate gene screening was performed and mutations in *SCN5A* were identified *(65)*.

Biophysical analysis of the mutants in *Xenopus* oocytes demonstrated a reduction in the number of functional sodium channels (which should promote development of reentrant arrhythmias) and, in some mutations, sodium channels that recover from inactivation more rapidly than normal *(64,65)*. Subsequent experiments revealed that, at physiological temperatures (37YC), reactivation of some channels was actually slower, whereas inactivation of the channel was importantly accelerated (i.e., the mutant is temperature sensitive) *(66)*. Kambouris et al. identified a mutation in essentially the same region of *SCN5A* as a Brugada syndrome-causing mutation (R1623Q), but the clinical and biophysical features of this mutation were found to be consistent with LQTS and not Brugada syndrome *(67)*. Subsequently, mutations have been identified in which some family members have Brugada syndrome, whereas other members of the same family have LQTS. It has also been shown that individual patients can demonstrate both entities over time.

3.4.3. Polymorphic Ventricular Tachycardia

Polymorphic ventricular tachycardia is characterized by the occurrence of salvoes of bidirectional and polymorphic ventricular tachycardias, typically in relation to adrenergic stimulation or physical exercise but without evidence of structural myocardial disease *(5)*. The clinical outcomes of these patients are reportedly poor, with estimates of mortality in the range of 30 to 50% by the age of 20 to 30 yr. The disorder is commonly inherited, with transmission in an autosomal-dominant pattern *(68,69)*.

The first gene identified for this disorder was mapped to chromosome 1q42–q43 *(68)*. The gene was shown to be the cardiac ryanodine receptor (*RyR2*), the same gene identified to cause the arrhythmogenic right ventricular dysplasia-type 2 phenotype *(67–72)*. Ryanodine receptors are the largest ion channels known to exist and RyR2 is abundantly expressed in myocardium, and, to a lesser extent, in the brain and gestational myometrium. This calcium-release channel is activated after stimulation of voltage-sensitive L-type calcium channels on the outer myocardial cell membrane, which permits the cellular entrance of tiny amounts of calcium ions but which activates RyR2. This activation enables large amounts of calcium ions to pass from the lumen of the sarcoplasmic reticulum into the cytoplasm, initiating myocardial contraction. Mutations in this gene lead to uncoupling of excitation–contraction coupling and to increased sensitivity of calcium-induced activation of the calcium-release channel complex.

A second gene causing this disorder was reported by Lahat et al. in autosomal-recessive polymorphic VT *(73)*. This gene, localized to chromosome 1p13–1p21, was identified as the gene encoding calsequestrin 2, which serves as the major calcium reservoir within the sarcoplasmic reticulum and interacts with RyR2 *(73,74)*.

3.5. Conclusion

Genetic screening to identify genes causing arrhythmia disorders has progressed from nearly impossible to *passé* in the past 15 yr because of the development of rapid, high-technology, and high-throughput methods for mutation screening. Fee-for-service laboratories are now offering genetic testing for these disorders.

4. Notes

1. Use deionized distilled water in all solutions and protocol steps.
2. A 2 *M* stock solution of TEAA, pH 7.0, for DHPLC buffers (**Subheadings 2.2.1.** and **2.2.2.**) is commercially available from ABI and is recommended because the pure base triethylamine, obtainable from vendors such as Fluka and J.T. Baker, is a flammable chemical that has an irritant effect on skin, eyes, and respiratory organs. If prepared in-house, make up a 1 *M* (rather than a 2 *M*) stock solution.

Briefly, weigh 202.38 g of triethylamine into a 2-L volumetric flask. Add 500 mL of water and stir with magnetic stirring bar at 300 rpm. Weigh 120.1 g of glacial acetic acid into a beaker and add the acid slowly to the triethylamine solution, which will heat up and form white fumes. Continue stirring and fill the flask with water to approx 1900 mL. Once the solution has cooled to room temperature, measure the pH value with the pH electrode. If the pH is less than 7.0, add drops of triethylamine, if the pH is greater than 7.0, add acetic acid, until the pH is adjusted. Remove stirring bar and fill with water to the 2-L mark on the volumetric flask. Add 100 mL of 1 *M* TEAA stock solution per liter of eluant. For eluant B, add 25% (v/v) of a grade of acetonitrile with the lowest obtainable UV cutoff (i.e., the wavelength at which the absorbance becomes high; an appropriate grade is available from J.T. Baker). EDTA is added (from 0.5 *M* stock) to prevent the interaction of DNA with divalent and trivalent metal cations that strongly bind the DNA to the stationary phase.

3. Provided that HPLC-grade reagents and an in-line vacuum degasser are used, it is unnecessary to filter and degas the buffers before use.
4. Store cycle-sequencing reaction buffer (10X) in aliquots at –20°C.
5. Store cycle-sequencing stop solution in aliquots at room temperature.
6. Store T4 polynucleotide kinase reaction buffer (10X) in aliquots at –20°C.
7. The initial denaturation inactivates AmpliTaq Gold. The incremental decrease in annealing temperature during the following 14 cycles improves the PCR specificity and minimizes the PCR optimization, provided that the melting temperatures of the primers are similar *(1)*.
8. This final denaturation and gradual reannealing regime ensures that equimolar amounts of heteroduplex and homoduplex molecules are formed.
9. Amplicons can be stored at 4°C for several weeks.
10. Successful mismatch detection requires the comparison of at least two chromosomes. Therefore, in the case of haploid genomes, PCR products have to be mixed with a reference. Determine yields for test and reference amplicons by agarose gel electrophoresis in UV tracings at roughly equimolar ratios. Because heteroduplexes are overrepresented in UV tracings because of the encased UV absorption of the single-stranded components constituting the "bubble" formed around the mismatch, heteroduplexes are successfully detected even when only one out of eight chromosomes is mutated.
11. Baseline resolution of the 257-bp and 267-bp, and the 434-bp and 458-bp fragments, respectively, should be obtained. If not, request replacement of the column.
12. Avoid direct contact between the stainless steel column and the hot metal surfaces of the column oven. The surfaces are warmer than the circulating air in the oven; hence, direct contact will heat the mobile phase in the column to a higher temperature than indicated on the column oven display. Such contact will also result in discrepancies between the predicted and observed temperatures.
13. Equilibration time is dependent on the dead volume of the chromatograph (i.e., the volume of liquid pathway between solvent mixer and column outlet); displace dead volume at least once, which typically takes 1 to 3 min.

14. For temperature optimization, start the gradient at 7% below the estimated percentage of buffer B at which the amplicion is expected to elute at 50ºC (to account for the shift in retention toward lower percentages of buffer B with increasing column temperatures). Once the optimum temperature has been determined, a gradient window as small as 4.5% during 2.5 min can be set. For amplicons up to 600 bp, increase the gradient by 1.8% of buffer B per minute. For larger amplicons, use a shallower gradient, e.g., 1.2% of buffer B per minute.
15. Chromatographic profiles of single PCR products that show more than one peak are indicative of the presence of mismatch.
16. Only 10 to 20 fmol of DNA template is needed per cycle-sequencing reaction. It is convenient to calculate the equivalent amount of double-stranded DNA (i.e., how much will constitute 10 fmol) as follows: nanograms of DNA template = 10 fmol × N × 6.6 × 10^{-3}, where N is the number of basepairs of the sequencing template.
17. Human genomic DNA cannot be analyzed directly by cycle sequencing. To screen genomic DNA for mutations, it is necessary to amplify the sequence of interest beforehand by a standard PCR reaction.
18. The oligonucleotide sequencing primer is derived from sequence immediately 5′ to the sequence being screened for mutations. Although either PCR primer can be used as a sequencing primer, clearer results can be obtained by using a nested primer.

References

1. Priori, S. G., Barhanin, J., Hauer, R. N. W., et al. (1999) Genetic and molecular basis of cardiac arrhythmias: impact on clinical management (Parts I and II). *Circulation* **99**, 518–528.
2. Schwartz, P. J., Priori, S. G., and Napolitano, C. (2000) The long QT syndrome, in *Cardiac Electrophysiology: From Cell to Bedside*. 3rd ed (Zipes DP, Jalife J, eds.), WB Saunders, Philadelphia, PA, pp. 597–615.
3. Scheinman, M. M. (2005) History of Wolff-Parkinson-White syndrome. *Pacing Clin. Electrophysiol.* **28**, 152–156.
4. Brugada, P. and Brugada, J. (1991) A distinct clinical and electrocardiographic syndrome: right bundle-branch block, persistent ST segment elevation with normal QT interval and sudden cardiac death. *PACE* **14**, 746.
5. Leenhardt, A., Lucet, V., Denjoy, I., Grau, F., Ngoc, D. D., and Coumel, P. (1995) Catecholaminergic polymorphic ventricular tachycardia in children: A 7 year follow-up of 21 patients. *Circulation* **91**, 1512–1519.
6. Chou, Q., Russell, M., Birch, D. E., Raymond, J., and Bloch, W. (1992) Prevention of pre-PCR, mispriming and primer dimerization improves low-copy-number amplifications. *Nucl. Acids. Res.* **20**, 1717–1723.
7. O'Donovan, M. C., Oefner, P. J., Austin, J., et al. (1998) Blind analysis of denaturing high performance liquid chromatography as a tool for mutation detection. *Genomics* **52**, 44–49.
8. Oefner, P. J., Huber, C. G., Umluuft, F., Berti, G.-N., Stimpfl, E., and Bonn, G. K. High resolution liquid chromatography of fluorescent dye-labeled nucleic acids. *Anal. Biochem.* 1994; 223:39–46.

9. Kuklin, A., Munson, K., Gjerde, D., Haefele, R., and Taylor, P. Detection of single-nucleotide polymorphisms with the WAVE DNA fragment analysis system. *Genet. Test.* 1998; 1:201–206.

10. Murray, V. (1989) Improved double-stranded DNA sequencing using the linear polymerase chain reaction. *Nucl. Acids. Res.* **17**, 8889.

11. Innis, M. A. and Gelfand, D. H. (1990) Optimization of PCRs, in *PCR Protocols: A Guide to Methods and Applications* (Innis, M. A., Gelfand, D. A., Sninsky, J. J., White, T. J., eds.), Academic, San Diego, CA, pp 3–12.

12. Priori, S. G., Napolitano, C., and Schwartz, P. J. (1999) Low penetrance in the long-QT syndrome: Clinical impact. *Circulation* **99**, 529–533.

13. Priori, S. G., Schwartz, P. J., Napolitano, C., et al. (1998) A recessive variant of the Romano–Ward long-QT syndrome. *Circulation* **97**, 2420–2425.

14. Keating, M. T., Atkinson, D., Dunn, C., Timothy, K., Vincent, G. M., and Leppert, M. (1991) Linkage of a cardiac arrhythmia, the long QT syndrome, and the Harvey ras-1 gene. *Science* **252**, 704–706.

15. Wang, Q., Curran, M. E., Splawski, I., et al. (1996) Positional cloning of a novel potassium channel gene: *KVLQT1* mutations cause cardiac arrhythmias. *Nat. Genet.* **12**, 17–23.

16. Splawski, I., Tristani-Firouzi, M., Lehmann, M. H., Sanguinetti, M. C., and Keating, M. T. (1997) Mutations in the *minK* gene cause long QT syndrome and suppress I_{Ks} function. *Nat. Genet.* **17**, 338–340.

17. Jiang, C., Atkinson, D., Towbin, J. A., et al. (1994) Two long QT syndrome loci map to chromosome 3 and 7 with evidence for further heterogeneity. *Nat. Genet.* **8**, 141–147.

18. Curran, M. E., Splawski, I., Timothy, K. W., Vincent, G. M., Green, E. D., and Keating, M. T. (1995) A molecular basis for cardiac arrhythmia: *HERG* mutations cause long QT syndrome. *Cell* **80**, 795–803.

19. Wang, Q., Shen, J., Splawski, I., et al. (1995) *SCN5A* mutations associated with an inherited cardiac arrhythmia, long QT syndrome. *Cell* **80**, 805–811.

20. Mohler, P. J., Schott, J. J., Gramolini, A. O., et al. (2003) Ankyrin-β mutation causes type 4 long-QT cardiac arrhythmia and sudden cardiac death. *Nature* **421**, 634–639.

21. Andersen, E. D., Krasilnikoff, P. A., and Overvad, H. (1971) Intermittent muscular weakness, extrasystoles, and multiple developmental anomalies: a new syndrome? *Acta Pediatr. Scand.* **60**, 559–564.

22. Andelfinger, G., Tapper, A. R., Welch, R. C., Vanoye, C. G., George, A. L., Jr., and Benson, D. W. (2002) KCNJ2 mutation results in Andersen syndrome with sex-specific cardiac and skeletal muscle phenotypes. *Am. J. Hum. Genet.* **71**, 663–668.

23. Plaster, N. M., Tawil, R., Tristani-Firouzi, M., et al. (2001) Mutations in Kir2.1 cause the developmental and episodic electrical phenotypes of Andersen's syndrome. *Cell* **105**, 511–519.

24. Tristani-Firouzi, M., Jensen, J. L., Donaldson, M. R., et al. (2002) Functional and clinical characterization of KCNJ2 mutations associated with LQT7 (Andersen syndrome). *J. Clin. Invest.* **222**, 381–388.

25. Li, H., Chen, Q., Moss, A. J., et al. (1998) New mutations in the *KVLQT1* potassium channel that cause long QT syndrome. *Circulation* **97,** 1264–1269.
26. Barhanin, J., Lesage, F., Guillemare, E., Finc, M., Lazdunski, M., and Romey, G. (1996) *KVLQT1* and IsK (*minK*) proteins associate to form the I$_{Ks}$ cardiac potassium current. *Nature* **384,** 78–80.
27. Sanguinetti, M. C., Curran, M. E., Zou, A., et al. (1996) Coassembly of *KvLQT1* and *minK* (IsK) proteins to form cardiac I$_{Ks}$ potassium channel. *Nature* **384,** 80–83.
28. Wollnick, B., Schreeder, B. C., Kubish, C., Esperer, H. D., Wieacker, P., and Jensch, T. J. (1997) Pathophysiological mechanisms of dominant and recessive *KVLQT1* K+ channel mutations found in inherited cardiac arrhythmias. *Hum. Molec. Genet.* **6,** 1943–1949.
29. Sanguinetti, M. C., Jiang, C., Curran, M. E., and Keating, M. T. (1995) A mechanistic link between an inherited and an acquired cardiac arrhythmia: *HERG* encodes the I$_{Kr}$ potassium channel. *Cell* **81,** 299–307.
30. Trudeau, M. C., Warmke, J., Ganetzky, B., and Robertson, G. (1995) *HERG*, a human inward rectifier in the voltage-gated potassium channel family. *Science* **269,** 92–95.
31. Sanguinetti, M. C., Curran, M. E., Spector, P. S., and Keating, M. T. (1996) Spectrum of *HERG* K+-channel dysfunction in an inherited cardiac arrhythmia. *Proc. Natl. Acad. Sci. USA* **93,** 2208–2212.
32. Furutani, M., Trudeau, M. C., Hagiwara, N., et al. (1999) Novel mechanism associated with an inherited cardiac arrhythmia. Defective protein trafficking by the mutant *HERG* (G601S) potassium channel. *Circulation* **99,** 2290–2294.
33. Zhou, Z., Gong, Q., and Epstein, M. L., and January, C. T. (1998) *HERG* channel dysfunction in human long QT syndrome. *J. Biol. Chem.* **263,** 21,061–21,066.
34. McDonald, T. V., Yu, Z., Ming, Z., et al. (1997) A *MinK-HERG* complex regulates the cardiac potassium current I$_{Kr}$. *Nature* **388,** 289–292.
35. Bianchi, L., Shen, Z., Dennis, A. T., et al. (1999) Cellular dysfunction of *LQT5-minK* mutants: abnormalities of I$_{Ks}$, I$_{Kr}$ and trafficking in long QT syndrome. *Hum. Molec. Genet.* **8,** 1499–1507.
36. Abbott, G. W., Sesti, F., Splawski, I., et al. (1999) *MiRP1* forms I$_{Kr}$ potassium channels with *HERG* and is associated with cardiac arrhythmia. *Cell* **97,** 175–187.
37. Moss, A. J., Zareba, W., Kaufman, E. S., et al. (2002) Increased risk of arrhythmic events in long-QT syndrome with mutations in the pore region of the human ether-a-go-go-related gene potassium channel. *Circulation* **105,** 794–799.
38. Gellens, M., George, A. l., Chen, L., et al. (1992) Primary structure and functional expression of the human cardiac tetrodotoxin-insensitive voltage-dependent sodium channel. *Proc. Natl. Acad. Sci. USA* **89,** 554–558.
39. Bennett, P. B., Yazawa, K., Makita, N., and George, A. L., Jr. (1995) Molecular mechanism for an inherited cardiac arrhythmia. *Nature* **376,** 683–685.
40. Dumaine, R., Wang, Q., Keating, M. T., et al. (1996) Multiple mechanisms of sodium channel-linked long QT syndrome. *Circ. Res.* **78,** 916–924.
41. An, R. H., Wang, X. L., Kerem, B., et al. (1998) Novel *LQT-3* mutation affects Na+ channel activity through interactions between alpha- and beta 1 -subunits. *Circ. Res.* **83,** 141–146.

42. Splawski, I., Timothy, K. W., Tateyama, M., et al. (2002) Variant of SCN5A so-dium channel implicated in risk of cardiac arrhythmia. *Science* **297**, 1333–1336.
43. Viswanathan, P. C., Benson, D. W., and Balser, J. R. (2003) A common SCN5A polymorphism modulates the biophysical effects of an SCN5A mutation. *J. Clin. Invest.* **111**, 341–346.
44. Schott, J. J., Charpentier, F., Peltier, S., et al. (1995) Mapping of a gene for long QT syndrome to chromosome 4q25-27. *Am. J. Hum. Genet.* **57**, 1114–1122.
45. Nattel, S. (2003) Lost anchors cost lives. *Nature* **421**, 588–590.
46. Honore, E., Attali, B., Heurteaux, C., et al. (1991) Cloning, expression, pharma-cology and regulation of a delayed rectifier K⁺ channel in mouse heart. *EMBO J.* **10**, 2805–2811.
47. Arena, J. P. and Kass, R. S. (1988) Block of heart potassium channels by clofilium and its tertiary analogs: relationship between drug structure and type of channel blocked. *Mol. Pharmacol.* **34**, 60–66.
48. Moss, A. J., Zareba, W., Hall, W. J., et al. (2000) Effectiveness and limitations of beta-blocker therapy in congenital long-QT syndrome. *Circulation* **101**, 616–623.
49. Schwartz, P. J., Priori, S. G., Locati, E. H., et al. (1995) Long QT syndrome pa-tients with mutations in the SCN5A and HERG genes have differential responses to Na⁺ channel blockade and to increases in heart rate: Implications for gene-specific therapy. *Circulation* **92**, 3381–3386.
50. Compton, S. J., Lux, R. L., Ramsey, M. R., et al. (1996) Genetically defined therapy of inherited long-QT syndrome. Correction of abnormal repolarization by potassium. *Circulation* **94**, 1018–1022.
51. Etheridge, S. P., Compton, S. J., Tristani-Firouzi, M., and Mason, J. W. (2003) A new oral therapy for long QT syndrome: Long-term oral potassium improves repolarization in patients with HERG mutations. *J. Am. Coll. Cardiol.* **42**, 1777–1782.
52. Zareba, W., Moss, A. J., Daubert, J. P., Hall, W. J., Robinson, J. L., and Andrews, M. (2003) Implantable cardioverter defibrillator in high-risk long QT syndrome patients. *J. Cardiovasc. Electrophysiol.* **14**, 337–341.
53. Schwartz, P. J., Priori, S. G., Spazzolini, C., et al. (2001) Genotype-phenotype correlation in the long-QT syndrome: Gene-specific triggers for life-threatening arrhythmias. *Circulation* **103**, 89–95.
54. Priori, S. G., Schwartz, P. J., Napolitano, C., et al. (2003) Risk stratification in the long-QT syndrome. *N. Engl. J. Med.* **348**, 1866–1874.
55. Neyroud, N., Tesson, F., Denjoy, I., et al. (1997) A novel mutation on the potas-sium channel gene *KVLQT1* causes the Jervell and Lange-Nielsen cardioauditory syndrome. *Nat. Genet.* **15**, 186–189.
56. Splawski, I., Timothy, K. W., Vincent, G. M., Atkinson, D. L., and Keating, M. T. (1997) Brief report: molecular basis of the long-QT syndrome associated with deafness. *N. Engl. J. Med.* **336**, 1562–1567.
57. Chen, Q., Zhang, D., Gingell, R. L., et al. (1999) Homozygous deletion in *KVLQT1* associated with Jervell and Lange-Nielsen syndrome. *Circulation* **99**, 1344–1347.
58. Schulze-Bahr, E., Wang, Q., Wedekind, H., et al. (1997) *KCNE1* mutations cause Jervell and Lange-Nielsen syndrome. *Nat. Genet.* **17**, 267–268.

59. Osher, H. L. and Wolff, L. (1953) Electrocardiographic pattern simulating acute myocardial injury. *Am. J. Med. Sci.* **226**, 541–545.
60. Edeiken, J. (1954) Elevation of RS-T segment, apparent or real in right precordial leads as probable normal variant. *Am. Heart. J.* **48**, 331–339.
61. Levine, H. D., Wanzer, S. H., and Merrill, J. P. (1956) Dialyzable currents of injury in potassium intoxication resembling acute myocardial infarction or pericarditis. *Circulation* **13**, 29–36.
62. Martini, B., Nava, A., Thiene, G., et al. (1989) Ventricular fibrillation without apparent heart disease. Description of six cases. *Am. Heart. J.* **118**, 1203–1209.
63. Aihara, N., Ohe, T., Kamakura, S., et al. (1990) Clinical and electrophysiologic characteristics of idiopathic ventricular fibrillation. *Shinzo* **22(Suppl 2)**, 80–86.
64. Gussak, I., Antzelevitch, C., Bjerregaard, P., Towbin, J. A., and Chaitman, B. R. (1999) The Brugada syndrome: clinical, electrophysiological, and genetic considerations. *J. Am. Coll. Cardiol.* **33**, 5–15.
65. Chen, Q., Kirsch, G. E., Zhang, D., et al. (1998) Genetic basis and molecular mechanism for idiopathic ventricular fibrillation. *Nature* **392**, 293–296.
66. Dumaine, R., Towbin, J. A., Brugada, P., et al. (1999) Ionic mechanisms responsible for the electrocardiographic phenotype of the Brugada syndrome are temperature dependent. *Circ. Res.* **85**, 803–809.
67. Kambouris, N. G., Nuss, H. B., Johns, D. C., Tomaselli, G. F., Marban, E., and Balser, J. R. (1998) Phenotypic characterization of a novel long-qt syndrome mutation (R1623Q) in the cardiac sodium channel. *Circulation* **97**, 640–644.
68. Priori, S. G., Napolitano, C., Memmi, M., et al. (2002) Clinical and molecular characterization of patients with catecholaminergic polymorphic ventricular tachycardia. *Circulation* **106**, 69–74.
69. Laitinen, P. J., Swan, H., Piippo, K., Viitasalo, M., Toivonen, L., and Kontula, K. (2004) Genes, exercise and sudden death: Molecular basis of familial catecholaminergic polymorphic ventricular tachycardia. *Ann. Med.* **1**, 81–86.
70. Swan, H., Piippo, K., Viitasalo, M., et al. (1999) Arrhythmic disorder mapped to chromosome 1q42-q43 causes malignant polymorphic ventricular tachycardia in structurally normal hearts. *J. Am. Coll. Cardiol.* **34**, 2035–2042.
71. Laitinen, P. J., Brown, K. M., Piippo, K. et al. (2001) Mutations of the cardiac ryanodine receptor (RyR2) gene in familial polymophic ventricular tachycardia. *Circulation* **103**, 485–490.
72. Marks, A. R., Priori, S., Memmi, M., Kontula, K., and Laitinen, P. J. (2002) Involvement of the cardiac ryanodine receptor/calcium release channel in catecholaminergic polymorphic ventricular tachycardia. *J. Cell. Physiol.* **190**, 1–6.
73. Lahat, H., Pras, E., and Eldar, M. (2004) A missense mutation in CASQ2 is associated with autosomal recessive catecholamine-induced polymorphic ventricular tachycardia in Bedouin families from Israel. *Ann. Med.* **1**, 87–91.
74. Laitinen, P. J., Swan, H., and Kontula, K. (2003) Molecular genetics of exercise-induced polymorphic ventricular tachycardia: Identification of three novel cardiac ryanodine receptor mutations and two common calsequestrin 2 amino-acid polymorphisms. *J. Hum. Genet.* **11**, 888–891.

5

Mutation Analysis of the *FBN1* Gene in Patients With Marfan Syndrome

Paul Coucke, Petra Van Acker, and Anne De Paepe

Summary

Marfan syndrome is an autosomal-dominant connective tissue disorder characterized by pleiotropic manifestations involving the skeletal, ocular, and cardiovascular systems and resulting from mutations in the gene for fibrillin, *FBN1*. The clinical diagnosis is based on a set of well-defined clinical criteria (Ghent nosology). Nevertheless, the age-related nature of some clinical manifestations and the variable phenotypic expression of the disorder may hamper the diagnosis. In those instances, molecular analysis of the *FBN1* gene is helpful to identify at-risk individuals. Mutations are spread over the entire *FBN1* gene and there are no particular hot spots. Different standard methodologies are available to identify these mutations, however, one of the most sensitive techniques is denaturing high-performance liquid chromatography. This approach allows the performance of the analysis in a semi-automated manner and has a mutation detection rate of approx 95%.

Key Words: Marfan syndrome; fibrillin-1; molecular diagnosis; mutation analysis; DHPLC.

1. Introduction

Marfan syndrome (MFS) (OMIM 154700) is an inherited disorder of connective tissue that affects mainly the skeleton, the eyes, and the cardiovascular system. The prevalence of the disease is approx 1 in 10,000 and the disease shows autosomal-dominant transmission *(1)*. The diagnosis of MFS is based primarily on clinical criteria and requires a combination of major and minor clinical manifestations in different organ systems. Major manifestations are highly specific for the condition and include ectopia lentis, dissection of the ascending aorta, dural ectasia, and presence of at least four of eight manifestations in the skeletal system *(2)*. Minor manifestations are numerous, but less specific because they are commonly found in many other conditions as well as in the general population. The presence of minor criteria only is insufficient to establish the clinical diagnosis of MFS, but indicates that the particular body

From: *Methods in Molecular Medicine, vol. 126: Congenital Heart Disease: Molecular Diagnostics*
Edited by: M. Kearns-Jonker © Humana Press Inc., Totowa, NJ

system is involved. According to the current nosological criteria (Ghent Nosology, 1996) the diagnosis of MFS in a sporadic patient requires the presence of a major manifestation in at least two different organ systems and the involvement of a third organ system *(3)*. In familial instances, a positive family history is considered a major diagnostic criterion. The diagnosis of MFS in a relative requires the presence of one additional major manifestation in one organ system and involvement of a second organ system. The clinical diagnosis can be challenging because of the striking inter- and intrafamilial variability in phenotypic expression and the age-related nature of several clinical manifestations. Therefore, molecular testing of the *FBN1* gene can be of value in the diagnostic work-up for MFS in specific situations.

The *FBN1* gene (OMIM 134797) involved in MFS was localized in 1990 on chromosome 15q21.1 and, 1 yr later, the gene was isolated *(4–6)*. The gene spans approx 200 kb of genomic DNA containing 65 exons. The coding region possesses 9663 nucleotides and, after translation, a protein of 350 kDa is formed *(7)*. FBN1, the protein product of *FBN1*, is a cysteine-rich monomeric glycoprotein containing 47 epidermal growth factor-like motifs, which are common in extracellular matrix proteins *(8)*. Each motif contains six highly conserved cysteine residues. Two other common motifs are the latent transforming growth factor-β1-binding protein motif, containing eight cysteine residues and a Fib-motif, which is a fusion of portions of the epidermal growth factor-like and latent transforming growth factor-β1-binding protein motifs *(9)*. Mutations causing changes in cysteine residues result in disturbances of intramolecular or intermolecular disulfide bonds. FBN1 is a major structural component of the extracellular microfibrils, providing numerous functions in the body, including scaffolding for elastic fibers. To date, more than 500 different *FBN1* mutations have been identified, including missense mutations (65%), mainly resulting in cysteine substitutions; premature termination mutations (20%); exon-skipping mutations (10%); and others, such as small insertions, deletions, or splice site mutations (http://www.umd.necker.fr) *(10)*. With a few exceptions, all known *FBN1* mutations identified to date are unique, and approx 25 to 30% of cases represent new mutations *(11)*. Because of the high interfamilial and intrafamilial variability, genotype–phenotype correlations for *FBN1* mutations are hard to identify, with the exception of neonatal MFS, which is caused by mutations clustered in exons 24 to 27 and exons 31 and 32 of the *FBN1* gene *(12)*.

Various mutation detection methods have been designed for the identification of sequence variations in the *FBN1* gene *(13,14)*. These techniques comprise single-strand conformation polymorphism analysis, heteroduplex analysis, and direct sequencing *(15,16)*. Denaturing high-performance liquid chromatography (DHPLC), a new mutation detection technique that was recently introduced, has allowed the automation of at least part of the laborious procedure *(17,18)*. DHPLC has several characteristics that makes it an attractive methodology to perform mutation analysis, especially for large genes with many exons. The advantages are the high sensitivity, rapid analysis time, on-line UV absorbance detection, and lack of a post-polymerase chain reaction (PCR) sample treatment requirement. The detection of mutations or polymorphisms, independent of the location within the fragment, is based on differential retention of double-stranded homo- and heteroduplex fragments under conditions of partial thermal denaturation *(19)*. Separation of DNA fragments is dependent on the elution strength of the organic solvent in the mobile phase and the number of ion pairs formed between the negatively charged DNA fragments and the positively charged triethylammonium acetate (TEAA) ions adsorbed to the stationary phase. The technique allows the detection of single base substitutions, small insertions, or deletions in 100- to 1000-bp DNA fragments by fractionation of heteroduplexes under partially denaturing conditions. The analysis by DHPLC is automated and very rapid, and nearly 95% of sequence alterations can be detected.

To perform mutation analysis of the *FBN1* gene, genomic DNA (gDNA) and/or complementary DNA (cDNA) is isolated from peripheral blood leukocytes or skin fibroblasts, respectively (*see* **Note 1**). Mutation screening of the genomic sequences is performed by amplification of 65 fragments, each representing 1 exon with flanking intron sequences, whereas 24 overlapping fragments are analyzed for the cDNA sequence. Mutation screening of the amplified product is performed with DHPLC. PCR products resulting in aberrant patterns are sequenced to determine the exact nature and position of the mutation.

2. Materials

1. Dulbecco's Modified Eagle's Medium (Invitrogen).
2. Fetal calf serum (FCS) (Invitrogen).
3. Penicillin G/streptomycin, kanamycine (Invitrogen).
4. Minimum Essential Medium (nonessential amino acids) (Invitrogen).
5. Easy DNA kit (Invitrogen).
6. Micro-To-Midi Total RNA Purification System (Invitrogen).
7. QIAmp DNA blood mini kit (Qiagen Inc, Valencia, CA).
8. PCR tubes.
9. PCR-quality water.
10. 10X PCR buffer (Invitrogen).
11. 25 mM $MgCl_2$ (Invitrogen).
12. dNTP solution (dCTP, dATP, dTTP, and dGTP) (Amersham Bioscience).
13. 10 pmol/µL amplification primer for gDNA and cDNA *FBN1* fragments (*see* **Subheading 3.3.**).
14. 5 U/µL platinum Taq polymerase (Invitrogen) or standard Taq DNA polymerase.

15. 100 ng/μL human gDNA.
16. Thermal cycler (e.g., Perkin–Elmer 9600 or equivalent).
17. HPLC instrumentation (e.g., WAVE DNA Fragment Analysis System, Transgenomic or similar systems from Varian or Hewlett–Packard).
    a. 0.1 *M* TEAA buffer, pH 7.0.
    b. Eluent A: 0.1 *M* TEAA.
    c. Eluent B: 25% acetonitrile in 0.1 *M* TEAA.
18. Equipment and reagents for agarose gel electrophoresis and ethidium bromide staining.
19. Additional equipment and reagents for sequencing analysis.
    a. BigDye terminator cycle sequencing reaction kit (Applied Biosystems or equivalent).
    b. ABI3100 DNA analysis system (Applied Biosystems or equivalent).

3. Methods

The methods described below outline:

1. Sampling and tissue culture.
2. DNA isolation procedures.
3. Amplification of DNA fragments.
4. Mutation analysis by DHPLC.
5. Characterization of the mutation by DNA sequencing.

3.1. Sampling and Tissue Culture

Fibroblast cultures are established from a skin biopsy, usually from the inner upper arm. The biopsy is mechanically diced and put into culture. The medium used is Dulbecco's Modified Eagle Medium supplemented with 10% FCS, 100 U/mL penicillin plus 100 μg/mL streptomycin, 100 μg/mL kanamycin, and 1X nonessential amino acids. The cells are grown at 37°C with 5% CO_2. Cells from the second passage are trypsinized and seeded in several different recipients for total RNA isolation (P60 cell culture disc) or for genomic DNA isolation (if no blood is available) (T80 flask). Cells from passage 3 are trypsinized, supplemented with 10% FCS and 10% dimethylsulfoxide, and stored in liquid nitrogen. If more RNA of DNA is necessary, cells are grown starting from the frozen stock.

3.2. Genomic DNA Isolation, Messenger RNA Isolation, and cDNA Production

Genomic DNA is isolated from the fibroblasts or from leukocytes using kits provided by Qiagen and Invitrogen. Before RNA extraction, cell cultures are incubated with 100 μg/mL cycloheximide (Sigma-Aldrich, St. Louis, MO) for 16 hr. Consequently, total RNA is obtained from the skin fibroblasts cultures using the Micro-to-Midi Total RNA Purification System (Invitrogen), as described by the manufacturer. First-strand cDNA is synthesized from total RNA (1 μg) using Moloney murine leukemia virus reverse transcriptase (Invitrogen), using random hexanucleotide primers. For some experiments, RNA samples are treated with RNase-free DNase (Invitrogen) before cDNA synthesis to avoid genomic DNA contamination in the reverse transcriptase PCR experiments.

3.3. Amplification of DNA Fragments

The complete cDNA analysis comprises amplification of 24 overlapping fragments with an average size of 450 bp. cDNA primers, together with their respective annealing temperature, are represented in **Table 1**.

Mutation screening of the *FBN1* genomic sequences is performed by amplification of 65 fragments, each representing 1 exon with flanking intron sequences, with an average size of 260 bp (**Table 2**).

1. Prepare mix for 20 reactions (*see* **Table 3** and **Note 2**).
2. Dispense 24 μL of mix into a PCR tube.
3. Add 1 μL of genomic DNA (100 ng/μL).
4. Set up negative control (1 μL water).

3.4. Amplification of DNA

Amplify using a touch-down PCR program on a thermal cycler, programmed according to **Table 4** (*see* **Note 3**).

PCR products are denatured at 96°C for 5 min and allowed to reanneal to form homoduplexes and heteroduplexes by cooling slowly to room temperature.

Analyze 5 μL of PCR product by electrophoresis on a 2%-agarose gel, and stain with ethidium bromide to confirm amplification of the desired fragment.

3.5. Mutation Analysis by DHPLC

DHPLC is performed on a WAVE system (Model 3500HT) using the Navigator™ software purchased from Transgenomic (Santa Clara, CA).

1. Before the analysis, column performance should be tested by injecting commercially available Mutation Control Standards (low and high range), according to the guidelines of the manufacturer.
2. A blank should be run (0 μL injection volume), using the method of the samples that will be analyzed, to equilibrate the column and preheat the oven.
3. Five microliters of crude PCR product is loaded into the system (*see* **Note 4**). Running conditions: flow rate of 1.5 mL/min.
   Both the column temperature and the acetonitrile gradient (Eluent A/Eluent B) are determined with the Navigator software for each DNA fragment. To achieve the best possible separation, the amplicon melting curves have to be located between 40 and 99% of the helical fraction. If more than one significant melting

Table1
FBN1 cDNA Primers and Annealing Temperatures
(Touch-Down PCR)

Exon no.	Direction	Primer sequence (5'→3' direction)	Annealing temperature
1	F	ATGCGTCGAGGGCGTCTGCT	60>48
	R	GCTACCTCCATTCATACAGCGA	
2	F	GATAGCTCCTTCCTGTGGCTCC	60>48
	R	CCGTGCGGATATTTGGAATG	
3	F	CCCCTGTGAGATGTGTCCTG	60>48
	R	TTGGTTATGGACTGTGGCAGC	
4	F	ACAGCTCTGACAAACGGGCG	60>48
	R	TGCAGCGTCCATTTTGACAG	
5	F	GCCAGTTGGTCCGCTATCTC	60>48
	R	ACATGAAAGCCCGCATTACAC	
6	F	AATGGCCGGATCTGCAATAA	60>48
	R	CTGGCCTCTCTTGTATCCACCA	
7	F	CTGGCTGTGGGTCTGGATGG	60>48
	R	GCAGTTTTTCCCAGTTGAATCC	
8	F	ATCTGTGAAAACCTTCGTGGGA	60>48
	R	AGGTGGCTCCATTGATGTTGA	
9	F	GTCTGCAAGAACAGCCCAGG	60>48
	R	TGGGACACTGACACTTGAATGA	
10	F	TACTCAAGAATTAAAGGAACA	60>48
	R	CGGCATTCGTCAATGTCTGTGC	
11	F	CATTGGCAGCTTTAAGTGCAGG	60>48
	R	ACCACCATTCATTATGCTGCA	
12	F	CCATTCAACTCCCGATAGGCT	60>48
	R	TTTTCACAGGTCCCACTTAGGC	
13	F	CAGGTGCTTGTGTTATGATG	60>48
	R	GCACAGACAGCGGTAAGA	
14	F	GATTGGAGATGGCATTAAGTGC	60>48
	R	TGTTGACACAGTTCCCACTGA	
15	F	CTACGAACTGGACAGAAGCGG	60>48
	R	ATACAGGTGTAGTTGCCAACGG	
16	F	ACTACCTGAATGAAGATACACG	60>48
	R	GACCTGTGGAGGTGAAGCGGTAG	
17	F	TCAACATGGTTGGCAGCTTCC	60>48
	R	AAAGATTCCCATTTCCACTTGC	
18	F	ACAATTGGTTCCTTCAACTG	60>48
	R	GCACAAATTTCTGGCTCTT	

(continued)

Table1 *(continued)*

Exon no.	Direction	Primer sequence (5'→3' direction)	Annealing temperature
19	F	CTTGGATGGGTCCTACAGATGC	60>48
	R	CACATTCTTGCAGGTTCCATT	
20	F	GGTTATACTCTAGCGGGAATG	60>48
	R	TCCCACGGGTGTTGAGGCAGCG	
21	F	AGCGGAGACCTGATGGAGAGG	60>48
	R	CAGTTGTGTTGCTTGGTTGCA	
22	F	CAAGAGGATGGAAGGAGCTGC	60>48
	R	GAACTGTTCATACTGGAAGCCG	
23	F	CTACCTCCAGCACTACCAGTGG	60>48
	R	GTAGCCATTGATCTTACACTCG	
24	F	CACCTGGTTACTTCCGCATAGG	60>48
	R	ATGATTCTGATTGGGGGAAAA	

F, forward; R, reverse.

domain is present in a fragment, additional analysis temperatures are selected, with a maximum of four temperatures. The Navigator software automatically calculates the corresponding gradient for each amplicon (*see* **Note 5**).

4. After eluting from the cartridge, the separated DNA fragments travel to the detector, where they are detected by UV absorption. The data collected from the detector are displayed in real-time on the computer monitor. Consequently, selected injections are aligned using mutation calling (Navigator Software). This allows the separation of the wild types from the mutations or polymorphisms (**Fig. 1**).

3.6. Characterization of Mutations by DNA Sequencing

Amplified fragments demonstrating alterations in DHPLC elution profile are confirmed in a repeat analysis. Sequence variation is identified by automated bidirectional sequencing using an ABI3100 sequencer (Applied Biosystems) with Big Dye terminator chemistry (Applied Biosystems), according to the guidelines of the company.

4. Notes

1. If fibroblasts are available, mutation screening is usually started at the cDNA level. Using this approach, only 24 cDNA amplicons have to be analyzed on the WAVE, which is significantly faster than the mutation analysis on genomic DNA, in which 65 exons need to be analyzed. Surprisingly, sequencing of cDNA fragments showing an aberrant WAVE pattern often fails to reveal the causal base change after sequencing. We assume that this is because of the uneven expression of the wild-type and mutant alleles, which is detectable by DHPLC but which

Table 2
FBN1 gDNA Primers and Annealing Temperatures (Touch-Down PCR)

Exon no.	Direction	Primer sequence (5'→3' direction)	Annealing temperature
1	F	CAGACCGAGCCCCGG	62>50
	R	CATCCTGCCCGTTGTTCT	+ 6%DMSO
2	F	TCTGCCAGGATTCATCTTGC	62>50
	R	CAACACAACAAAAGAAGGAC	
3	F	AAATCCATGTGCTAACAGAC	54>42
	R	GGTATAACCACATAAAATAA	
4	F	AAAGCGTCTCAGCTCTCTCC	60>58
	R	AAAATCCATCAGCACTTATCTC	
5	F	AAAGCGTCTCAGCTCTCTCC	62>50
	R	AGGTACCAGCATGTCTTTAC	
6	F	TCTGCATGATGGTTCCTGC	56>44
	R	CCATAGCAAATAAGATTAATCC	
7	F	TCACATTTTATTCTGCAATGAA	60>48
	R	TTTCTAATGTTGAGTTTTGCCT	
8	F	CCAGGGACATGATTTGACTAG	62>50
	R	TATGTGCTCCTTAACAAGCTTG	
9	F	GTTACAAGTATTATCTCAGCG	62>50
	R	GCTGGGATGGGATATTCTG	
10	F	AAATAAGGATGACTTCTGTGG	58>46
	R	AACTTATTTAATGACTAAAGTAGC	
11	F	ACTGATGAAAGATACCATAGTT	58>46
	R	AGGAACAGAATTACAACAGAC	
12	F	AGAATTATGAGGTATTGCTATG	60>48
	R	CAGTTAGCATATATGTCCCAC	
13	F	TCCCCTAAATAAAGCTATTTC	62>50
	R	AGACCCCTGATATTGAAACTG	
14	F	TTGGTTTCCTTCGTAAGCTT	56>44
	R	GGCACGTGAAGAACATGAT	
15	F	TTTTCAAGGGTTAAAACATAATTG	56>44
	R	GAGCGTTTGTTACCATTG	
16	F	CTCATCTGTTTGAAGTGACAG	60>48
	R	GCCAGCCTTCTGCCACC	
17	F	ACTTTGGAGGAAATGATGTGTGC	62>50
	R	GCCAGCCTTCTGCCACC	
18	F	TCAGAATATCTTACAGTGAG	60>48
	R	GCCAGCCTTCTGCCACC	
19	F	AGCAAAGTAGATACAGGCAAA	62>50
	R	AGTCTTATGGTTTTCTAATGGC	

(continued)

Table 2 *(continued)*

Exon no.	Direction	Primer sequence (5'→3' direction)	Annealing temperature
20	F	TTAGCCCAGCTTTACTGTGTGG	58>46
	R	TTGATAAACATAGAAAAATCATTCTC	
21	F	TATAATTCCAAGGTGTATGTTTG	54>42
	R	AGATAAATGAAATACTAGGCTTC	
22	F	CTACTTCATGTTCCAGGTC	60>48
	R	CTGTTCCGTTTTGTAGTTCTC	
23	F	TATGAACTTACCAGGTTCAAAAT	54>42
	R	TTGGGTGTGTGTCTGTACC	
24	F	ACAGCAAATTATTATGTGTGCAG	65>53
	R	ATCAAGTAGAGTGCTGAGATC	
25	F	CAAGAACTTCCAACCTTCATG	58>46
	R	GTCTCAGGACAGCCTTAATT	
26	F	AATTAAGGCTGTCCTGAGACT	62>50
	R	GCTTCATGGAATCCTTCTCTT	
27	F	AAGATGGACACCCAGCAATG	62>50
	R	CACCCAAACATAAGCTTCCAAC	
28	F	AGTTGTTTGAATGACATCATTG	54>42
	R	TAACATAACATAACATAAAATAAAG	
29	F	CAGACATCCAAACCATATCAG	62>50
	R	GAACCTACTGAGAGATTCAAC	
30	F	AATAGTCTTATGCTAGTAGGC	62>50
	R	ACAGTGCTTATGACTAACAAG	
31	F	GGAAAGTACTCAATGATATCAAATAG	60>48
	R	ATCTATAATTATGATACCAATCTC	
32	F	CCAAAAGACATTTGTGCTGAG	62>50
	R	GTGTAATCTATGCAGTCCTTG	
33	F	GTGAGTAGGAAAGTAACAGAGG	56>44
	R	CTGACCCAGTCTTCAAAAAAG	
34	F	CGAGGAAGAGTAACGTGT	54>42
	R	TCATCAAGCCCAGCAAGGCTC	
35	F	TTGCCTAATTATATTTGGCAGGTTTT	65>53
	R	CTTGTCTTCTGTGACGGCCC	
36	F	CTCTAGATTGGGCCCTGTTC	58>46
	R	TTGAGAATGGAATGTTTGGTGC	
37	F	GTAGAAAGATTCTGCCTGATG	62>50
	R	GAACTGGCTGGAGTTGAAAT	
38	F	GGTGTTAACTTACTTCAGACG	62>50
	R	CCTGGTAGCTCCTGGCACTC	
39	F	CCTTGGGTTTATTTACAATGC	54>42
	R	TCTGCAAGACCTTATCATCCT	

(continued)

Table 2 *(continued)*

Exon no.	Direction	Primer sequence (5'→3' direction)	Annealing temperature
40	F	AAGTTTTCATATTCACATACCACTT	62>50
	R	GATGAGAACCAAACATGCATTA	
41	F	GCTTGTTGAGTATCCACTTAG	62>50
	R	GCTTCCTTCGCTAAGACTG	
42	F	CCAATTATTGTTCTTTGCTGAC	60>48
	R	ACCAGAAAGTTCTGACAATG	
43	F	ACACGCACGCACTTTCCAT	62>50
	R	TGTGAAATTCGCCAAGTGTG	
44	F	TGCTGTACACATCTATGTTGTC	56>44
	R	TATTCTTCAGCTTAACTAATCTG	
45	F	GAGCTAGGATTACTCCTGAG	62>50
	R	TGCTGCATATCTGTCTGTG	
46	F	AAGTTCTCAGCCTATGGATG	60>48
	R	TAATTACAAAGAACACATATAAAAC	
47	F	TGATTATTGCTGGGATTATGAC	62>50
	R	CTGCATGATTCCTTGAGTGG	
48	F	GATGGAAGTCATGCCAGTG	62>50
	R	GGACACCCGACACTCCTC	
49	F	TGTGTTTGGTACCTGATGATG	62>50
	R	ACAAAGAAACAGAGCTTTGCC	
50	F	CTATGGTGCAATACGGACTC	62>50
	R	AAGGCCTACAGTCTTACTTAC	
51	F	AGCTTGTAATGAATTGCTATTG	60>48
	R	AAGCAGATTGAGAATACTGAG	
52	F	TTGTCCCTTCATTTAGATAGC	56>44
	R	CCTGATGGTGACTCACTAG	
53	F	TCTGATAGAATAAAAGGTATTATC	56>44
	R	TAAGACTTGTAATCAACCAATTG	
54	F	TTGGTAGGTTCCCTTTTGTTG	62>50
	R	AATTCCCAGCCTTCTCCTAC	
55	F	AACATTTTATGTTTAAAAGTCAGG	56>44
	R	AGCCCAGGTTCCTTCTGTCCACTGTC	
56	F	GCTCCATCCTCTATAAAATGG	62>50
	R	AAGTCTGGGTTTCCAGCATC	
57	F	GACCAAATTTTTAATATTTTGTTTG	62>50
	R	CCATATTTTCATCTGTGTTTCAC	
58	F	CATATTAATGTTGTCAATTTTATGA	62>50
	R	CCATAATCTAAATTTCCACTTG	

(continued)

Table 2 *(continued)*

Exon no.	Direction	Primer sequence (5'→3' direction)	Annealing temperature
59	F	GCGTGTACACATCATTTTTAG	56>44
	R	CTGTGGAGTTCTTACAGGCC	
60	F	ATCCTGTTTTGTTGGCTTGAC	62>50
	R	GAATCGCTACAATCCATGTAC	
61	F	TGATACAAAGAGAGCTTTGGG	62>50
	R	GCCAATAGCCACACAGGCCAC	
62	F	AGATTCTTGAAGTTTTTGGTGGTA	62>50
	R	CAGAAAGCAAGCAGTGTTTTG	
63	F	CAAGTGGCCAGATCCAATG	65>53
	R	GGTTCTCCTCTGCTAGGAC	
64	F	AGAACTCTTGTACCACCTAC	62>50
	R	AGTTTCTCCCTGGGGAGC	
65	F	TTTAATATGAGAGCTAAGTGGC	60>48
	R	TTGTACCTATGATATGATGATTC	

Table 3
Preparing PCR Mixes

	Volume (μL)	Final concentration
dNTPs (1 mM)	3	0.12 mM
10X PCR buffer	2.5	1X
25 mM MgCl$_2$	0.75	1.5 mM
Forward primer (30 μM)	0.5	0.6 μM
Reverse primer (30 μM)	0.5	0.6 μM
5 U/μL Taq polymerase	0.1	0.02 U/μL
PCR water	16.65	
Total	**24**	

Table 4
DNA Amplification Using a Touch-Down PCR Program on a Thermal Cycler

1 cycle	1 min	94°C (denaturation)
12 cycles	20 s	94°C (denaturation)
	15 s	62°C (annealing)[a]
	1 min	72°C (extension)
24 cycles	40 s	94°C (denaturation)
	40 s	50°C (annealing)
	30 s	72°C (extension)
1 cycle	10 min	72°C (extension)

[a]1°C decrease per PCR cycle (62°C → 50°C).

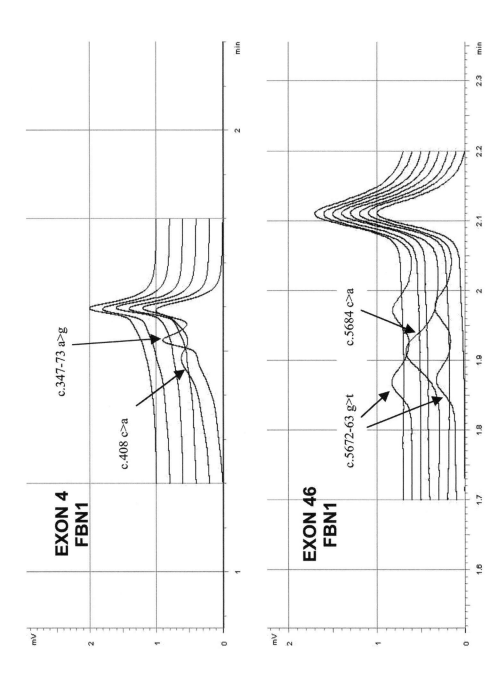

EXON 4
FBN1

c.347-73 a>g

c.408 c>a

EXON 46
FBN1

c.5684 c>a

c.5672-63 g>t

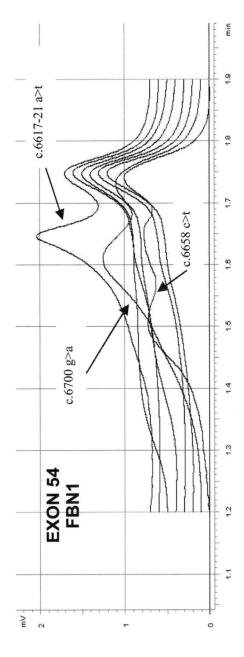

Fig. 1. Sample chromatograms. The three figures display aligned chromatograms from different patients. The aberrant pattern is indicated with an arrow and the corresponding base change in the *FBN1* gene is indicated.

is often more difficult to identify by direct sequencing. To identify the base change responsible for the aberrant WAVE pattern, the corresponding exons located within the cDNA fragment are then separately analyzed by DHPLC. Consequently, the exon containing the aberrant WAVE pattern is sequenced.

2. During the set up of the PCR reaction, it is important to avoid additives often present in commercially available polymerase mixtures and reaction buffers, such as gelatin, bovine serum albumin, Triton, and so on. These components can damage the separation cartridge severely or reduce the amount of runs.

3. A touch-down PCR is not mandatory, however, by using this approach, it is possible to reduce the amount of different PCR programs. This allows amplification of several amplicons in a single PCR run, making the total procedure much faster.

4. It is recommended that high-yield PCR product be loaded on the WAVE system if UV absorbance is used as detection method. This is necessary to obtain clear peaks in the chromatograms produced by the WAVE analysis. Low-yield PCR products result in aberrant WAVE patterns that do not contain base changes.

5. To avoid elution of the fragment outside of the separation window during DHPLC analysis, time shifts are adjusted in the method designed for each exon at each oven temperature. This is done when the oven temperature differs at least 3°C (plus or minus) from the predicted melting temperature of the amplicon by the Navigator software.

Acknowledgments

The authors thank Dr. D. Milewicz and Dr. E. Putman for providing the *FBN1* cDNA primer sequences. This work was supported by grant G.0290.02 from the Fund for Scientific Research-Flanders to ADP.

References

1. Gray, J. R., Bridges, A. B., Faed, M. J, et al. (1994) Ascertainment and severity of Marfan syndrome in a Scottish population. *J. Med. Genet.* **31**, 51–54.
2. Pyeritz, R. E. (2000) The Marfan syndrome. *Annu. Rev. Med.* **51**, 481–510.
3. De Paepe, A., Devereux, R. B., Dietz, H. C., Hennekam, R. C., and Pyeritz, R. E. (1996) Revised diagnostic criteria for the Marfan syndrome. *Am. J. Med. Genet.* **62**, 417–426.
4. Kainulainen, K., Pulkkinen, L., Savolainen, A., Kaitila, I., and Peltonen, L. (1990) Location on chromosome 15 of the gene defect causing Marfan syndrome. *N. Engl. J. Med.* **323**, 935–939.
5. Lee, B., Godfrey, M., Vitale, E., et al. (1991) Linkage of Marfan syndrome and a phenotypically related disorder to two different fibrillin genes. *Nature* **352**, 330–334.
6. Dietz, H. C., Cutting, G. R., Pyeritz, R. E., et al. (1991) Marfan syndrome caused by a recurrent de novo missense mutation in the fibrillin gene. *Nature* **352**, 337–339.

7. Sakai, L. Y., Keene, D. R., and Engvall, E. (1986) Fibrillin, a new 350-kD glyco-protein, is a component of extracellular microfibrils. *J. Cell Biol.* **103,** 2499–2509.
8. Handford, P. A., Mayhew, M., and Brownlee, G. G. (1991) Calcium binding to fibrillin? *Nature* **353,** 395.
9. Pereira, L., D'Alessio, M., Ramirez, F., et al. (1993) Genomic organization of the sequence coding for fibrillin, the defective gene product in Marfan syndrome. *Hum. Mol. Genet.* **2,** 1762.
10. Collod-Beroud, G. and Boileau, C. (2002) Marfan syndrome in the third Millennium. *Eur. J. Hum. Genet.* **10,** 673–681.
11. Gray, J. R., Bridges, A. B., Faed, M. J., et al. (1994) Ascertainment and severity of Marfan syndrome in a Scottish population. *J. Med. Genet.* **31,** 51–54.
12. Park, E. S., Putnam, E. A., Chitayat, D., Child, A., and Milewicz, D. M. (1998) Clustering of FBN2 mutations in patients with congenital contractural arachno-dactyly indicates an important role of the domains encoded by exons 24 through 34 during human development. *Am. J. Med. Genet.* **78,** 350–355.
13. Ganguly, A., Rock, M. J., and Prockop, D. J. (1993) Conformation-sensitive gel electrophoresis for rapid detection of single-base differences in double-stranded PCR products and DNA fragments: evidence for solvent-induced bends in DNA heteroduplexes. *Proc. Natl. Acad. Sci. USA* **90,** 10,325–10,429.
14. Pepe, G., Giusti, B., Evangelisti, L., et al. (2001) Fibrillin-1 (*FBN1*) gene frame-shift mutations in Marfan patients: genotype–phenotype correlation. *Clin. Genet.* **59,** 444–450.
15. Tynan, K., Comeau, K., Pearson, M., et al. (1993) Mutation screening of complete fibrillin-1 coding sequence: report of five new mutations, including two in 8-cys-teine domains. *Hum. Mol. Genet.* **2,** 1813–1821.
16. Comeglio, P., Evans, A. L., Brice, G. W., and Child, A. H. (2001) Detection of six novel *FBN1* mutations in British patients affected by Marfan syndrome. *Hum. Mutat.* **18,** 251.
17. Xiao, W. and Oefner, P. J. (2001) Denaturing high-performance liquid chromatog-raphy: a review. *Hum. Mutat.* **17,** 439–474.
18. Liu, W. O., Oefner, P. J., Qian, C., Odom, R. S., and Francke, U. (1997) Denaturing HPLC-identified novel *FBN1* mutations, polymorphisms, and sequence vari-ants in Marfan syndrome and related connective tissue disorders. *Genet. Test.* **1,** 237–242.
19. Frueh, F. W. and Noyer-Weidner, M. (2003) The use of denaturing high-perfor-mance liquid chromatography (DHPLC) for the analysis of genetic variations: impact for diagnostics and pharmacogenetics. *Clin. Chem. Lab. Med.* **41,** 452–461.

6

Mutation Analysis of *PTPN11* in Noonan Syndrome by WAVE

Navaratnam Elanko and Steve Jeffery

Summary

The chapter details the methodology for polymerase chain reaction amplification and WAVE denaturing high-performance liquid chromatography (DHPLC) analysis for all coding exons for the gene *PTPN11*, which is mutated in approx 50% of cases of Noonan Syndrome. Although DNA sequencing is initially required to determine the mutation(s) detected by WAVE (sequencing methods are not described in this chapter), each mutation has its own DHPLC signature, and experienced operatives can determine known mutations on this basis. The new Navigator software has made this process more reliable.

Key Words: Noonan syndrome; WAVE; DHPLC; mutation analysis.

1. Introduction

Noonan Syndrome (NS) is a genetic disorder with an autosomal-dominant manner of inheritance, although approx 50% of cases are sporadic new mutations *(1)*. The primary clinical features include a typical facial appearance with widely spaced eyes and low-set ears, sparse curly hair, pectus deformities, and often a cardiac lesion (most commonly pulmonary valve stenosis but sometimes hypertrophic cardiomyopathy). A gene locus for NS was identified at 12q24 in 1994 *(2)*, but it was clear that the condition was heterogeneous. A collaborative approach between three laboratories eventually found the gene that was located at 12q24 to be *PTPN11* *(3)*. This gene encodes the protein, src-homology region 2-domain phosphatase-2 (SHP-2), which is a nonreceptor tyrosine phosphatase involved in a variety of cellular pathways *(3)*, including semilunar valvulogenesis *(4)*. An interesting genotype–phenotype correlation, with pulmonary valve stenosis more common in cases with a *PTPN11* mutation and hypertrophic cardiomyopathy more common in those without the *PTPN11* mutation, has been suggested by some groups *(5–7)*. One publication

From: *Methods in Molecular Medicine, vol. 126: Congenital Heart Disease: Molecular Diagnostics*
Edited by: M. Kearns-Jonker © Humana Press Inc., Totowa, NJ

found no difference in the distribution of cardiac defects between those with
and without *PTPN11* mutations *(8)*. **Table 1** presents a list of the distribution
of mutations found to date in *PTPN11* for a diagnosis of NS.

There is a variety of methods for screening for mutations in *PTN11*; the
method chosen depends partly on available funding and equipment. Although
direct sequencing is clearly the most likely to give the closest to 100% accuracy, it is possible to miss heterozygous changes even with this technology, and
it is comparatively expensive. Single-stranded conformational polymorphism
(SSCP) analysis, even if run on an automated sequencer, is only approx 95%
accurate *(9)* and requires fluorescently tagged primers, but WAVE analysis is
inexpensive, rapid, with 95 to 100% sensitivity reported *(10,11)*. The initial
outlay expense for the equipment is clearly a problem for smaller laboratories,
in which SSCP slab gel analysis (sensitivity, 69–85%) is likely to be the favored
option, followed by direct sequencing of abnormal conformers. For SSCP, the
single-stranded DNA fragments produce the variously sized bands on a gel,
whereas, in denaturing high-performance liquid chromatography (DHPLC), the
heterozygous duplex of the normal and mutant DNA polymerase chain reaction
(PCR) fragments is detected on a column. DHPLC has the added advantage
over SSCP that larger fragments can be used (the largest fragment that has been
successfully analyzed in our lab was 743 bp). Because DHPLC is far superior
to SSCP in our hands, we detail the DHPLC methodology for the first step in
mutation detection. Any conformer that differs from the normal DHPLC pattern is suggestive of a sequence variation, and direct sequencing should be performed using an automated DNA sequencer, if available, or manually, if an
automated DNA sequencer is not available. Sequencing reactions are not detailed in this chapter.

2. Materials

1. PCR machine (various suppliers, such as Techne, Hybaid, MJ Research, and
   Applied Biosystems).
2. WAVE Nucleic Acid Fragment Analysis System (or WAVE System) 3500HT
   (Transgenomics, Cheshire, UK or Omaha, NE).
3. DNA extraction kits (there are several on the market).
4. For PCR reactions: Taq polymerase plus buffer. There are a huge number on the
   market and the WAVE user must be cautious in choosing because there are sub-
   stances that are incompatible with the technology (*see* **Note 1**). Amplitaq Gold
   with PCR Buffer 11 or Amplitaq Gold buffer and MgCl$_2$ (Applied Biosystems,
   cat. no. 8080241) are very robust, as is FastStart Taq (Roche).
5. dATP, dCTP, dGTP, and dTTP.
6. 20 pmol of each primer (*see* **Table 2**).
7. 50 ng DNA.

Table 1
***PTPN11* Mutations in NS[a]**

Exon	No. of cases	Nucleotide substitution	Amino acid substitution	Domain
1	1	C5T	Thr2Ile	N-SH2
2	3	A124G	Thr42Ala	N-SH2
3	1	C174G	Asn58Lys	N-SH2
3	2	G179C	Gly60Ala	N-SH2
3	2	G181A	Asp61Asn	N-SH2
3	4	A182G	Asp61Gly	N-SH2
3	5	T184G	Tyr62Asp	N-SH2
3	11	A188G	Tyr63Cys	N-SH2
3	1	G205C	Glu69Gln	N-SH2
3	1	T211C	Phe71Leu	N-SH2
3	2	G214T	Ala72Ser	N-SH2
3	2	C215G	Ala72Gly	N-SH2
3	21	C218T	Thr73Ile	N-SH2
3	2	G228C	Glu76Asp	N-SH2
3	3	G228T	Glu76Asp	N-SH2
3	6	A236G	Gln79Arg	N-SH2
3	2	A236C	Gln79Pro	N-SH2
3	4	A317C	Asp106Ala	N-SH2/C-SH2 linker
4	1	G417C	Glu139Asp	C-SH2
4	1	G417T	Glu139Asp	C-SH2
4	1	G417A	Glu139Asp	C-SH2
7	1	A767G	Gln256Arg	PTP
7	1	A836G	Tyr279Cys	PTP
7	2	A844G	Ile282Val	PTP
7	1	T853C	Phe285Leu	PTP
8	1	T854C	Phe285Ser	PTP
8	28	A922G	Asn308Asp	PTP
8	4	A923G	Asn308Ser	PTP
8	1	A925G	Ile309Val	PTP
13	1	G1502A	Arg501Lys	PTP
13	2	G1505C	Ser502Thr	PTP
13	1	G1508C	Gly503Arg	PTP
13	4	A1510G	Met504Val	PTP
14	1	C1678T	Leu560Phe	PTP

[a]From **refs. 5–8**. Index cases only.

Table 2
**Primer Pairs and T$_{ann}$ to Amplify the *PTPN11* Coding Sequence,
and Sizes of PCR Products**[a]

Product Exon		Primer sequence	T$_{ann}$	Length
1[b]	Forward	5'-gctgacgggaagcaggaagtgg-3'	60°C	589 bp
	Reverse	5'-CTGGCACCCGTGGTTCCCTC-3'		
2	Forward	5'-ACTGAATCCCAGGTCTCTACCAAG-3'	60°C	405 bp
	Reverse	5'-cagcaagctatccaagcatggt-3'		
3	Forward	5'-cgacgtggaagatgagatctga-3'	60°C	384 bp
	Reverse	5'-CAGTCACAAGCCTTTGGAGTCAG-3'		
4	Forward	5'-aggagagctgactgtatacagtag-3'	58°C	447 bp
	Reverse	5'-catctgtaggtgatagagcaaga-3'		
5	Forward	5'-ctgcagtgaacatgagagtgcttg-3'	60°C	329 bp
	Reverse	5'-GTTGAAGCTGCAATGGGTACATG-3'		
6	Forward	5'-tgcattaacaccgttttctgt-3'	54°C	282 bp
	Reverse	5'-GTCAGTTTCAAGTCTCTCAGGTC-3'		
7	Forward	5'-GAACATTTCCTAGGATGAATTCC-3'	56°C	271 bp
	Reverse	5'-GGTACAGAGGTGCTAGGAATCA-3'		
8	Forward	5'-GACATCAGGCAGTGTTCACGTTAC-3'	57°C	350 bp
	Reverse	5'-CCTTAAAGTTACTTTCAGGACATG-3'		
9	Forward	5'-GTAAGCTTTGCTTTTCACAGTG-3'	56°C	357 bp
	Reverse	5'-CTAAACATGGCCAATCTGACATGTC-3'		
10	Forward	5'-GCAAGACTTGAACATTTGTTTGTTGC-3'	60°C	284 bp
	Reverse	5'-GACCCTGAATTCCTACACACCATC-3'		
11	Forward	5'-CAAAAGGAGACGAGTTCTGGGAAC-3'	60°C	453 bp
	Reverse	5'-GCAGTTGCTCTATGCCTCAAACAG-3'		
12	Forward	5'-GCTCCAAAGAGTAGACATTGTTTC-3'	56°C	250 bp
	Reverse	5'-GACTGTTTTCGTGAGCACTTTC-3'		
13	Forward	5'-CAACACTGTAGCCATTGCAACA-3'	60°C	356 bp
	Reverse	5'-CGTATCCAAGAGGCCTAGCAAG-3'		
14[c]	Forward	5'-ACCATTGTCCCTCACATGTGC-3'	60°C	259 bp
	Reverse	5'-CAGTGAAAGGCATGTGCTACAAAC-3'		
15	Forward	5'-CAGGTCCTAGGCACAGGAACTG-3'	60°C	321 bp
	Reverse	5'-ACATTCCCAAATTGCTTGCCT-3'		

[a]Reproduced from **ref. 5.**

[b]Because of the high GC content of the exon 1 sequence, a PCR buffer designed for GC-rich sequences is needed. There are several on the market. One effective buffer is the GC-rich PCR System from Roche.

[c]GC-clamps were added at the 5' for DHPLC analysis: forward primer, 5'-CCCGCCGCCCCCGCCG-3'; reverse primer, 5'-CCGCGCCCCCGCCCG-3' (product length, 290 bp).

T$_{ann}$, annealing temperature.

8. 96-well PCR plates that fit the PCR machine. We use PCR Plate, Thermo-Fast 96 (ABgene, cat. no. AB-0600). The plates used are important because they determine the Z-value (depth of the well) of the rack parameter setting of the autosampler.
9. Adhesive PCR film (ABgene, cat. no. AB-0558).
10. WAVE-optimized DHPLC buffers and DNASep column from Transgenomic:
    a. Buffer A: 0.1 *M* triethylammonium acetate (TEAA) in water, pH 7.0.
    b. Buffer B: 0.1 *M* TEAA, 25% acetonitrile (ACN), pH 7.0.
11. Syringe wash solution: 8% ACN, in water.
12. Solution D: 75% ACN, 25% water.
13. DHPLC column: DNASep HT cartridge.

The solutions in **steps 11** and **12** can easily made in-house with HPLC-grade ACN and 18.2 MΩ-cm quality water.

3. Methods

Because there are areas of the gene in which mutations are more frequent, there has to be a strategy for exon analysis. Exons 3, 8, and 13 should be analyzed first. Any samples in which there is a change detected by WAVE should then be investigated by direct sequencing to determine whether the change is a polymorphism or a mutation. Those samples with no base changes should then have exons 7, 4, and 2 analyzed. Those samples still negative for any base change would then be investigated for the remainder of the coding region of *PTPN11*.

3.1. Polymerase Chain Reaction

For exons 2 to 15, each 25-µL reaction contains approx 50 ng DNA, 1 U of AmpliTaq Gold DNA polymerase, and 20 pmol of each primer (*see* **Table 2**). WAVE analysis is extremely sensitive and can detect a base change even if adjacent to the primer. Therefore, primers should be designed to avoid any unwanted intronic polymorphisms, if possible. For each reaction, use 75 µ*M* each dNTP and the standard PCR buffer for the polymerase used, with a final concentration of $MgCl_2$ of 1.5 m*M*. Primer sequences, product lengths, and annealing temperatures are shown in **Table 2**.

1. A master mix containing all components except for DNA should be prepared just before starting the PCR reaction. There should be sufficient volume for all of the samples, plus three extra (in case of error), and a negative control with no DNA, to ensure that there is no contamination of the mix.
2. DNA should be diluted to give approx 50 ng/µL.
3. The master mix (24 µL) is added to as many wells as required in the PCR plate, plus one well for the negative control, and one well for the positive control (a known mutation), if a positive control is available. The plate is placed on the PCR machine and an adhesive PCR film placed over the plate.

4. All PCRs are performed using the same time parameters but varying annealing temperatures. For the first cycle, an 8-min denaturing step at 94°C is used, followed by 33 cycles of 94°C for 45 s; 54°C to 60°C for 30 s (*see* **Table 2** for relevant temperature for each exon); and 72°C for 45 s; with a final extension step of 10 min at 72°C. The primers are designed to include intron–exon boundaries plus consensus sequences (*see* **Note 2**).
5. After PCR amplification, the plate is removed from the PCR machine and transferred to the WAVE analyzer.

3.2. WAVE (DHPLC) Analysis

The transgenomic WAVE machine operates using the principle of HPLC, a chromatographic separation technique that was far more familiar to protein biochemists than molecular biologists until recently. It uses a DHPLC column packed with a nonporous hydrophobic separation matrix (polystyrene–divinylbenzene copolymer beads) that detects the presence of heteroduplexes that are formed by the hybridization between the wild-type and the variant strands.

Proper maintenance of the WAVE system is crucial for reliable and reproducible results.

Running a mutation standard (and a sizing standard) before analyzing a batch of test samples is highly recommended (*see* **Note 3**). Any heterozygous sequence variation in the target DNA produces a mixture of wild-type and mutant PCR products when amplified. To enhance the formation of heteroduplexes, the PCR products (in the sealed PCR plate) are heated at 94°C for 5 min and cooled slowly to 20°C at a rate of 1.2°C/min. A method can be set up in a PCR machine to achieve this. Crude PCR product is used in the DHPLC analysis and no post-PCR handling, other than this heteroduplexing process, is involved (*see* **Note 4**).

The autosampler of the WAVE 3500HT system can accommodate two 96-well plates on a temperature-controlled rack (*see* **Note 5**). Heteroduplexed samples are automatically injected through the DNASep column that is sited in a temperature-controlled oven. Oven temperature for analysis, which causes partial denaturation of the DNA fragments, is predicted by the Navigator software (Transgenomic), and the user is also able to choose alternate temperatures depending on the melting profile of the DNA fragment (*see* **Note 6**). Partially denatured homoduplexes and heteroduplexes have differential affinities (mediated by the ion-pairing reagent, TEAA) toward the column and are subsequently eluted by a linear ACN gradient formed by the automated mixing of buffers A and B. The Navigator software also predicts the necessary gradient for this temperature-mediated heteroduplex analysis. More than one temperature is required in most of the cases to push the sensitivity toward 100%. The number of temperatures needed for a thorough analysis varies, depending on the melting properties predicted by the Navigator software and on the size of the DNA fragment. Choosing the right temperature is important for successful screening (*see* **Note 6**).

The flow rate during analysis is 1.5 mL/min and the gradient duration is 2.0 min. Each sample can be analyzed in approx 3.5 min (turn-around time).

The UV detector identifies the eluted products at 260 nm, and the progress of analysis is displayed by the Navigator software as a real-time chromatogram, in which the peak height is measured in mV. Any peak that falls below 1 mV is considered invalid because this may lead to a false-positive assessment. In these cases, a larger volume is reinjected or the PCR is repeated.

The peaks that differ in shape or width from the normal sample are scored as possible sequence variants and are confirmed by direct sequencing. As opposed to the previous software (WAVEMAKER), the Navigator software has the capability to normalize the peaks of different heights and, hence, any peak broadening can be readily identified.

DHPLC analysis is fast and inexpensive and the cost per injection can be brought close to 45 cents when the resources are used sensibly.

3.2.1. Practical Procedure

The Buffer B percentages and temperature(s) used for all 15 exons of *PTPN11* are shown in **Table 3** (when using the latest Navigator software, percentage of Buffer B is automatically calculated for the predicted temperature; here, the buffer B gradient is 10% over 2 min, i.e., a 5% slope). We will use exon 8 as an example for the WAVE analysis process, using a WAVE DNA Fragment Analysis System 3500HT equipped with an accelerator module.

The DNA sequence (252 bp) that includes *PTPN11* exon 8 is: **Ttggactaggctggggagta**actgatttgaactgttttttcctgaagcagtccaggacttatgtgac*C*gtgg tctcttttcttctagTTGATCATACCAGGGTTGTCCTACACGATGGTGATCCCAAT GAGCCTGTTTCAGATTACATCAATGCA*AATA*TCATCATGgtaagctttgctttt cacagtgttttctgaccatacatttctagcctattttgtattttaaa**tccttcctcatgtcctgaaag**.

The primer sequences are in boldface type. Three known coding mutations (922A>G, 923A>G, and 925A>G), and one intronic polymorphism (−21C>T), are also shown in bold in the sequence, with the intronic polymorphism in upper case bold italic type.

Launch the Navigator Software by double clicking the shortcut from the desktop. In the Navigator Connection window, there are five tabs to access primary pages. Three tabs, "DNA," "Injection," and "Analysis," are necessary to run samples.

Table 3
Percentage of Buffer B and Temperatures Used
in DHPLC Analysis for *PTPN11* Mutation Detection[a]

Exon	Buffer B Loading (%)	Initial (%)	Final (%)	Temperature[b]
1	56	61	67	67°C
2	55	60	66	56°C, 57°C
3	54	59	65	57°C, 58°C
4	53	58	64	56°C, 57°C
5	51	56	62	56°C, 58°C
6	50	55	61	56°C, 57°C
7	50	55	61	56°C, 57°C
8	51	56	62	57°C, 58°C
9	52	57	63	56°C, 57°C
10	50	55	61	57°C, 58°C
11	54	59	65	59°C
	49	54	60	64°C
12	48	53	59	58°C, 59°C
13	51	56	62	59°C
	50	55	61	60°C
14	52	57	63	57°C
	49	54	60	60°C
15	51	56	62	56°C, 57°C

Reproduced from **ref. 5**.
[a]Percentage of buffer A = 100% − % of Buffer B.
[b]Where two temperatures are given, both are used.

3.2.2. DNA Page

1. Select the "DNA" tab to open the DNA page.
2. Under "Amplicons," select the "+" button to create a new amplicon. Enter or paste the sequence, and enter a name for the sequence (e.g., *PTPN11* exon 8). Right click at the entered sequence and select "Format Sequence." The melting profiles for the predicted analysis temperature and four additional temperatures (which are changeable) are displayed. Usually, we keep the predicted temperature and choose at least one additional (higher than predicted) temperature for analysis, based on the melting profile (*see* **Note 6** for guidance on temperature selection). Select only the predicted temperature at this point.
3. Click the "Method" tab, then click the green "+" button to create a new method. In the "Method Setup" dialog box, enter a name for the method (e.g., PTPN11 exon 8). Select "Rapid DNA" as the "Application Type" from the drop-down menu, and select "Generate" to create the new method, with the temperature as suffix (e.g., PTPN11 exon 8~56.8). If more than one temperature is selected, that

number of methods will be created. From the list of methods displayed, double click the newly generated method to open the "Edit Method" window. (However, the method generated by Navigator for predicted temperature hardly requires editing).

4. Select "Rapid Method" from the drop-down menu within "Application Type." This is applicable to the WAVE models with an accelerator module (e.g., 3500HT). Enter 2.0 min for "Gradient Duration," 5% for "Slope," 3 for "Drop for Loading;" Navigator calculates the buffer gradient automatically. Save the method. If another temperature analysis is needed, tick the "Manual Mode" in the "Edit Method" window and enter the required "Time Shift" with a + or − sign to elute the peak to the right or left, respectively. Save as a different method (*see* **Note 6**).

3.2.3. Injection Page

Select the "Injection" tab to open the Injection Page.

1. To create a "New Project," select "File," then "New Project" to open the "New Project" dialog box and enter a new project name (e.g., March05) and save. Open "Project Defaults" within the "Setup" dialog box and tick "Fast Clean" and "Disable Tray Change Request." Projects can be opened via the "File" menu.
2. Click the "+" button in the "Tray Type" area and enter a new tray name (e.g., Noonan 24Mar05) and specify the tray type using the drop-down menu (e.g., "96-well tray column-back" means that a 96-well plate is used in the back or inside tray and the injections are performed column by column).
3. On the speed plate, select (click and drag down and across) the vials to be injected. A right click on the highlighted area opens the "Speed Plate Injections" window. Choose the relevant "Method Name" from the drop down menu. Enter the injection volume (if different from the default volume of 5 μL) and click "Generate" to create injections in the injection table. Here:
   a. Vial number and volume to be injected can be altered.
   b. The name of the sample can be entered or a list of names can be pasted, e.g., from Microsoft Excel®.
   c. Another method could be chosen from the list to run injections.
   d. Analysis (oven) temperature can be changed, with other injection or analysis parameters, such as percentage of buffer B remaining the same. This facility enables testing of other temperatures chosen in **Subheading 3.2.2., item 2.**
   e. It is recommended that two blank runs (by entering zero as the volume) are performed before the mutation standard or samples are injected.
4. Check the performance of the system by running a "Low temperature mutation standard" before a batch of sample injections (*see* **Note 3**).
5. Place the samples in the autosampler and highlight the injections to be run (e.g., two blanks and two *PTPN11* exon 8 normal samples) in the injection table, and send them to the "Queue Transactions" table by clicking the green arrowhead ("Run Injection") button at the top. The computer takes control of the WAVE system and injection starts after a brief equilibration period. As soon as each sample run is completed, the injection row is grayed out; highlight these data and send them to the "Analysis" page.

Generate a second set of four injections; this time, enter the second temperature to be tested in the injection table. As in **Subheading 3.2.3., step 5**, queue the injections. If the peak is not eluted between 1.5 and 2 min, note the necessary time shift with a + or – sign (e.g., +0.6 min) to shift the peak to the right or left, respectively. A new method has to be created including the second temperature and the time shift in the "Edit Method" dialog box (*see* **Subheading 3.2.2.**), if necessary (also *see* **Note 6**).

3.2.4. Analysis Page

Select the "Analysis" tab.

1. The traces can be displayed either individually or in groups, with an adjustable offset, and compared with a normal trace (*see* **Fig. 1A**). Ticking the "Show" squares will display the traces, and selecting "Show All" displays all of the ticked traces. A test trace is compared with a known normal trace. Any noticeable discrepancy should be followed up by direct sequencing, unless the signature of the Waveform suggests a particular base change that can be detected using a restriction enzyme.
2. The Navigator software has a sophisticated "Normalizing" capability that makes the analysis accurate and rapid (*see* **Fig 1B**). This facility was not available with the previous WAVE software, WAVEMAKER, and is extremely useful in allowing peak broadening to be distinguished. However, we did not find "Mutation Calling" very useful (*see* **Note 7**).
3. To print traces (pdf files), highlight the rows, then select "File," "Reports," "Analysis," and "Build Report" (text can be added here).

4. Notes

1. Compatibility. Bovine serum albumin, autoclaved water, mineral oil, formamide, proteinase K, undisclosed PCR ingredients (enhancers, stabilizers, or other additives), and gelatin are some of the substances that are not compatible with the column in any magnitude. At levels higher than 1% in the PCR reaction mixture, polyethylene glycol, Triton X-100, Nonidet P-40, Tween-20, sodium dodecyl sulphate, and sodium lauryl sulphate are found to cause cartridge degradation. The following PCR additives are allowed up to the limits shown in parentheses; selecting the active clean option at the end of each injection and performing a hot wash after 96 injections are recommended: dimethylsulfoxide (10%), glycerol (2%), and betaine (2.5 M).
2. The PCR temperatures shown in **Table 2** (from **ref. 5**) were transferred without problem to our laboratory. However, it does sometimes happen that different PCR machines in different laboratories do not produce the expected results. If the amplimers produced are not clean enough or strong enough, it may be necessary to carry out a temperature or Mg^{2+} optimization to improve the procedure.
3. WAVE Mutation Standard (8 µL) analyzed at 56°C shows peaks corresponding to homoduplexes and heteroduplexes. Four distinct peaks should be observed each time (*see* **Fig. 2**), and the retention time difference between the two hetero-

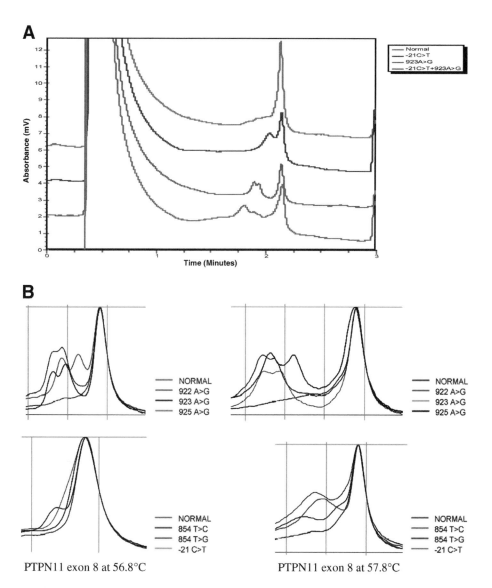

A

B

PTPN11 exon 8 at 56.8°C   PTPN11 exon 8 at 57.8°C

Fig. 1. (**A**) *PTPN11* exon 8 at 57.8°C. The presence of more than one sequence variation, for example a mutation and a polymorphism, as shown here (as analyzed by the WAVEMAKER software), results in an elution profile significantly different from those produced individually. This characteristic feature allows the signature-based identification of polymorphisms, which can be confirmed by an appropriate restriction enzyme analysis, or by sequencing if no restriction site is produced or destroyed. The Navigator software makes this kind of recognition even easier, as shown in (**B**). Chromatograms analyzed using the normalizing function of the Navigator software. In this mode (which was not included in the previous software versions, namely, HSM and WAVEMAKER), the peaks are brought to the same height; hence, the analysis becomes simple. It also allows the user to predict the change (using previous knowledge), based on the specific signatures (*see* **Note 6**).

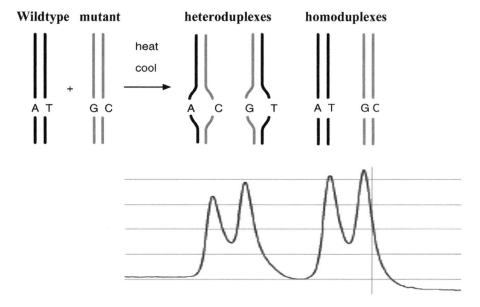

Fig. 2. Peaks that would be expected from the low-temperature mutation standard at 56°C for hetero- and homoduplexes.

duplexes should be approximately equal to that of the homoduplexes. Any substantial deviation from the WAVE form should be corrected by performing a hot wash, using fresh buffers and/or washing the column with a Transgenomic DNASep wash solution (the in-line filter can also be changed). If this fails to fix the problem, oven calibration should be performed (further advice available from the Transgenomic Help Desk).

Hot wash: Reverse the column in the oven compartment, set the oven temperature to 80°C, pump 100% wash solution D through the column for 20 to 30 min (flow rate, 0.9 mL/min), and equilibrate the column by passing 50% buffer A and 50% buffer B through the column for 20 to 30 min (at a rate of 0.9 mL/min). It is not necessary to turn the column back. After the hot wash, retest the mutation standard.

4. Soon after heteroduplexing, the PCR plate can be frozen until the analysis. The plate seal should not be removed while the plate is still cold; this will lead to residual adhesive material left on the plate and may cause the PCR plate to be dislodged from the autosampler tray! Use the hot lid (of the PCR machine) to heat the plate seal and peel the seal off while it is hot.

5. Autosampler. The tray in the autosampler is usually set to 10°C. If condensation is noticed, the temperature could be raised just enough to stop the condensation. Samples can be injected by columns or by rows. The correct option should be selected when a new tray is set up.

6. WAVE analysis temperature selection. The analysis temperature recommended by the Navigator software is 56.8°C. DHPLC analysis is carried out at partial

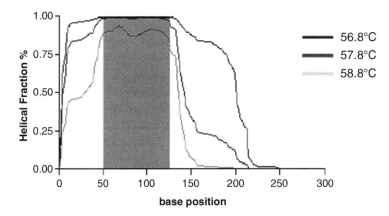

Fig. 3. *PTPN11* exon 8 (252 bp) melting profile.

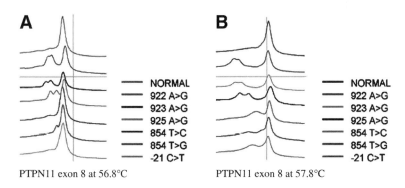

Fig. 4. PCR products (5 μL) analyzed by WAVE at two different temperatures; both temperatures detected the –21C>T sequence variations in the region, which was 100% helical at these temperatures. WAVE forms, which are reproducible, correspond to each variation.

melting temperatures at which the helical fraction falls between 40 and 99%. In theory, any sequence variation in the region, which is 100% helix (shaded region at 56.8°C), is likely to be missed. Hence, a second temperature, such as 58.8°C, may be necessary (**Fig. 3**). However, it is common that a sequence variation is detected even if the region is 100% helical (**Fig. 4**).

Using a second or even third temperature is common in the case of larger DNA fragments. When using temperatures 2 or 3°C higher or lower than the predicted temperature, addition of a positive or negative time shift to the method may be necessary to increase or decrease the retention time of the peak. Testing is recommended for all of the available samples with mutations or polymorphisms at different temperatures. Temperatures of less than 1°C difference are normally not helpful. Higher temperatures tend to generate broad peaks, which could create difficulties when analyzing the data. Using the highest possible temperature without jeopardizing the quality of the peak is very useful.

7. The "Mutation Calling" software should align the waveforms into groups of similarity, but we did not find that it worked reproducibly, or that it separated the groups properly. Hence, we instead use the "Normalizing" capability for this purpose, and identify the variants by eye.

Acknowledgments

We thank Prof. Michael Patton, Dr. Andrew Crosby, Dr. Kamini Kalidas, John Short, Dr. Adam Shaw, and Gayathri Sivapalan for their part in the NS research at St George's Hospital Medical School. We also thank Dr. Bruce Gelb and Dr. Marco Tartaglia, who performed the initial WAVE analysis on *PTPN11* and shared their methodology with us.

References

1. Sharland, M., Morgan, M., Smith, G., Burch, M., and Patton, M. A. (1993) Genetic counseling in Noonan syndrome. *Am. J. Med. Genet.* **45**, 437–440.
2. Jamieson, R., van der Burgt, I., Brady, A., et al. (1994) Mapping a gene for Noonan Syndrome to the long arm of chromosome 12. *Nat. Genet.* **8**, 357–360.
3. Tartaglia, M., Mehler, E. L., Goldberg, R., et al. (2001) Mutations in *PTPN11*, encoding the protein tyrosine phosphatase SHP-2, cause Noonan syndrome. *Nat. Genet.* **29**, 465–468.
4. Chen, B., Bronson, R. T., Klaman, L. D., et al. (2000) Mice mutants for Egfr and Shp2 have defective cardiac semilunar valvulogenesis. *Nat. Genet.* **24**, 296–299.
5. Tartaglia, M., Kalidas, K., Shaw, A., et al. (2002) *PTPN11* Mutations in Noonan Syndrome: Molecular Spectrum, Genotype-Phenotype Correlation, and Phenotypic Heterogeneity. *Am. J. Hum. Genet.* **70**, 1555–1563.
6. Musante, L., Kehl, H. G., Majewski, F., et al. (2003) Spectrum of mutations in PTPN11 and genotype–phenotype correlation in 96 patients with Noonan syndrome and five patients with cardio–facio–cutaneous syndrome. *Eur. J. Hum. Genet.* **11**, 201–206.
7. Maheshwari, M., Belmont, J., Fernbach, S., et al. (2002) PTPN11 mutations in Noonan syndrome type I: detection of recurrent mutations in exons 3 and 13. *Hum. Mutat.* **20**, 298–304.
8. Sarkozy, A., Conti, E., Seripa, D., et al. (2203) Correlation between PTPN11 gene mutations and congenital heart defects in Noonan and LEOPARD syndromes. *J. Med. Genet.* **40**, 704–708.
9. Mogensen, J., Bahl, A., Kubo, T., Elanko, N., Taylor, R., and McKenna, W. J. (2003). Comparison of fluorescent SSCP and denaturing HPLC analysis with direct sequencing for mutation screening in hypertrophic cardiomyopathy. *J. Med. Genet.* **40**, e59.
10. Jones, A. C., Austin, J., Hansen, N., et al. (1999) Optimal temperature selection for mutation detection by denaturing HPLC and comparison to single-stranded

conformation polymorphism and heteroduplex analysis. *Clin. Chem.* **45**, 1133–1140.

11. Choy, Y. S., Dabora, S. L., Hall, F., et al. (1999) Superiority of denaturing high performance liquid chromatography over single-stranded conformation and conformation-sensitive gel electrophoresis for mutation detection in TSC2. *Ann. Hum. Genet.* **63**, 383–391.

7

Williams–Beuren Syndrome Diagnosis Using Fluorescence *In Situ* Hybridization

Lucy R. Osborne, Ann M. Joseph-George, and Stephen W. Scherer

Summary

Williams–Beuren syndrome (WBS) is most commonly caused by a 1.5-Mb hemizygous deletion of chromosome 7q11.23. Other genomic rearrangements of this region have also been described, some as polymorphisms and others as rare variants, the latter often being directly associated with clinical symptoms. Fluorescence *in situ* hybridization of either metaphase or interphase nuclei can be used to detect all of these chromosomal rearrangements, providing the ability to test this segment of chromosome 7 in families with a suspected diagnosis of WBS.

Key Words: Chromosome 7; fluorescence *in situ* hybridization (FISH); deletion; inversion; interphase; metaphase.

1. Introduction

Williams–Beuren syndrome (WBS) is a complex disorder, caused by deletion of approx 1.5 Mb of DNA, spanning at least 25 genes, on one copy of chromosome 7 *(1,2)*. The incidence of WBS is estimated at between 1 in 7500 people and 1 in 20,000 people *(3,4)*, and it is usually sporadic, although cases of autosomal-dominant transmission have been described *(5)*. WBS is almost always associated with a recognizable facies and characteristic cardiovascular lesions, most frequently, stenosis of the ascending aorta is found (in ~80% of individuals); other symptoms occur less frequently *(6)*. A unique cognitive and behavioral profile is also associated with this disorder, involving mild mental retardation, friendliness, anxiety, and developmental motor disabilities *(7)*.

Although the vast majority (>95%) of individuals presenting with classic features of WBS have a common 1.5-Mb deletion at band q11.23 on one copy of chromosome 7, some individuals have a translocation, partial deletion, or an inversion of the same genomic region that may result in a less severe phenotype *(8–11)*. The use of a now well-defined DNA sequence assembly of the

From: *Methods in Molecular Medicine, vol. 126: Congenital Heart Disease: Molecular Diagnostics*
Edited by: M. Kearns-Jonker © Humana Press Inc., Totowa, NJ

human genome along with fluorescence *in situ* hybridization (FISH) mapping technology makes it possible to clearly define rearrangements of the WBS region in families with a suspected WBS proband. The flow chart shown in **Fig. 1** outlines a general step-wise order in which specific tests can be performed on an individual with a suspected diagnosis of WBS. The initial screen would examine for the common deletion using commercially available (quality assured) probes. Karyotyping (performed in parallel to or after the standard diagnostic FISH test) and targeted FISH analyses could then be used to detect macroscopic changes, such as translocations or smaller deletions/inversions, respectively. Each type of analysis varies in the number of probes used and in the cell stage analyzed after hybridization.

Alternative methods for the detection of deletions are available and are described in Chapter 8. For example, genotyping of DNA from the proband and parents with polymorphic markers can be used to search for loss of heterozygosity, indicating the absence of a parental allele. Commonly used polymorphic markers spanning the deletion region are listed in **Fig. 2**. Quantitative polymerase chain reaction is also used to detect the reduction in probe copy number associated with the deletion. This method requires more fine-tuning to generate a panel of probes that amplify consistently, but is very useful when DNA but no cells are available from the proband. Array comparative genomic hybridization is another new powerful methodology that is being developed, but is not discussed here because it is not yet in standard practice.

2. Materials

2.1. Preparation of Target DNA

1. Thermotron.
2. CO_2 incubator.
3. Low-speed centrifuge.
4. Vacutainer blood collection tubes containing sodium heparin.
5. 8-mL flat-bottomed tubes.
6. T25 vented tissue culture flasks.
7. Cell culture medium 1: α-Minimum Essential Medium, 15% fetal calf serum (FCS), 4 U/mL sodium heparin, 100 mg/mL streptomycin plus 100 U/mL penicillin, and 2 mL/100 mL phytohemagglutinin (M-form [Invitrogen] reconstituted in 10 mL water).
8. Cell culture medium 2: RPMI-1640 medium with pyruvate, 10% FCS, 100 mg/mL streptomycin plus 100 U/mL penicillin, and 2 mM L-glutamine.
9. Cell culture medium 3: RPMI-1640 medium with pyruvate, 20% FCS, 100 mg/mL streptomycin plus 100 U/mL penicillin, 2 mM L-glutamine, and 10 µg/mL colcemid.
11. 0.075 M KCl, prewarmed to 37°C.

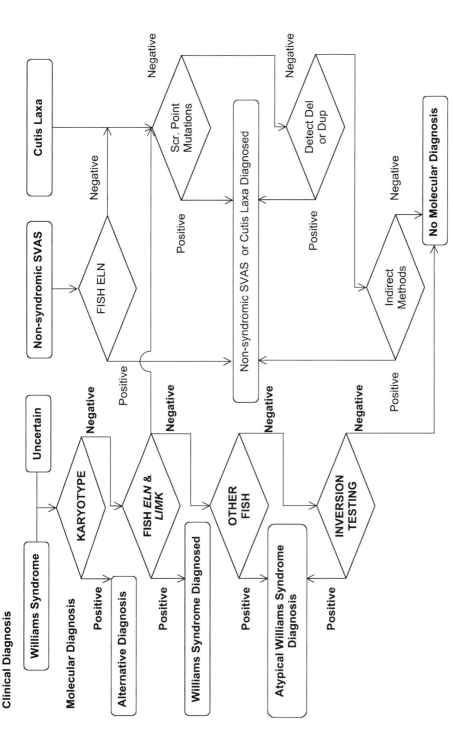

Fig. 1. Flow chart of the molecular analysis of individuals with a possible clinical diagnosis of WBS. ELN, elastin; Scr, screen; Del, deletion; Dup, duplication.

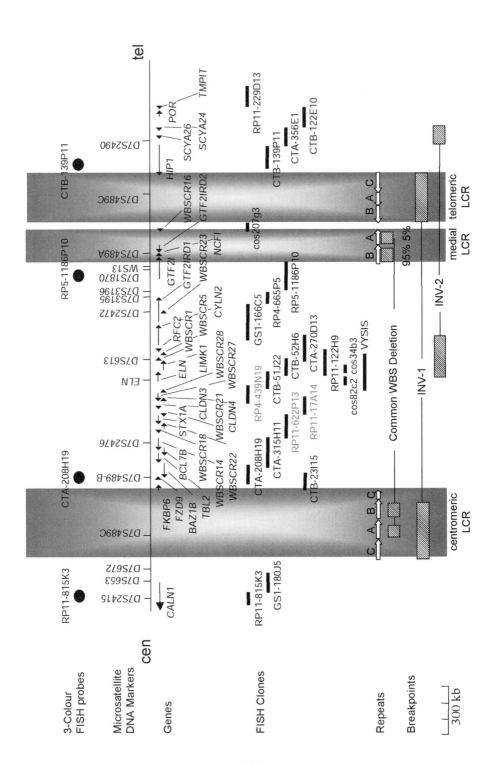

12. Fixative (3:1, methanol:acetic acid; prepare same day and store at –20°C).
13. Glass microscope slides (precleaned, frosted).

2.2. Preparation of Probes for FISH Analysis

1. Luria Bertani broth.
2. Appropriate antibiotic (e.g., 20 µg/mL chloramphenicol; 20 µg/mL kanamycin; or 100 µg/mL ampicillin).
3. Solutions for standard alkaline lysis DNA extraction.
4. DIG-Nick Translation Mix (Roche, cat. no. 1745816).
5. BioNick Labeling System (Invitrogen, cat. no. 18247-015).
6. Nick Translation Kit (Vysis, cat. no. 32-801300).
7. Spectrum Green dUTP (Vysis, cat. no. 30-803200).
8. 10 mg/mL salmon sperm DNA (Invitrogen, cat no. 15632-011).
9. 3 M sodium acetate.
10. TE buffer: 10 mM Tris-HCl, pH 7.5, 1 mM EDTA .
11. 100% ethanol.
12. Agarose gel electrophoresis equipment.

2.3. DNA Denaturation and Hybridization

1. Water baths at 37, 42, 62, and 75°C.
2. Hybridization buffer: 31% deionized formamide, 2.5% w/v dextran sulphate, 2.5X standard sodium citrate (SSC).
3. 1 mg/mL human Cot DNA (Invitrogen, cat. no. 15279-011).
4. Denaturing solution: 70% deionized formamide, 2X SSC, pH 5.5.
5. 70, 90, and 100% ethanol at –20°C.
6. 70, 90, and 100% ethanol at room temperature in Coplin jars.
7. 2X SSC, pH 7.0, 0.1% Tween-20.
8. 22 × 22-mm glass cover slips.

Fig. 2. *(opposite page)* WBS region at 7q11.23 and diagnostic reagents. Genomic clones used for FISH analysis are shown above and below the annotated genes (orientation of gene transcription indicated by direction of arrows). The clones given in the darker font give strong single-copy signals under FISH examination. The exception is CTA-208H19, which sometimes gives a second, fainter signal. Microsatellite DNA markers are also shown. The WBS low-copy repeats (LCRs) are indicated by the vertical shaded blocks and have been divided into segments of nearly identical sequence (**A–C**) shown in their correct orientation in relation to the centromere and telomere. The breakpoints of the common deletion and the two inversions (inv-1 and inv-2) are shown at the bottom of the figure. The common deletion breakpoints cluster within the hatched boxes, with 95% of the deletions residing in the B block and the remaining 5% residing in the A block of the medial LCR. The inversion breakpoints have not yet been fine-mapped at the nucleotide level, but have been localized within the regions marked by hatched boxes.

9. Rubber cement.
10. Coplin jars.
11. Wash solution 1: 1:1, deionized formamide: 2X SSC at 42°C; must always be freshly prepared.
12. Wash solution 2: 0.05% SSC at 62°C.

2.4. Immunodetection

1. Water baths at 37 and 40°C.
2. Blocking solution: 0.5% bovine serum albumin (BSA).
3. 2X SSC.
4. Wash solution 3: 4X SSC, 0.1% Tween-20 at 40°C.
5. Anti-digoxigenin–rhodamine antibody, for detection of digoxigenin-labeled probe (anti-digoxigenin–rhodamine FAb fragments [Roche, cat. no. 1207750] reconstituted in double-distilled water; working concentration, 1 μg conjugate/mL; 0.5% BSA).
6. Avidin, Alexa Fluor 488 antibody, for detection of biotin labeled probe—green signal (Molecular Probes, cat. no. A-21370; reconstituted in phosphate-buffered saline; working concentration, 10 μg conjugate/mL; 0.5% BSA).
7. Avidin-Cy5 antibody, for detection of biotin labeled probe—yellow signal (MetaSystems, *B*-tect, cat. no. 0901-060-NI; working solution, detection 1 + 3 solution and blocking reagent solution, 1 μL: 50 μL).

2.5. Chromosome Counterstaining and DAPI Staining

1. Coplin jars.
2. 22 × 40-mm glass cover slips.
3. DAPI solution (0.2 μg DAPI/mL; 2X SSC).
4. 2X SSC.
5. Antifade solution.

3. Methods

Outline of methods:
1. Preparation of target DNA.
2. Preparation of probes for FISH analysis.
3. Denaturation and hybridization of the target DNA and the probes.
4. Immunodetection.
5. Counterstaining.
6. Visualization and interpretation of the results.

3.1. Preparation of Target DNA

Metaphase chromosomes should be prepared for standard WBS deletion testing or partial deletion testing, and interphase nuclei prepared for WBS inversion testing. Both preparations can be made from either peripheral blood or lymphoblastoid cell lines and they can be safely stored at –20°C until they are required for making slides.

3.1.1. Peripheral Blood Lymphocyte Culture and Harvest

1. Collect venous blood into a Vacutainer tube containing sodium heparin. If blood is collected in a Vacutainer tube containing anticoagulant citrate-dextrose, increase the sodium heparin in the medium to 6 U/mL.
2. Dispense 6 mL of cell culture medium 1 into 8-mL flat-bottomed tubes and add 5 to 8 drops of blood to each tube.
3. Incubate horizontally in a 37°C CO_2 incubator for 70–72 h.
4. 25 min before harvesting, add 83 ng/mL colcemid and reincubate at 37°C.
5. Pellet cells at low speed ($120g$) for 10 min, remove supernatant, resuspend, add 8 mL of prewarmed hypotonic solution, and incubate for 15 min at 37°C.
6. Pellet cells again, remove supernatant, resuspend, and add 1 mL of cold fixative, drop-by-drop, using a Pasteur pipet, while agitating the tube.
7. Add 7 mL of cold fixative and incubate at –20°C for at least 1 h.
8. Pellet cells again, remove all but 1 mL of supernatant, resuspend pellet.
9. Make a test slide to ensure that metaphases are present.
10. Add 7 mL of cold fixative to the resuspended cells. Repeat **Subheading 3.1.1., step 8** three times.

3.1.2. Lymphoblastoid Cell Line Culture and Harvest

When receiving lymphoblast cell lines cultures for cytogenetic preparations, check for cell concentration using an inverted phase–contrast microscope. As the cells grow, the color of the medium progressively changes from orange to yellow, indicating they have reached confluence (2–3 d). Cells are then grown upright in T25 vented tissue culture flasks, using cell culture medium 2, at 37°C in a CO_2 incubator. The final volume of culture should not exceed 20 mL in this size flask. To obtain a high mitotic index, it is important to feed and to harvest the cells at the same time on each consecutive day (days 1, 2, and 3).

1. Allow cells to reach confluence, then split 1:1 with fresh cell culture medium 2.
2. Allow cells to reach confluence and perform the following procedures at the same time each day:
    Day 1: Inoculate 5 mL of prewarmed culture medium 2 with 5 mL of culture.
    Day 2: Feed cultures 1:1 using prewarmed culture medium 3.
    Day 3: Half an hour before harvesting, add 0.5 µg of colcemid and reincubate for 15 min.
3. Transfer the contents of each flask to a 15-mL conical, screw-cap tube, pellet the cells ($120g$) for 10 min, remove the supernatant, and resuspend by gentle agitation.
4. Add 8 mL of prewarmed hypotonic KCl. Mix by inverting tubes and place at 37°C for 15 min.
5. Pellet the cells, remove the supernatant, resuspend by gentle agitation, and add ice-cold fix, drop-by-drop, with shaking, to approx 1 mL. Bring volume up to 10 mL with fixative.

6. Place at –20°C overnight.
7. The next day, repeat **Subheading 3.1.2., step 5** and change fixative twice.

3.1.3. Slide Preparation

1. Turn on the Thermotron and allow to equilibrate at required conditions of temperature and humidity (empirically determined).
2. Pellet cell preparation (120*g*) for 10 min, remove supernatant and resuspend in enough fresh fixative so that the cell suspension appears faintly turbid.
3. Clean the slide surface using a few drops of fixative (3:1, methanol:acetic acid) and wipe dry using a lint-free tissue. Place slide on the flat surface of the Thermotron, add one drop of cell suspension onto the center of the slide and leave to dry.
4. Check the slides under the phase contrast microscope to ensure good chromosome quality and to assess the cell density. Metaphases should be 3 to 4 per field (at 10X magnification), well-spread, and have minimal or no visible cytoplasm present.
5. If slides are being used for interphase FISH procedures, it is important to have a much higher density of cells per field to facilitate more efficient data acquisition, especially when a scanning microscope is being used. To accomplish this without compromising the quality of the spread, cell concentration of the cell suspension is retained, but the number of drops per slide on the same spot is increased until the desired density is reached. Nuclei should be close together, but without their walls touching.
6. Slides can be stored at room temperature for up to 3 wk.

3.2. Preparation of Probes for FISH Analysis

3.2.1. Selection of FISH Probes

3.2.1.1. CLONE SELECTION

The locations of specific probes in relation to the WBS deletion are shown in **Fig. 2**. These clones are all in the public domain and are available through a number of sources, including our own genome resource center (available at: www.tcag.ca).

3.2.1.2. DETECTION OF THE COMMON WBS DELETION

For standard WBS-deletion FISH testing, the commercially available Williams Syndrome Region Probe from Vysis may be used. This probe is dual-color and prelabeled, and consists of a probe (~180 kb in size) spanning the elastin gene locus, the *LIMK1* gene, and microsatellite marker D7S613 (*see* **Fig. 2** for locations). The probe also contains a control probe for the region containing loci D7S486 and D7S522 (7q31). Alternatively, the P1 artificial chromosome (PAC) clone RP11-122H9 is equivalent to the Vysis WBS probe; we use RP1-13N03, which maps to 7p22.3, as a chromosome 7 short-arm control.

3.2.1.3. Detection of Smaller Deletions

Probes used for detecting smaller deletions may be chosen from the panel shown in **Fig. 2**. We routinely use the cosmid clones 34b3 and 82c2 from the LL07NC01 chromosome 7-specific cosmid library to check for partial deletions of the elastin gene, and RP5-1186P10 and CTA-208H19 to check for deletions that do not include elastin.

3.2.1.4. Detection of Larger Deletions

We routinely use RP11-815K3 to assay for deletions extending in a centromeric direction and CTB-139P11 to detect deletions extending in a telomeric direction from the common deletion interval (**Fig. 2**).

3.2.1.5. Detection of Inversions

Three-color interphase FISH analysis is used for inversion detection. Because of the proximity of the probes (<2 Mb apart), their order can only be readily determined when visualized in interphase nuclei. The three probes are labeled individually with red, green, and yellow labels, then mixed and hybridized to interphase nuclei preparations. The three probes consist of two within the common deletion region and another outside just to the telomeric side. The probes we use are CTA-208H19, RP5-1186P10, and CTB-139P11 because this combination will detect both inversion-1 and inversion-2 (shown in **Fig. 2**) (*see* **Note 1**).

3.2.2. Genomic Clone Propagation, Amplification, and Isolation of DNA

1. Inoculate a single bacterial colony containing the cloned DNA of interest into 5 mL of Luria Bertani broth supplemented with the appropriate antibiotic in a 15-mL snap-cap tube and incubate at 37°C overnight, with shaking.
2. Pellet cells (1700*g* for 10 min), discard supernatant, and extract the plasmid DNA using a standard alkaline column-based lysis protocol (e.g., QIAprep kit from Qiagen) as follows:
3. Resuspend the cell pellet in 300 μL of P1 solution using the vortex.
4. Lyse cells by adding 300 μL of P2 solution and mix gently. Incubate at room temperature for 5 min. The appearance of the suspension should turn change from turbid to translucent.
5. Neutralize by slowly adding 300 μL of P3 solution, shaking while adding. A thick white precipitate will form. Place tubes on ice for at least 5 min.
6. Centrifuge tubes at 1700*g* for 10 min. Transfer the supernatant to a 1.5-mL eppendorf tube and discard pellet.
7. Centrifuge the eppendorf tubes at 18,000*g* for 10 min.
8. Precipitate DNA: transfer 750 μL of supernatant to another eppendorf tube containing 800 μL of isopropanol. Avoid transferring any of the white precipitate

material. Mix by inverting the tubes several times. Place the tubes at –20°C for at least 30 min (tubes can be left at –20°C overnight at this stage).

9. Centrifuge the tubes for 15 min at 18,000*g* at 4°C. Discard supernatant.
10. Wash the DNA pellet by adding 800 µL of 70% ethanol. Invert tubes several times to mix. Centrifuge at 14,000 rpm for 5 min at 4°C.
11. Carefully remove the supernatant by pipetting.
12. Allow pellets to dry at room temperature (10–20 min). Pellets will turn from white to translucent when most of the ethanol has evaporated.
13. Resuspend the DNA in 30 µL of double-distilled, autoclaved water and allow to sit at room temperature for 1 h to ensure complete resuspension.

3.2.3. Probe Labeling

3.2.3.1. DIGOXIGENIN (RED SIGNAL)

Use 300 to 400 ng bacterial artificial chromosome (BAC)/P1 artificial chromosome (PAC) clone DNA in 16 µL of sterile ddH$_2$O and label using the DIG-Nick Translation Mix (Roche), according to the manufacturer's instructions, with the following modifications:

Add 4 µL DIG-Nick Translation Mix, mix and centrifuge briefly.
Incubate for 5–7 h at 15°C.
Place reaction on ice and proceed with steps in **Subheading 3.2.4.**
Stop the reaction with 2 µL of 0.5 *M* EDTA (pH 8.0) and add 6 µL of salmon sperm DNA.

Separate the unincorporated nucleotides from the labeled DNA probe by repeated ethanol precipitation. Add 0.1 volume of 3 *M* sodium acetate and 2.5 volumes of cold (–20°C) ethanol, mix and freeze at –20°C for 30 min. Pellet at 18,000*g* for 10 min. Remove supernatant and dry pellet. Resuspend the pellet in 20 µL autoclaved ddH$_2$O.

3.2.3.2. BIOTIN (GREEN SIGNAL)

Mix the components in a microcentrifuge tube on ice and spin briefly.

5 µL 10X dNTP mix
600–750 ng BAC clone DNA
5 µL 10X enzyme mix
Distilled water to 45 µL
Incubate at 15°C for 3–5 h

Place the reaction on ice and proceed with steps in **Subheading 3.2.4.** to check the size of fragments.

Add 5 µL stop buffer and 6 µL salmon sperm DNA. Separate the unincorporated nucleotides from the labeled DNA probe by repeated ethanol precipitation. Add 0.1 volume of 3 *M* sodium acetate and 2.5 volumes of cold (–20°C) ethanol, mix and freeze at –20°C for 30 min. Pellet at 20,000g for 10 min. Remove supernatant and dry the pellet. Resuspend the pellet in 20 μL of autoclaved ddH$_2$O. Biotinylated probes are very stable and can be stored at –20°C for at least 1 yr.

3.2.3.3. DIGOXIGENIN AND BIOTIN COMBINED (YELLOW SIGNAL)

Label two sets of DNA separately with digoxigenin and biotin, as described in **Subheadings 3.2.3.1.** and **3.2.3.2.** and mix in a ratio of 3 parts digoxigenin to 2 parts biotin.

3.2.3.4. SPECTRUM GREEN (DIRECT LABEL)

Mix the components in a microcentrifuge tube on ice and spin briefly.

1 μg BAC clone DNA
2.5 μL of 0.2 mM Spectrum Green
5 μL of 0.1 mM dTTP
10 μL of dNTP mix
5 μL of 10X nick translation buffer
10 μL nick translation enzyme
Nuclease-free water to 50 μL
Incubate 8–16 h at 15°C

Stop the reaction by heating in a 70°C water bath for 10 min and chill on ice. Add 6 μL of salmon sperm DNA. Separate the unincorporated nucleotides from the labeled DNA probe by repeated ethanol precipitation. Add 0.1 volume of 3 M sodium acetate and 2.5 volumes of cold (–20°C) ethanol, mix, and freeze at – 20°C for 30 min. Pellet at 18,000g for 10 min. Remove supernatant and dry the pellet. Resuspend the pellet in 20 μL of autoclaved ddH$_2$O and store at –20°C.

3.2.4. Determination of Labeled Fragment Length

The length of the labeled fragments should be checked after the labeling reaction is complete, but before the probe is cleaned and precipitated ready for use. At the appropriate step during the labeling process (*see* **Subheading x.x.**), place the reaction on ice and take a 3 μL aliquot for testing. Add gel-loading buffer, place sample on ice for 3 min, and run the sample on an agarose minigel, along with a DNA molecular weight marker. The probe should range between 200 and 500 nucleotides in length. If necessary, reincubate the reaction at 15°C and check the fragment size again.

3.3. DNA Denaturation and Hybridization

Ready the slides and appropriate probes that have been labeled with different fluorochromes. At least 2 μL of labeled probe is required for each slide.

Place a Coplin jar containing denaturing solution in a water bath at 75°C. Label eppendorf tubes, one for every probe being used (to avoid confusion, it is best to use different colored tubes for different probes) and prepare the probe mix, which consists of:

> 1 μL human Cot DNA (1 mg/mL)
> 7 μL hybridization buffer
> 2 μL required labeled probe

Vortex probe mixes briefly and then spin down (when hybridizing using three probes, use the same volumes as **Subheading 3.3.** for each probe, and use a 22 × 40-mm cover slip).

3.3.1. Probe Denaturation

Ensure that the temperature in the water bath is at 75°C, then immerse probes for exactly 5 min. Remove samples and place samples into water bath at 37°C for 20–30 min to reanneal.

3.3.2. Pretreatment and Denaturation of Target DNA

1. Before pretreatment, slides are aged for 2–3 h at 55°C.
2. Pretreat slides with 2X SSC plus 0.1% Tween-20 at 37°C for 30 min.
3. Removes slides, drain briefly, and dehydrate (for 2 min each) through an ethanol series at room temperature.
4. Have a 70, 90, and 100% ethanol series ready at –20°C.
5. Place slides in denaturing solution (70% deionized formamide in 0.6X SSC) at 75°C.
6. Drain denaturing solution into waste beaker, using forceps to retain slides in jar.
7. Immediately add ice-cold 70% ethanol to jar and discard ethanol at once.
8. Add ice-cold 70% ethanol to jar and leave for 3 min.
9. Drain slides briefly on a paper towel, and submerge in ice-cold 90% ethanol for 3 min.
10. Drain slides briefly on a paper towel, and submerge in ice-cold 100% ethanol for 3 min; remove slides, drain, and air-dry slides on rack.

3.3.3. Hybridization

1. Label slides with the probe names to be used.
2. Combine the chosen probes, mix by flicking the tube, and spin down.
3. Place the probe solution on the cells and drop on a 22 × 22-mm cover slip. Seal with rubber cement and mark the area covered by the cover slip on the back of slide with a diamond pencil.
4. Place slides in a moist, dark chamber and leave at 37°C overnight.

3.3.4. Washing

It is extremely important to ensure that the slides do not dry out during the washing process, because this will cause excessive background fluorescence.

1. Prewarm the Coplin jar containing 200 mL of Wash solution 1 at 42°C and 500 mL of Wash solution 2 at 62°C.
2. Remove cover slips from the hybridized slides and clean any residual rubber cement.
3. Place slides into Wash solution 1 at 42°C and shake for 5 min. Repeat two times.
4. Repeat twice with Wash solution 2; after removing the last wash, let the slides cool for a few minutes before adding 2X SSC.

3.4. Immunodetection

The following **steps 1**, **2**, and **3** are only necessary in interphase FISH testing, when using a combination of FISH probes including one that is labeled with biotin and being detected with Avidin-Cy5. For all other probes, begin at **step 4** (*see* **Note 2**). The following procedures must be performed in the dark because the detection process is light sensitive.

1. Remove slides from 2X SSC and blot excess liquid from edges without allowing slides to dry out. Apply 40 μL of blocking solution (0.5% BSA) to each slide and cover with a plastic cover slip.
2. Incubate at 37°C for 30 min in a dark, humidified chamber.
3. Remove cover slips and rinse slides in Wash solution 3 at 40°C with shaking for 5 min. Transfer slides to a Coplin jar containing fresh 2X SSC at room temperature.
4. Each slide requires 20 μL each of anti-digoxingenin and avidin, and Alexa Fluor 488, premixed.
5. Take one slide at a time out of the SSC, drain by shaking, blot the back of slide, but do not allow the slide to dry out.
6. Add detection solution to each slide, drop a plastic cover slip over the slide, and remove any air bubbles.
7. Place slides in moist, dark chamber and incubate at 37°C for 30–60 min. Be very careful not to let the slides dry out.
8. Remove the plastic cover slip and put slides in a Coplin jar with Wash solution 3 preheated to 40°C. Place the Coplin jar containing the slides on a shaker for 5 min. Repeat twice.

3.5. Chromosome Counterstaining and DAPI Banding

Successful FISH mapping of DNA probes requires identification of both the specific chromosome as well as the banding localization. In our laboratory, we use DAPI banding as a routine method of staining when analyzing the relational mapping of two or more probes.

1. After the last wash, drain the slides and place them in DAPI solution for 5 min.
2. Drain the slides and place them back into jar of 2X SSC to prevent drying.
3. One slide at a time, drain briefly, add 15 μL of Antifade solution to the area, and place a cover slip on the slide.

Slides are now ready for viewing and can be stored in the dark at –20°C to preserve the signal.

3.6. Image Capture and Analysis

3.6.1. Microscopy

The images of the DAPI-stained chromosomes and hybridized, fluorescently labeled probes are captured on an epifluorescence microscope (e.g., Zeiss, Leitz, Nikon, or Olympus). The microscope should be equipped with a high-intensity mercury arc lamp source and objectives that include lenses of high numerical aperture and low self-fluorescing, UV-transmitting light. For scanning metaphases and interphase nuclei, dry objective magnifications of ×10 and ×20 are appropriate. The visualization and localization of fluorescent probe signals requires oil objectives of ×63 and ×100 (*see* **Note 3**).

3.6.2. Image Capture

The filter sets chosen for viewing fluorescent signals and counterstained chromosomes will depend on which fluorochromes are used and the type of mapping being performed. A narrow bandpass filter can be used for viewing a single fluorochrome, but the detection of multiple fluorochromes simultaneously requires a wide bandpass filter. The use of such filters (from Chroma or Omega Optical) often results in a loss of signal intensity, necessitating the use of a high-resolution cooled-charged couple device camera. These cameras capture each fluorescent signal in grayscale and the individual fluorochrome images are then transferred to an image analysis software program, such as Adobe Photoshop, for the addition of color and merging of the signals.

Registration is critical when capturing images using two or more different filters. Even slight changes in registration when switching between filters can potentially result in error in signal localization. Automatic computer-controlled filter wheels and software packages that enable the capture of real-time images are now available and can minimize this problem.

3.6.3. Analysis

3.6.3.1. DELETION DETECTION

For the detection of deletions of the WBS region on metaphase chromosomes, it is advisable to score at least 20 nuclei in which the signals on both chromosome 7 copies are clear.

3.6.3.2. INVERSION DETECTION

For three-color inversion testing, it is necessary to score a larger number of interphase nuclei because of the three-dimensional nature of the molecules being viewed in the cell. Only chromosomes in which the three probe signals are clearly visible and are aligned in a linear orientation with respect to each other should be scored. At least 50 to 60 chromosomes are needed to reliably determine whether an inversion of the WBS region is present. It is also advisable to have the scoring performed independently by two people to remove any bias regarding the interpretation of the probe order.

The large number of chromosomes scored is necessary because an altered order of probes will be seen on some chromosomes, even if an inversion is not present. This is because of the orientation of the chromosomal DNA on the slide not corresponding to its actual orientation in the genome.

When scoring the interphase nuclei, we report the number of chromosomes with the following probe order (*see* **Fig. 2**):

> Expected: CTA-208H19 to RP5-1186P10 to CTB-139P11
> Inversion-1: RP5-1186P10 to CTA-208H19 to CTB-139P11 (first described in **ref. 10**)
> Inversion-2: CTA-208H19 to CTB-139P11 to RP5-1186P10 (first described in **ref. 11**)

When an inversion is truly present on one chromosome 7, approx 50% of chromosome 7s will be scored as such, with 50% being scored as normal. The occurrence of less than 20% of chromosomes scored as Inv-1 or Inv-2 is considered within normal experimental variation.

4. Notes

1. The three probes used for interphase inversion testing may be labeled individually in two ways:
   Red signal: labeled with digoxigenin, detected with anti-digoxigenin–rhodamine

Green signal: labeled with biotin, detected with avidin, Alexa Fluor 488
Yellow signal: probe labeled with digoxigenin and biotin separately and mixed
or,
Red signal: labeled with digoxigenin, detected with anti-digoxigenin–rhodamine
Green signal: labeled with Spectrum Green
Yellow signal: labeled with biotin, detected with avidin–Cy5
2. When using a combination that includes a probe directly labeled with Spectrum Green, the additional steps are needed to block nonspecific hybridization of Avidin–Cy5 and prevent generation of a high background signal.
3. The oil used for high-power objectives should be nonfluorescing.

References

1. Ewart, A. K., Morris, C. A., Atkinson, D., et al. (1993) Hemizygosity at the elastin locus in a developmental disorder, Williams syndrome. *Nat. Genet.* **5,** 11–16.
2. Peoples, R., Franke, Y., Wang, Y. K., et al. (2000) A physical map, including a BAC/PAC clone contig, of the Williams-Beuren syndrome—deletion region at 7q11.23. *Am. J. Hum. Genet.* **66,** 47–68.
3. Greenberg, F. (1990) Williams syndrome professional symposium. *Am. J. Med. Genet.* **37,** 85–88.
4. Stromme, P., Bjornstad, P. G., and Ramstad, K. (2002) Prevalence estimation of Williams syndrome. *J. Child Neurol.* **17,** 269–271.
5. Morris, C. A., Thomas, I. T., and Greenberg, F. (1993) Williams syndrome: autosomal dominant inheritance. *Am. J. Med. Genet.* **47,** 478–481.
6. Morris, C. A., Demsey, S. A., Leonard, C. O., Dilts, C., and Blackburn, B. L. (1988) Natural history of Williams syndrome: physical characteristics. *J. Pediatr.* **113,** 318–326.
7. Pober, B. R. and Dykens, E. M. (1996) Williams syndrome: an overview of medical, cognitive, and behavioral features. *Child Adolesc. Psych. Clinics N. Am.* **5,** 929–943.
8. Frangiskakis, J. M., Ewart, A. K., Morris, C. A., et al. (1996) LIM-kinase 1 hemizygosity implicated in impaired visuospatial constructive cognition. *Cell* **86,** 59–69.
9. Tassabehji, M., Metcalfe, K., Karmiloff-Smith, A., et al. (1999) Williams syndrome: use of chromosomal microdeletions as a tool to dissect cognitive and physical phenotypes. *Am. J. Hum. Genet.* **64,** 118–125.
10. Osborne, L. R., Li, M., Pober, B., et al. (2001) A 1.5 million-base pair inversion polymorphism in families with Williams–Beuren syndrome. *Nat. Genet.* **29,** 321–325.
11. Scherer, S. W., Cheung, J., MacDonald, J. R., et al. (2003) Human chromosome 7: DNA sequence and biology. *Science* **300,** 767–772.

8

Congenital Heart Disease

Molecular Diagnostics of Supravalvular Aortic Stenosis

May Tassabehji and Zsolt Urban

Summary

Supravalvular aortic stenosis (SVAS) is a congenital heart disease that can occur as an iso-lated autosomal-dominant condition or as part of the developmental disorder Williams–Beuren syndrome (WBS) and is caused by heterozygous genetic lesions involving the *elastin* (*ELN*) gene locus on chromosome 7q11.23. SVAS is one of many phenotypic features associated with the contiguous gene microdeletion disorder, WBS, and is caused by deletion of the *ELN* locus on one chromosome 7 homolog. Point mutations, chromosomal deletions, and translocation involving *ELN* have also been described in individuals with nonsyndromic SVAS. In addition, *ELN* is involved in the connective tissue disorder, autosomal-dominant cutis laxa, and has been implicated as a susceptibility gene for hypertension and intracranial aneurysms. The molecular analysis of *ELN* defects is, therefore, an area of significant interest. Genetic screening can be achieved using a variety of techniques to detect both mutations and gross chromosome rear-rangements involving the *ELN* locus, providing the ability to screen families and individuals with SVAS and associated elastinopathies.

Key Words: Supravalvular aortic stenosis (SVAS); autosomal-dominant cutis laxa (ADCL); elastin; chromosome 7; mutation; deletion.

1. Introduction

The characteristic elastic properties of many tissues are caused by the pres-ence of the protein ELN. Tissues rich in ELN include major arteries (28–32% dry weight), aorta (50%), lungs (3–7%), elastic ligaments (50%), tendons (4%), and skin (2–3%). ELN itself is a major component (~90%) of elastic fibers, which endow connective tissues with the critical properties of elasticity and resilience, and complement collagen fibrils, which provide tensile strength *(1)*. Smooth muscle cells, endothelial cells, fibroblasts, and chondrocytes all syn-thesize ELN. ELN (initially synthesized as a 72-kDa soluble monomer,

From: *Methods in Molecular Medicine, vol. 126: Congenital Heart Disease: Molecular Diagnostics*
Edited by: M. Kearns-Jonker © Humana Press Inc., Totowa, NJ

tropoelastin [TE]) is a very hydrophobic protein and has a characteristic primary structure of alternating hydrophobic and crosslinking domains. The hydrophobic domains are thought to be responsible for the resilience of the protein. After secretion, individual TE molecules are covalently crosslinked by the enzyme, lysyl oxidase, to form an insoluble network of elastic fibers. ELN is synthesized mainly during development, and has an extremely slow turnover (half-life approaching the age of the organism), so little remodeling of elastic fibers occurs during adult life. The human *ELN* (NM_000501) maps to chromosome 7q11.2. Comparative studies show that *ELN* has 34 exons compared with the bovine *eln*, and that human exon 34 is homologous to bovine exon 36 *(2,3)*. Functionally distinct hydrophobic and crosslinking domains of the protein are encoded in separate alternating exons in the gene (**Fig. 1**). The exon-to-intron ratio is unusually large (20:1) and the introns contain large amounts of repetitive sequences that seem to predispose this region to genetic instability. Molecular defects in *ELN* have been described in two conditions: supravalvular aortic stenosis (SVAS) and autosomal-dominant cutis laxa (ADCL).

1.1. Elastinopathies

SVAS (MIM 185500) is a congenital narrowing of the ascending aorta that is frequently progressive and can lead to heart failure and death if not treated early, therefore patients often need corrective surgery in early infancy *(4)* (**Fig. 2**). SVAS can occur sporadically, as a familial condition with autosomal-dominant inheritance *(5)* or as a component of Williams–Beuren syndrome (WBS) *(4)*. The expression of SVAS is highly variable, both in familial SVAS and among patients with WBS. This chapter focuses on isolated or nonsyndromic SVAS. SVAS is caused by point mutations *(3,6–11)* or gross chromosomal abnormalities (large deletions or translocations) involving *ELN (12–15)* that abolish the function of one copy of the gene. It seems that most, if not all, SVAS mutations described result in functional haploinsufficiency for ELN *(8–11)*. Affected individuals, therefore, express only 50% of the normal amount of TE during development, which results in reduced arterial ELN content and, consequently, abnormally increased proliferation of vascular smooth muscle cells *(11)*. This manifests as the characteristic marked media thickening in great arteries seen in SVAS patients.

ADCL (MIM 123700) is a connective tissue disorder characterized by lax inelastic skin and other internal organ involvement (often hernias) *(15)*. The skin of ADCL patients tends to hang in loose folds, giving an appearance of premature aging. *ELN* mutations associated with ADCL are generally single nucleotide deletions near the end of the gene that result in in-frame frameshifts, predicted to replace the C-terminal amino acids with novel ones *(16–*

Elastin gene on human chromosome 7q11.23 ~ 40.52 Kb

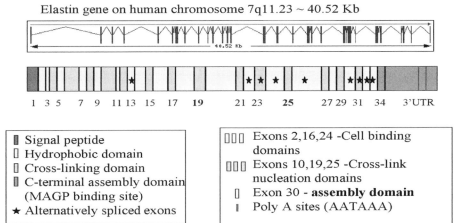

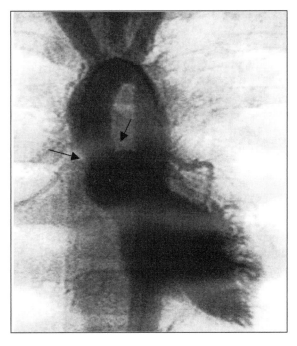

Fig. 1. *ELN* structure and functional domains. MAGP, microfibril-associated glycoprotein.

Fig. 2. Angiogram of a patient with SVAS. Note the typical hourglass-shaped narrowing of the ascending aorta.

18). However, recently, a partial tandem duplication in *ELN* was also described to cause ADCL *(19)*. Unlike SVAS, in ADCL, mutant TE protein is produced that is thought to alter the architecture of elastic fibers, resulting in a different pathomechanism to SVAS *(16,19)*.

In addition to its involvement in SVAS and ADCL, *ELN* has been suggested to be a susceptibility gene for hypertension and intracranial aneurysms *(20)*. Thus, mutational molecular analysis of *ELN* defects has become an area of significant interest.

1.2. Genetic Lesions Involving ELN

Previous studies have described the point mutations in *ELN* that cause nonsyndromic (isolated) SVAS or ADCL. In most cases, unrelated families have different molecular defects. More than 50 different *ELN* mutations have been described in patients with SVAS, and 5 *ELN* mutations have been described in patients with ADCL *(16–19)*. Most mutations (>85%) are truncating, caused by nonsense or frameshift mutations (which result in premature stop codons) or by splicing mutations, both at the consensus acceptor and donor splice junctions as well as in introns, which lead to truncated protein because of aberrant splicing. Missense mutations are not common (~10% of cases) and their contribution to the SVAS pathology is yet to be comprehensively defined *(7,10)*. The defect in *ELN* generally seems to be quantitative, with insufficient levels of ELN being produced. In fact truncating mutations in *ELN*, caused by mutations that introduce premature termination codons, have been shown to result in haploinsufficiency for ELN as a consequence of nonsense-mediated decay (a cell surveillance mechanism in place to ensure that only error-free messenger RNAs [mRNAs] are accurately translated) of the mutant mRNA *(9–11)*. This confirms that functional haploinsufficiency is the most likely pathological mechanism underlying SVAS.

Recurrent mutations have been described in *ELN*, some of which include the truncating Y150X (exon 9), Q442X (exon 21), and K176X (exon 10) mutations and splice mutations at the acceptor splice junction of exon 16. However, given that most families have unique *ELN* defects, screening for known mutations or hot spots is unlikely to be an efficient approach for molecular diagnosis. When screening for mutations, it is important to be aware that common intragenic polymorphisms exist in the *ELN* gene. Those described within or near exons include:

1. 196+71G>A in intron 4 (allele frequencies: G, 0.96; A, 0.04).
2. 233–94G>A in intron 5 (G, 0.92; A, 0.08).
3. 326–59G>A in intron 6 (G, 0.93; A, 0.07).
4. 1264G>A in exon 20, giving the expressed polymorphism of G442S (G, 0.62; A, 0.38).

5. 1315+17T>C in intron 20 (T, 0.80; C, 0.20).
6. 1501–24T>C in intron 23 (T, 0.64; C, 0.36).
7. 1828G>C in exon 26, giving the expressed polymorphism G610R (G, 0.93; C, 0.07).
8. 2273–34C>T in intron 32 (C, 0.73; T, 0.27).
9. *502_*503insA in the 3'-untranslated region (A–, 0.76; A+, 0.24).
10. *659G>C in the 3'-untranslated region (G, 0.61; C, 0.39).

This chapter proposes a flow chart for the molecular analysis of suspected ELN-related pathologies (**Fig. 1** in Chapter 7 on WBS) and discusses methods for the discovery and analysis of point mutations and single nucleotide polymorphisms (SNPs) and for detecting large deletions and rearrangements involving the *ELN* locus. Finally, methods for indirect analysis of inherited *ELN* defects are discussed.

2. Materials

2.1. Polymerase Chain Reaction

1. Vortex mixer.
2. Bench-top centrifuge.
3. Thermal-cycling machine.
4. Agarose gel electrophoresis equipment (horizontal electrophoresis tank and power pack, gel tray, and combs).
5. Short-wavelength UV transilluminator (254–300 nm).
6. 0.5-mL thin-walled eppendorf tubes or 96-well polymerase chain reaction (PCR) plates.
7. Sterile deionized water (dH$_2$O).
8. dNTPs (20 mM stock; the final concentration of each dNTP [dATP, dCTP, dGTP, and dTTP] is 5 mM). Add 25 µL of each 100-mM stock dNTP to 400 µL of dH$_2$0 to make 20 mM stock. Store at –20°C.
9. Taq DNA polymerase and 10X PCR buffer (provided by manufacturer). For increased specificity, use Ampli*taq* gold™ DNA polymerase (PerkinElmer LAS, UK, cat. no. N808-0145) with the 10X PCR buffer supplied with the Taq polymerase (100 mM Tris-HCl, pH 8.3, 500 mM KCl, and 0.01% w/v gelatin) for "hot-start" specificity.
10. Oligonucleotides resuspended with sterile water to 5 µM stocks.
11. 25 mM MgCl$_2$.
12. Target DNA: 50–100 ng of total genomic DNA.
13. 10X TBE electrophoresis buffer: 108 g Tris-base, 55 g boric acid, and 20 mL of 0.5 M EDTA, distilled water to a final volume of 1 L).
14. Molecular weight marker (1-kb ladder).
15. High-quality mineral oil.
16. Ethidium bromide.
17. 5X gel-loading buffer: 1X TBE containing 20% glycerol and 0.1 g of bromophenol blue tracking dye.
18. Molecular biology-grade agarose solid.

2.2. Single-Strand Conformation Polymorphism/Heteroduplex Analysis

1. Vertical polyacrylamide gel electrophoresis (PAGE) and gel casting apparatus (e.g., Gibco-BRL SA32 gel system with a metal cooling plate).
2. 1-mm gel spacers.
3. Heating block.
4. Acrylamide plus methylene *bis*-acrylamide at a 49:1 ratio (Sigma–Aldrich Company, Dorset, UK, cat. no. A-0924). A 40% stock solution mixture is made using deionized water and stored at 4°C.
5. TEMED.
6. 10% (w/v) ammonium persulphate solution.
7. 1X TBE electrophoresis buffer (dilute 10X stock TBE 1:9 with distilled water).
8. Formamide loading buffer: 10 mL of molecular biology-grade formamide; 200 µL of 0.5 M EDTA; 5–10 mg of xylene cyanol; and 5–10 mg of bromophenol blue.

2.3. Silver Staining of PAGE Gels

1. Gel shaker.
2. Hoefer SE 1200 Easy Breeze™ Air Gel Dryer (Amersham Biosciences).
3. Porous cellophane sheets.
4. Solution I: 10% (v/v) ethanol and 0.5% (v/v) acetic acid.
5. Solution II: 0.1% aqueous solution of silver nitrate ($AgNO_3$).
6. Solution III: aqueous solution of 1.5% (w/v) sodium hydroxide and 0.1% (v/v) formaldehyde (stock 37% [v/v]). This solution must be prepared immediately before use. Add 1.6 mL of 37% (v/v) formaldehyde stock solution to 400 mL of 1.5% (w/v) sodium hydroxide.
7. Solution IV: 0.75% (w/v) aqueous solution of sodium carbonate (Na_2CO_3).

Warning: Formaldehyde has high toxicity, is a severe irritant, and is a carcinogen.

2.4. Denaturing High-Performance Liquid Chromatography

All solutions and water used must be at least high-performance liquid chromatography (HPLC) grade.

1. WAVE denaturing HPLC (DHPLC) system (Transgenomic, Omaha, NE).
2. DNASep 4.8 mm × 50-mm cartridge.
3. Buffer A: 0.1 M triethylammonium acetate solution, pH 7.0.
4. Buffer B: 0.1 M triethylammonium acetate, 25% (v/v) acetonitrile, pH 7.0.
5. Syringe wash solution: 8% (v/v) acetonitrile, aqueous solution.
6. Solution D: 75% (v/v) acetonitrile, aqueous solution.

2.5. Cycle Sequencing

1. Thermal-cycling machine with a heated lid (e.g., PE Applied Biosystems [ABI], Warrington, UK; or GeneAmp PCR System 9700 thermal cycler).

2. ABI PRISM® 3100 Genetic Analyzer or ABI PRISM 377 automated DNA sequencer.
3. 0.2-mL thin-walled eppendorf tubes or 96-well plates.
4. Quickstep 2 kit (Edge BioSystems, Gaithersburg, MD, cat. no. 33617).
5. ABI PRISM BigDye Terminator Cycle Sequencing Kit v3.1.
6. Microspin G50 columns (Pharmacia Amersham, cat. no. 275330-01).
7. 3 *M* sodium acetate, pH 5.0.
8. Ethanol (100%).
9. Formamide sequencing loading buffer: five parts molecular biology-grade deionized formamide to one part 25 m*M* EDTA, pH 8.0; with 50 mg/mL blue dextran can be purchased from ABI (HiDi loading buffer, ABI, cat. no. 4311320).

2.6. Microsatellite Genotyping

1. Vertical PAGE gel electrophoresis apparatus.
2. Bench-top microcentrifuge.
3. Heating block (at 95°C).
4. Phenol plus chloroform (1:1).
5. Formamide loading buffer.
6. 40% (19:1) acrylamide:*bis*-acrylamide solution (Sigma-Aldrich, cat. no. A2917).
7. TEMED.
8. 10X TBE electrophoresis buffer.
9. Sucrose loading buffer: 4.0 g sucrose, 1.0 mL 10X TBE buffer, bring up to 10 mL with dH$_2$O. Heat to 68°C to dissolve the sucrose. Add 5 mg xylene cyanol and 5 mg bromophenol blue.
10. 10% (w/v) ammonium persulphate solution.
11. ABI PRISM 377 automated DNA sequencer (or automatic sampling on an ABI PRISM 3100 Genetic Analyzer).
12. Loading buffer: 12.0 μL formamide + 3.0 μL blue dextran (50 mg/mL in 25 m*M* EDTA) + 0.3 μL Genescan®-350 TAMRA marker.
13. HiDi loading buffer (ABI, cat. no. 4311320).

2.7. RNA Preparation

1. Bench-top microcentrifuge.
2. Sterile, disposable plasticware is required throughout.
3. Confluent cultured human fibroblast cell lines in 25- or 75-cm^2 flasks.
4. TRIzol® reagent (Invitrogen Life Technologies, Paisley, UK, cat. no. 15596-018).
5. 10 U/μL DNase I, RNase-free.
6. RNase-free water for resuspension of RNA pellets (e.g., Gibco Ultrapure, Invitrogen, cat. no. 10977-015).
7. Diethylpyrocarbonate (DEPC)-treated double-distilled water. Add 0.1% DEPC to double-distilled water. The mixture is strongly agitated and left to stand overnight in a fume cabinet before autoclaving to inactivate the DEPC before use.
8. Chloroform, analytical quality.

9. Phenol plus chloroform plus isoamyl alcohol, 25:24:1 (v/v), molecular biology grade.
10. Chloroform plus isoamyl alcohol, 24:1 (v/v), molecular biology grade.
11. Isopropyl alcohol, molecular biology grade.
12. Absolute ethanol, analytical grade.
13. 75% ethanol prepared with DEPC-treated water.
14. RNase-free Tris-EDTA buffer. Prepared either with commercially available RNase-free stock solutions of Tris-HCl and EDTA or with DEPC-treated stock solutions. However, because Tris-HCl contains an amino group that interacts with DEPC and makes it unavailable for RNase inactivation, it must be treated with 1% DEPC.
15. 200 mM Tris-HCl, pH 8.0 (1% DEPC-treated; *see* **Subheading 2.7., item 14**).
16. 25 mM MgCl$_2$.
17. 3 N NaCl prepared with DEPC-treated water.
18. DNase I, amplification grade, with buffer.

2.8. First-Strand Complementary DNA Synthesis and Reverse Transcriptase PCR

1. Thermal-cycling machine with a heated lid.
2. Oligo(dT)20.
3. Total RNA.
4. 25 mM MgCl$_2$.
5. 0.1 mM dithiothreitol.
6. 10 mM dNTP.
7. 200 U/μL SuperScript III reverse transcriptase (RT) and 10X RT buffer (Invitrogen).
8. 40 U/μL RNaseOUT Recombinant RNase Inhibitor (Invitrogen).
9. *Escherichia coli* RNase H (2 U/μL).
10. DEPC-treated water.
11. 10 μM control primers.
12. 200 mM Tris-HCl (pH 8.4), and 500 mM KCl.
13. Platinum® *Taq* DNA Polymerase (Invitrogen).

3. Methods

High-throughput low-cost technologies are often required to detect disease-causing SNPs and mutations. The large size of *ELN* requires a reliable method for the identification of disease-causing variants. Several different technologies can be used for *ELN* mutation screening and detection; in this chapter, we describe three technologies that are currently in use and discuss their advantages and limitations:

1. Single-strand conformation polymorphism (SSCP)/heteroduplex (HD) analysis.
2. DHPLC.
3. Direct sequencing.

SSCP/HD is a comparatively inexpensive and accessible technique. It is, however, time consuming, with limited throughput, and is less sensitive compared with other techniques. Alternatively, DHPLC or direct-sequence analysis are sensitive and high-throughput techniques for the detection of point mutations and SNPs in genes. Although direct DNA sequencing is potentially both a high-throughput and a sensitive method, limitations include the relatively high cost of screening a large gene such as *ELN*, and the necessity of reviewing sequence chromatograms to avoid missing putative sequence changes. In addition, detection of mosaics (the presence of two populations of cells with different genotypes in one patient, in which usually one of the two is affected by a genetic disorder, resulting from a mutation during development that is propagated to only a subset of the adult cells) is difficult. In contrast, DHPLC provides a sensitive, rapid, and low-cost method for the analysis of sequence variants. The presence of HDs can be readily recognized by quick visual inspection of the chromatograms. Disadvantages of DHPLC are that the presence of a common SNP in the same DNA fragment may obscure the detection of a gene defect and the expense of the equipment required.

Therefore, each technique has advantages and disadvantages, but by using combinations of these techniques more than 95% mutation detection can be achieved.

3.1. SSCP/HD Analysis

The combined SSCP/HD analysis technique is widely used for mutation detection (schematic depicted in **Fig. 3A**). SSCP is based on the principle that the electrophoretic mobility of nucleic acids in a nondenaturing gel depends on both shape and size. The secondary structure conformation adopted by single-stranded DNA is flexible, unlike double-stranded DNA, and is determined by intramolecular interactions and base stacking, which depends on sequence composition. The secondary structure of single-stranded DNA can, therefore, be altered by a single nucleotide base change resulting in measurable differences in electrophoretic mobility under nondenaturing conditions. HDs are formed when a mixture of wild-type and mutant double-stranded DNA molecules are denatured by heating followed by slow reannealing. HD DNA exhibits distinct slower electrophoretic mobility compared with the corresponding homoduplex, because a double-stranded configuration that is more open is adopted surrounding the mismatched bases. The position and the type of nucleotide mismatch determine the conformation of HD. Although SSCP is largely empirical (no theory is available for predicting the dependence of conformation on sequence, and of mobility on conformation), in combination with HD mutation screening, SSCP provides a more efficient mutation-screening method, with detection rates of up to 90% and detection sensitivity limits of approx 1 mutant cell in the presence of 10 normal cells.

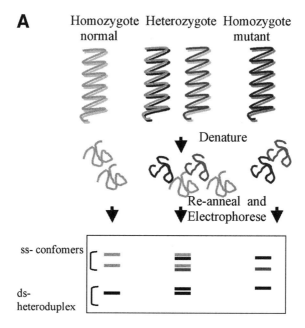

Fig. 3. SSCP/HD *ELN* mutation screening technique. **(A)** Schematic of the SSCP/ HD technique. ss, single strand; ds, double strand.

For SSCP/HD, the protocol involves:

1. Amplifying the target sequence from genomic DNA by PCR.
2. Denaturing the amplicon to single-stranded DNA and performing electrophoresis on a nondenaturing polyacrylamide gel.

Bands of the single-stranded DNA migrating in the gel at positions different from the wild type indicate the presence of a mutation (*see* **Fig. 3B**). The sensitivity of PCR SSCP tends to decrease as the fragment length increases. For fragments of approx 200 bp, more than 90% of single base changes can be detected; whereas for fragments of 400 bp, the detection rate is lowered to 80%. Sequences larger than 350 bp can be divided into shorter segments by generating overlapping fragments or digesting the amplicon (if suitable restriction sites reside within it) before analysis. HDs will form during PCR if the DNA has two different alleles that result in a mixed population of wild-type and mutant DNA. After denaturation and reannealing (by heating and cooling), four distinct species can form in nondenaturing polyacrylamide gels: wild-type homoduplex, mutant homoduplex, and two HDs. The formation and stability of the HDs depends on the type of mutation in the fragment; for example, deletions and insertions create relatively stable heteroplexes, whereas single base missense changes are less stable because of their sensitivity to temperature,

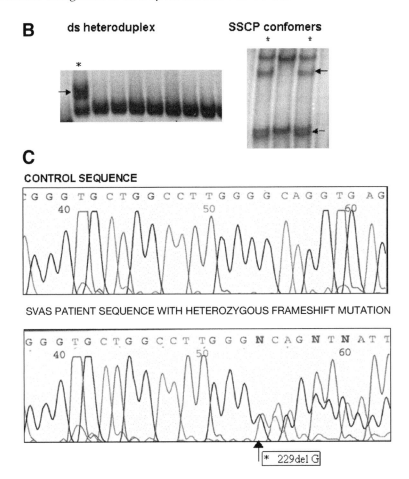

Fig. 3. *(continued)* SSCP/HD *ELN* mutation screening technique. **(B)** Examples of mutations which result in HD formation and abnormal ss conformers using SSCP/HD screening (* indicates SVAS patients with *ELN* gene mutations). **(C)** Sequence trace showing the sequence frameshift that occurs in an SVAS patient with a heterozygous deletion of 1 bp in exon 5 (229delG).

solvents, and ionic strength of the buffer; therefore, electrophoresis conditions must be optimized to detect all changes.

This combined SSCP/HD technique represents a simple but efficient method for point mutation analysis and can detect missense, frameshift, nonsense, and splice-site mutations *(3,6,8–10,16)*.

3.1.1. PCR Amplification of ELN Gene Exons

Exons comprising *ELN* are amplified from human genomic DNA using PCR. The primers used to amplify the *ELN* exons and the PCR amplification annealing conditions are summarized in **Table 1**.

1. Prepare a 10X stock of the oligonucleotides at a concentration of 5 μ*M*, using the following equation to calculate oligonucleotide stock concentrations:

$$\mu M \text{ (pmoles/}\mu\text{L)} = \frac{OD^{260nm} \times 100}{N}$$

   OD^{260nm} = optical density at 260 nm of the undiluted primer stock; N = number of bases in the oligonucleotide.
2. For each 10 μL PCR reaction add:
   a. 1 μL 10X PCR buffer: 166 m*M* ammonium sulphate; 670 m*M* Tris-HCl (pH 8.0 at 25°C); 37 m*M* magnesium chloride; 67 μ*M* EDTA; and 0.85 mg/mL bovine serum albumin (PCR buffers are provided with the Taq polymerase supplied by manufacturers and have different formulae).
   b. 1.5 μL of 20-m*M* dNTP stock (5 m*M* of each dATP, dCTP, dTTP, and dGTP).
   c. 1 μL of 5-μ*M* forward primer.
   d. 1 μL of 5-μ*M* reverse primer.
   e. 5.4 μL distilled sterile water.
   f. 0.1 μL of 5-U/μL Taq polymerase.
   g. 1 μL of 50-ng/μL genomic DNA (50–100 ng genomic template).
3. If using a thermal-cycling machine without a heated lid, add a drop of mineral oil to avoid evaporation. The melting temperature (T_m) of a specific oligonucleotide primer can be calculated using the formula: $T_m = 2(A + T) + 4(G + C)$, where A, C, G, and T are the nucleotides in the primer (formula developed for hybridization assays with oligonucleotides at a salt concentration of 1 *M*) *(21)*. Usually, the chosen annealing temperature is calculated as $T_m -5°C$. The parameters for thermal cycling, including annealing temperatures, have been determined empirically for each pair of *ELN* oligonucleotide primers (summarized in **Tables 1** and **2**).
   Cycling parameters: initial denaturation: 94°C for 3 min; followed by 30 cycles of:
   a. Denaturation: 94°C for 1 min.
   b. Annealing: annealing temperature for 1 min.
   c. Extension: 72°C for 1 min.
   d. Final extension: 72°C for 5 min.
4. Monitor 2 μL of the amplified PCR products by electrophoresis on ethidium bromide-stained agarose gels (1% w/v containing 0.5 μg/mL of ethidium bromide) in 1X TBE buffer. Alternatively, the gel can be stained after electrophoresis by soaking for 30 min in a dilute solution of ethidium bromide (0.5 μg/mL in 1X TBE) and visualized on a short-wavelength UV transilluminator.

3.1.2. SSCP/HD Electrophoresis

Samples for combined SSCP/HD analysis can be unprocessed PCR products ranging from 100 to 400 bp in size. It is important that the PCR product is clear of nonspecific artifacts before mutation screening to avoid interference with the assay. SSCP/HD analysis is performed by upright PAGE in a cold room

Table 1
Primer Sequences for the *ELN* Gene for Mutation Screening and Microsatellite Markers for Genotyping[a]

ELN exons	Forward PCR primer 5' to 3'	Reverse PCR primer 5' to 3'	PCR amplicon size (bp)	Anneal temperature (°C)
1	CAGCCGACGAGGCAACAATTAGGC	TGAGCGTCTAGTCACCTGGCCCA	228	60
2	TCCATGTAATTGTGGGTTTTGCC	CAATGTTCCTACCTTCTGTAGTG	261	60
3	CTTGCCCAAGGTCACGTAGTTAG	ATGAGGGAGTCCTTGATGCTCGG	259	60
4	GGTTGGATAAGTAGTAGATGGAT	AGGCTAATCGGTGTCCACACCTC	249	60
5	TCCAGGAGACATTTCCCACTCTG	GGCAGTTGGTATCAGCATCAGTC	255	60
6	AGGCAGGGCCAGAGCGTAGGAGT	AAGCCTGAGTTGAGGGAAGGTTC	254	60
7–8	TACGCAATGCCTCACCTGTCCTG	TGCCCTCTGTCCTCCAGCCCCAG	255	60
9	CTGCCTGGGTGGGAAGGGCTG	GGCCTTACTATGATGCCCAGGCT	273	65
10	GTTCCCAGCAGGGCCTGCAAGGC	GGCCCTGAGCCAGTCCAGGATCC	231	65
11	CGCAGCATGCGATGACTGGTCTG	GGAGAAATTGGGCAGGCTTGGAT	258	60
12	GAGATTCAGGGAGTCCCTCGAAG	CACCCGGCCGAGTGGTGCATCTT	255	60
13	TGGTGGGAGCCCAGCAAGGCATG	AGATTCCCACTCCAAGACCCCAA	235	60
14	AGTGTGATGTCTGCACAGATGAC	ACCAGGGTCTGGATGCAGGGTG	227	65
15	CTGAAGCTCCCATGTATACCCAC	GTCAATAGTAATGGGAATGGAG	245	60
16–17	CGTCTAAGTGGCCATCCTGCCTG	TTGCGGCTAGGGTCTCCGAGGTC	378	65
18	ATACTCTACTAACCACCCTTCTA	TGGCAATAGTCTCAATATTTCTC	300	60
19	GCATGAAAGGAGATGGCCCAAC	TTTAGTTCTGGCAAGTAAAGGC	223	60
20	CTCTTTCCCAATCCATCAGCATC	CCCATCCCTTCTCAACCCATGTC	297	60
21	GAGGTCGTATCCATGCCTTACAG	TCCAGGCCATTTCAGTCCTGGAG	253	60
22	AAAGTGAGTACTGGGAGGGGCAA	CGACCTTGGTCAACTCCAGGGAC	208	65
23	GTCCCTGGAGTTGACCAAGGTCG	CCCAGAATGTGACAGCTTAAGTG	300	60
24	AGCTTCTGTCCTCTTTGATCAGG	GGGCCCCTCAGGCTCATTGACTC	254	60
25	TGGCTCCCGGCATTGGCCCTGGTG	CCTGGCTGTTGCCCCTAACCAGC	239	60
26	GGCATGCTCCCTGCCTGCTGTCG	CCCAGATGCTTAGGAGAACCTAA	313	60
27	CAGCTTCAGGGCTTTGAGGAAGC	GTGACCACCCCAGTCCTGTGCTG	242	65
28–29	AACACTCATTTTCCCTCCTCTCC	GCCTGGGGGCCTGGCGGCAGCTC	290	60
30	CCATCGAAGGCCAGGGGAGACC	CCATCTCTGTCTCGCATACACAC	261	60
31	GGTGGCATTGGCATTCCTGAGCCG	GTTAAGGAATGTCCCAGACAAGAT	220	65
32	TTCCTTAACCCAGAACCCAGCAG	CCTTGTGTGGACATGGGCTCTGG	242	60
33	CCAGACAGAGGTCTTGGGTGAGC	CCCTTCTGAGCAGGAGATGGCAC	233	60
34	CTTCTTGGAGCCTCCATTCGAG	TTCTCCACCAAGCAGTAGCACC	244	55

Microsatellite markers

| *ELN*i1 | GCCCACATGGGCAGATTGCT | CCCTCATCCACAGACAGGTC | 254–286 | 60 |
| *ELN* Helg18/19 | ATGAGACGTGGTCAAGGGTAT | GGGATCCCAGGTGCTGCGGTT | 161–175 | 60 |

(continued)

Table 1 *(continued)*

ELN exons	Forward PCR primer 5' to 3'	Reverse PCR primer 5' to 3'	PCR amplicon size (bp)	Anneal temperature (°C)
*LIMK1*GT D7S613	TGGGGCAGGAGAATGATGTG	AGTCTTCTTTGCGGGCTATGTTA	180	60
G18333 D7S2472	CCTGAAGGTAGGTAGTTTAACC	CTGGGTTCAACCGATTCTCC	147	60
Z53057 D7S3195	TCTAAAGTCTGCCAGGCTAC	GCAGCGAGACTCCATC	83–103	55
G68161 D7S3196	TTGCAGGGCTGTGAGGATTAAC	TCTGGTCATAAATTGGAACTCCATAGA	405	60
G68162 D7S1870	AGGCTGTCTCTAAATAAATTCCGTCAA	TGTCCTCCCACAAGTCCGTAAA	225	60
Z51768 D7S2490	TTCACTCAGGAAGTGGC	TGGTGATGTGCTTTACTACG	108–132	60
Z53428 D7S2476	TGTAAGCCACCGCACCT	AGCACCCGGCATAGATGT	134–156	55
Z53107 D7S672	GGGCAACATAGCACGATT	CAGGAGTCAGTTAGATAAGGTCAC	128–160	60
Z24075	ACATGAAGGTCTACCAGTAGCC	CACTTTGGTTGGAGCAAGG	132–160	60
RT-PCR primers				
ELN 5'–3' ELN	CATTCCTGGTGGAGTTCCTG	TGGGAAAATGGGAGACAATC	2224	55–60
X18–21	GGGATCCCAGGTGCTGCGGTT	ACCGTACTTGGCAGCCTT	287	55
Γ-*ACTIN*	GCTCG TCGTCGACAACGGCTC	CAAACATGATCTGGGTCATCTTCTC	353	60

[a]Genbank accession numbers for the sequences are included.

(~4°C) to control temperature and the DNA bands are visualized using silver staining. Alternatively, temperature-controlled electrophoretic units run at 4°C can be used. Because the conformation adopted by single-stranded DNA is sensitive to a range of parameters (e.g., fragment length, gel matrix composition, ionic strength, and temperature) achieving high detection rates by SSCP/HD requires running gels under the conditions specified here for *ELN*.

1. An upright PAGE gel electrophoresis system that can accommodate glass plates approx 33.8 cm long is required for SSCP/HD analysis with 1-mm-thick spacers to aid gel handling for subsequent staining. The acrylamide used has a 49:1 ratio of acrylamide to crosslinking reagent (methylene *bis*-acrylamide). The percentage of the gel depends on the molecular weight of the sample product, for ex-

able 2
CR and Chromatography Conditions for DHPLC[a]

mplicon	Primer 1	Primer 2	Size	Temp	Oven	Buffer B
LNe01	CTCTTTCCCTCACAGCCGAC	GTCTAGTCACCTGCCAAAGGG	238	58	66.0°C	52%
LNe02	TTCTTGTTTCCATGTAATTGTGG	GGCGTGTCAATGTTCCTACC	268	56	60°C	53%
LNe03	CAAGGTCACGTAGTTAGGCA	GCCTCCTCCCACCGCCTGGA	286	60	62.4°C	54%
LNe04	GTGATTCCACACTGCCCACA	GTTGCCTTGTCCTGTTCCTA	241	54	61.1°C, 62.5°C	52%
LNe05	GATCGACCCTGAGCATCACA	GTCCCCGTCAGTGCCCAGGA	308	60	61.5°C, 63.0°C	54%
LNe06	GTCTGGCAGAGAGCGGAAGA	GGAGGGCCCCACGGAAGCCA	274	60	63.0°C, 64.0°C	53%
LNe07	GCTAGCTGTGCCCAGTCTGA	CTCCGGCTCCAGGCTGAGGA	298	60	63.5°C, 63.9°C	54%
LNe08	GCAAGGCTTGGTGGAGCCAA	CGCAGGCACCAGCCTGGCTA	249	60	63.5°C, 64.7°C	52%
LNe09	CTGCCCCTGTCGGGCACAGA	GCCTCAGTCTCCCAAAGCAA	262	60	62.5°C	53%
LNe10	GAGGGGAGGGGTTCCCAGCA	GGATCCCACCCCATTTCACA	224	58	63.7°C, 64.1°C	51%
LNe11	CCTTGGTGCTGTCTGGCCCA	GGGTGCCACTTTGTGCTACA	252	60	61.0°C, 61.8°C, 63.8°C	53%
LNe12	GAAGCAGGATGGTTTCTGGA	GAACCACCACACCCGGCCGA	245	63	62.4°C	52%
LNe13	CTTTAGCACCTGTGGGGGTA	CGAGGTGCTCTCCTGGCCCA	238	60	62.9°C	52%
LNe14	GGTGATGTCTGCACAGATGA	CTGGAGCCTGGAAGATCAGT	161	58	62.5°C, 63.5°C, 64.5°C	48%
LNe15	GAAGCTCCCATGTATACCCA	CTTTGGAGGCAGGCTGTCAA	258	58	62.5°C, 64.0°C	53%
LNe16	CCCAGACAGGCCCATCTGGA	GTGGCCATCTCAAGGACACA	280	58	62.6°C, 63.1°C	54%
LNe17	GTGTCCTTGAGATGGCCACA	CCCGAGCCGTGGACTTACCA	153	58	64.8°C, 65.2°C	47%
LNe18	CTCTGAGGTTCCCATAGGTT	CACACACACGCCCAGCTCA	215	60	59.2°C, 63.9°C	51%
LNe19	CCAACACACAGATGGGTAGA	GGCAAGTAAAGGCCAGGACA	197	63	60.7°C, 62.2°C	50%
LNe20	CTTTCCCAATCCATCAGCAT	CATCCCTTCTCAACCCATGT	293	60	direct sequencing[b]	
LNe21	CCTTACAGGCAGAAGAGCTT	CAGTTTGCCCTGAGGTTGGA	205	58	63.3°C, 64.6°C	50%
LNe22	CCATTCTCTTCTTCCTCCGA	CTCCAGGGACCCTTCCATGA	242	58	62.0°C, 65.3°C	52%
LNe23	GGAAGACTGAGCCTAGAGAT	CACAGGAGAAAGCAGTTCTC	188	60	62.0°C, 64.0°C	50%
LNe24	GCTTCTGTCCTCTTTGATCA	AGAGAGGGGGATTAGAGATG	298	54	59.0°C, 63.5°C, 64.4°C	54%
LNe25	CCCGCCTCCATCTCTAATC	AACCAGCTCTGAGATCGTTG	139	58	62.9°C, 64.6°C	46%
LNe26	TGCCTGCTGTCGCCACCACT	GCTTAGGAGAACCTAACAAG	295	62	63.8°C	54%
LNe27	CAATAGAGGCCAAGGAAGTC	CAAGGGAGCCACAAGTGGTT	179	60	62.5°C	49%
LNe28	GTCTGCTTGCCTTGTGTCC	GAACACAGACCGAGTTCAGG	180	56	61.6°C, 64.9°C	49%
LNe29	GGAGGGAATCTAACCAGTAC	GCAGGGACTCTGAGTCTACA	212	56	63.5°C, 65.5°C, 66.8°C	51%
LNe30	ACAGGCCGAGGCTTCAGTC	TCCATCTCTGTCTCGCATAC	199	56	61.0°C, 62.5°C, 64.0°C	50%
LNe31	CAGGTGGCATTGGCATTC	GTCCCAGACAAGATCTTCAG	212	56	62.6°C, 64.0°C	51%
LNe32	GAACCCAGCAGGGATATCA	CCCACTGCTAGATGGACA	202	60	62.0°C, 63.6°C	50%
LNe33	TGCAGGCAGAAAGTGATGAG	GCCCTTCTGAGCAGGAGAT	208	60	62.3°C, 63.2°C	51%
LNe36	GATTAGAGCCGAAACTGAG	TGCCCTGTGGATCTGCAAG	257	54	62.6°C	53%

[a]Temp, annealing temperature; Oven, DHPLC oven temperature; Buffer B, Buffer B mixing ratio with uffer A at the start of the elution gradient.

[b]Not screened by DHPLC because analysis of chromatograms is complicated by varying allelic combinations for common polymorphisms 1264G>A and 1315+17T>C.

ample: 500 bp, 7% (w/v); 300 bp, 7.75% (w/v); and 200 bp, 8% (w/v).

2. Prepare an 8% (w/v) nondenaturing PAGE gel that has been allowed to polymerize for at least 1 h:

   a. 15 mL of 40% (49:1) acrylamide:*bis*-acrylamide solution.
   b. 7.5 mL of 10X TBE.
   c. 62.5 μL TEMED.
   d. dH$_2$O to a final volume of 52 mL.
   e. Add 500 μL of freshly made 10% (w/v) ammonium persulphate solution.

3. Make up 1 L of electrophoresis buffer (1X TBE) and refrigerate at 4°C for at least 1 h before use.

4. Rinse unpolymerized acrylamide out of the PAGE gel wells, add cold electrophoresis buffer (1X TBE) to the buffer chambers and allow the gel to refrigerate in a cold room at 4°C for 2 h before loading.

5. Prepare the PCR samples (*ELN* amplicons) for loading by mixing with an equal volume of formamide loading buffer, then denature by heating at 94°C for 3 min and immediately snap-cool on ice. Load between 5 and 10 μL (depending on amplification efficiency). Some PCRs do not form HDs readily in formamide. If this is the case, preload the wells with 1–2 μL of the PCR sample before heat denaturation.

6. Electrophorese at 300 V constant voltage overnight (~16–18 h); the xylene cyanol dye front will have run a distance of approx 25 cm. Note that smaller PCR products may require a reduced electrophoresis voltage.

7. Remove the top glass plate from the PAGE gel and gently peel the gel off of the plate into a tray for visualization by silver staining (modified from **ref. 22**).

3.1.3. Silver Staining of DNA in PAGE Gels

1. Carefully transfer the polyacrylamide gel into a plastic tray. Fix the gel in 400 mL of solution I for 6 min, then add solution II and incubate for 15 min.

2. Decant off the solution, rinse the gel with distilled water, and add 400 mL of solution III and incubate for 20 min in a fume cabinet.

3. Pour off the solution and rinse the gel twice with distilled water, then fix with 400 mL of solution IV for 10 min.

4. The gel can be stored permanently by drying between two sheets of porous cellophane soaked in distilled water and locked into the drying frame (Easy Breeze gel drying system) to air-dry.

3.2. Denaturing High-Performance Liquid Chromatography

DHPLC detects mutations on the basis of mismatches between amplified DNA fragments that result in the formation of HDs. These are thermally less stable than their corresponding homoduplexes, and are resolved by means of ion-pair reversed-phase liquid chromatography at elevated column temperatures, typically in the range of 50 to 70°C, depending on the GC-content of the sequences. Temperature is the most important parameter that affects the sensitivity of DHPLC in detecting mutations.

1. PCR amplification of genomic amplimers is essentially conducted as described in **Subheading 3.1.**, using the oligonucleotide primers and annealing temperatures described in **Table 2**. The final volume of the PCR reactions is generally 25 µL (*see* **Note 1**). To facilitate the formation of HDs, the amplimers are denatured and slowly ramped to room temperature in 30 min. For the GeneAmp 9700 PCR machine (ABI), the following incubation regimen is used: 95°C, 3 min; 3% ramp to 37°C; 37°C, 20 min; 25°C, 20 min.
2. For all amplicons, the following DHPLC conditions are used:
   a. Percentage of buffer B for loading = indicated buffer B concentration (**Table 2**) – 5%.
   b. Loading volume = 8 µL; loading duration = 0.5 min.
   c. Gradient slope = 2%/min (starting at the indicated **Table 1** buffer B concentration).
   d. Gradient duration = 4.5 min.
   e. Clean duration = 0.5 min (with 100% buffer D).
   f. Percentage of buffer B for equilibration = indicated buffer B concentration (**Table 2**) – 5% (same as for loading).
   g. Equilibration duration = 0.9 min.
   Several amplimers contain more than one melting domain. Thus, for complete coverage of the amplimers, it is necessary to conduct DHPLC screening at multiple oven temperatures, as indicated in **Table 2**. An example of DHPLC conditions is shown in **Table 3**.
3. At the conclusion of the DHPLC, chromatograms are reviewed using the Navigator (Transgenomic, v1.5.3) software or equivalent, and compared with normal control chromatograms (**Fig. 4A**). Amplimers with altered chromatograms are further analyzed by direct DNA sequencing (**Fig. 4B**, **Subheading 3.3.**). Chromatograms are often allele specific and can be directly used for genotyping of known variants. This characteristic is particularly useful in investigating the occurrence of patient-derived variants in collections of normal control DNA.

3.3. Mutation Detection by Direct Sequencing

Mutations can be identified in PCR-amplified DNA fragments by direct sequencing using fluorescence-based cycle-sequencing technology (ABI BigDye Terminator v3.1 kit). Essentially, all of the exons are amplified from the patient's genomic DNA and sequenced in both the forward and reverse orientation, using the *ELN* PCR primers. A normal control individual is sequenced alongside the patient's DNA, so that the sequence traces can be compared for heterozygous mismatches. In addition, mutations detected by the mutation-screening techniques identified in **Subheadings 3.1.** and **3.2.** are

Table 3
**Example of DHPLC Running Conditions for Amplimer
hELN01**

	Time (min)	Buffer A (%)	Buffer B (%)	Buffer D (%)
Loading	0.0	53	47	0
Start gradient	0.5	48	52	0
Stop gradient	5.0	39	61	0
Start clean	5.1	0	0	100
Stop clean	5.6	0	0	100
Start equilibration	5.7	53	47	0
Stop equilibration	6.6	53	47	0

characterized by sequencing using this method. Generally, PCR reactions should be strong and specific, because nonspecific products in the PCR reaction (including primer–dimer) will be sequenced using this method and generate a high background interference.

1. Set up a 40-μL PCR reaction using primers specific to the region requiring sequencing from the patient DNA sample and a normal control sample.
2. Monitor 3 μL of the PCR-amplified product on a 1% ethidium bromide agarose gel to confirm successful amplification, then purify the PCR products before sequencing to remove primers and unincorporated dNTPs, using the Quickstep 2 kit or any other commercially available PCR clean-up kit.
3. The Quickstep 2 kit protocol involves briefly vortexing the poly(4-hydroxystyren) (SOPE) resin and adding one-fifth of the volume of the PCR reactions to be purified to the SOPE resin and vortexing to mix.
4. Centrifuge the Performa Gel Cartridges for 3 min at 750*g*, then add the PCR product onto the center of the column and centrifuge for 3 min at 750*g*. To determine the concentration of DNA recovered, 2 to 3 μL of the eluate is monitored, and can then be used directly in BigDye sequencing reactions.
5. Set up the BigDye terminator cycle sequencing reactions as follows:
   a. x μL of purified PCR reaction (~300–600 ng of product).
   b. 4 μL of BigDye terminator mix.
   c. 0.32 μL of 10-μ*M* sequencing primer.
   d. Milli-Q water to give a final volume of 10 μL.
6. Use the following cycling sequence conditions with a PE ABI GeneAmp PCR System 9700 thermal cycler. If you have a different thermal cycler, please consult ABI (www.appliedbiosystems.com) for the cycling conditions.
   a. 96°C, 1 min.
   b. 96°C, 10 s.
   c. 50°C, 20 s.

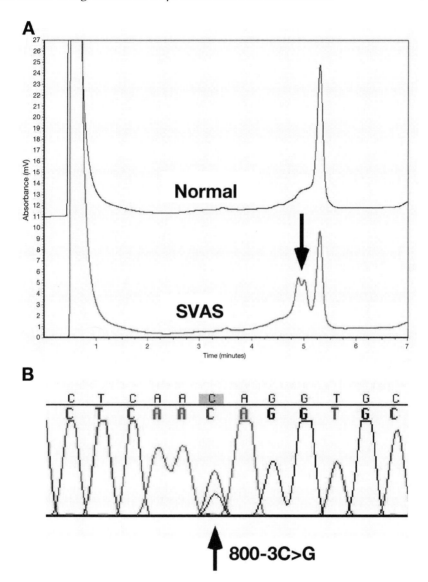

Fig. 4. Mutation detection using DHPLC. (**A**) Chromatogram of DHPLC analysis at 62.6°C of exon 16 amplicons obtained from a normal control and a SVAS patient. Arrow indicates HD peaks in the SVAS sample. (**B**) Sequence analysis confirmed the presence of a splice-site mutation (800–3C>G) in the same SVAS patient.

   d. 60°C, 4 min.
   e. 25 cycles or **step 6, b–d**.
   f. 4°C.
 7. Unincorporated dye-labeled terminators must be removed by Sephadex G-50 column purification (Micro-spin G50 columns) or by ethanol precipitation. Do not use ethanol precipitation to clean up samples that will be run on a sequencing apparatus that uses capillary electrophoresis columns (e.g., ABI PRISM 3100 Genetic Analyzer), because the high salt concentrations retained in the samples affect the output quality significantly.
 8. For G50 column purification: resuspend the Sephadex resin in the columns by gentle vortexing, then snap off the bottom closure. Prespin the columns for 1 min at 735*g* (4000 rpm for a MSE Micro Centaur microcentrifuge). Place the columns in a clean 1.5-mL tube and apply the sample to the center of the compacted resin bed. Spin the columns for 2 min at 735*g* (4000 rpm for a MSE Micro Centaur microcentrifuge). The purified samples are collected in the bottom of the support tube. Discard the columns and retain the flow-through samples.
 9. For ethanol precipitation, add 0.1 volume of 3 *M* sodium acetate and 2.5 volumes of cold (–20°C) ethanol to the sequence reaction. Leave at room temperature for 20 min and pellet by centrifugation at 13,000 rpm for 15 min. Remove the supernatant and wash the pellet by adding 150 µL of 70% ethanol. Centrifuge at 13,000 rpm for 5 min, discard the supernatant, and allow the pellet to air-dry for 5 min at room temperature.
10. Resuspend the pellet in 15 µL of formamide sequencing loading buffer (for the ABI PRISM 3100 Genetic Analyzer) or 0.8 µL formamide loading buffer (for ABI PRISM 377 automated DNA sequencer) by vortexing. Centrifuge samples briefly, then denature for 2 min at 95°C and immediately store on ice until ready to load (to avoid reannealing of the DNA). Load the samples (automatic sampling on a 96-well plate format for the ABI PRISM 3100 Genetic Analyzer and 0.4 µL for the ABI PRISM 377 automated DNA sequencer) and sequence on the appropriate sequencing platform using the conditions recommended by the manufacturer. Data is subsequently analyzed using the installed DNA Sequencing Analysis Software (*see* **Fig. 4B**).

3.4. Analysis of Partial Deletions and Translocations at the ELN *Locus*

   Some SVAS cases occur because of gross chromosome rearrangements, such as translocations or deletions, which involve *ELN* and can be detected by cytogenetic analysis through karyotyping (in the case of translocations) *(11)* and by fluorescent *in situ* hybridization (FISH) analysis (for microdeletions at the *ELN* locus) *(6)*. The methodology for FISH analysis is described in Chapter 7, when applied to diagnose the microdeletion condition, WBS. For nonsyndromic SVAS cases with partial deletions in the region including *ELN*, the FISH probe cosmids 82c2 and 34b3 can be used to detect microdeletion using the protocols described in Chapter 7.

3.5. Indirect Methods of Molecular Diagnosis

3.5.1. Genotyping With Microsatellite Markers or SNPs

Microsatellites or dinucleotide repeat polymorphisms are short, tandemly repeated, consensus sequences that, because of their high allelic diversity, are popular and simple markers for molecular genotyping and linkage analysis. An informative dinucleotide (dG-dT)n repeat polymorphism resides in intron 18 (11 bases downstream of *ELN* exon 18) of the human *ELN* gene and consists of eight alleles with sizes ranging between 161 and 175 bp (Genbank accession number L01989) *(23)*. In addition, a highly polymorphic tetranucleotide repeat marker is located in intron 1 of ELN *(24)*. This microsatellite marker (alongside others, such as *LIMK1GT*, D7S1870, and others shown in **Fig. 2** of Chapter 7) can be used for determining the parental origin of a WBS deletion, and aids diagnosis when FISH analysis is not available. In addition, this microsatellite marker can be used in linkage analysis to track the mutant allele in autosomal-dominant SVAS families in which the mutations have not been defined, or to establish the *ELN* deletion status in sporadic SVAS patients with ELN deletions when FISH analysis is not possible because of lack of the appropriate samples or resources. The technique involves PCR amplification of DNA using oligonucleotide primers complementary to a region flanking the microsatellite locus, size fractionation of the amplified product on a nondenaturing polyacrylamide gel, and detection of DNA fragments either by silver staining of the gel or using a fluorescent detection system (if a fluorescent PCR primer is used). Typical molecular genotypes from SVAS and WBS families using the nonfluorescent technique are shown in **Fig. 5**.

3.5.2. Nonfluorescent ELN $(GT)_n$ Polymorphism Genotyping

1. All amplifications are carried out as described in **Subheading 3.1.1.**, apart from a reduction in the number of cycles to 27 cycles. Product sizes vary from 128 to 154 bp.
2. PCR products are purified by phenol extraction. An equal volume of buffer-saturated phenol plus chloroform (1:1) is added to the DNA solution, mixed by vortexing, then separating the phases by centrifugation at 12,000g for 5 min.
3. Carefully remove the aqueous (top) layer to a new tube, being careful to avoid the interface. Mix 4 µL with an equal volume of sucrose loading buffer and load onto an 8% polyacrylamide nondenaturing gel prepared using the following reagents (for a 16-cm gel):
   a. 5 mL of 40% (19:1) acrylamide:*bis*-acrylamide solution.
   b. 2.5 mL 10X TBE.
   c. 30 µL TEMED.
   d. Deionized H$_2$O to a final volume of 25 mL.
   e. Add 200 µL of freshly made 10% (w/v) ammonium persulphate solution.
   f. Allow to polymerize for 1 h at room temperature.

4. Electrophoresis is performed at 300 V constant voltage for 3 h (room temperature) on a vertical PAGE apparatus setup. The DNA bands are visualized by silver staining (**Subheading 3.1.3.**).

3.5.3. Fluorescent Nonfluorescent ELN (GT)$_n$ Polymorphism Genotyping

Fluorescent microsatellite analysis can also be preformed using primers that have been commercially fluorescently tagged at the 5'-end with 6-FAM, HEX, NED, or TET phosphoramidites. These should be stored in the dark at –20°C.

1. Make up the following PCR cocktail:
   a. Forward plus reverse primer mix (10 μM stocks)   2.0 μL
   b. 10X PCR buffer*:   2.0 μL
   c. 2 mM dNTP mix   2.0 μL
   d. 25 mM MgCl$_2$ 1.6 μL
   e. *Taq* polymerase (5 U/μL)   0.16 μL
   f. dH$_2$O   10.84 μL
   g. DNA (20–50 ng/μL)   2.0 μL
   h. Total   20.0 μL

   *100 mM Tris-HCL, pH 8.3; 500 mM KCl; and 0.01% w/v gelatin (Perkin-Elmer buffer). Ampli*taq* gold DNA polymerase. This enzyme confers a "hot-start" that improves the efficiency and specificity of PCR reactions.
2. Conditions for PCR amplification are: 94°C (4 min), then 30 cycles at (94°C, 30 s; 60°C, 45 s; 72°C, 45 s), and a final extension at 72°C for 10 min.
3. PCR amplimers are diluted 1:10, and 1 to 2 μL are added to 15.3 μL of standard or loading buffer (12.0 μL formamide + 3.0 μL blue dextran [50 mg/mL in 25 mM EDTA] + 0.3 μL Genescan-350 TAMRA) or HiDi loading buffer.
4. Denature samples at 96°C for 2 min, and place on ice. Load 0.4 to 0.8 μL of each sample mix on an ABI PRISM 377 automated DNA sequencer (or automatic sampling on an ABI PRISM 3100 Genetic Analyzer) using the Genetic Analyzer and Genescan software to analyze the alleles, according to the manufacturer's instructions.

3.5.4. Analysis of ELN Expression in Cultured Fibroblast Cells

RNA isolation and RT-PCR protocol:

1. To look for any mutations not detected using techniques given in **Subheadings 3.1.–3.4.** (e.g., intronic or whole exon deletions) that may affect the *ELN* mRNA transcript.
2. To examine the consequences of any intronic mutations detected residing outside of the consensus donor or acceptor splice junctions, or missense mutations that may affect normal splicing but do not have obvious pathological features *(10)*. Established skin fibroblast cultures from the affected and a normal control individual are required for RNA expression studies.

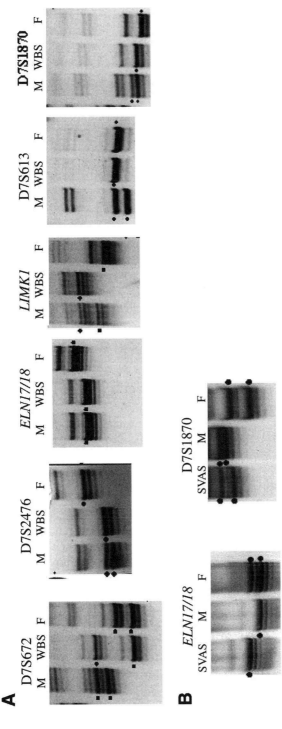

Fig. 5. Linkage analysis using polymorphic microsatellite repeats at 7q11.23. (**A**) WBS family. The WBS child shows monoallelic inheritance for all of the markers except for D7S672, which lies outside of the commonly deleted region in WBS. (**B**) An individual with sporadic SVAS showing a hemizygous deletion of the *ELN* but not the D7S1870 marker. M, mother; F, father. Alleles are highlighted with a black dot.

3.5.5. Total RNA Preparation

A number of procedures are available for preparation of total RNA from tissues or cultured cells. A reliable and simple method involves the use of a modified 14 *M* solution of guanidine salts and urea (Chaosolv) that act as denaturing agents. The isolated RNA should be treated with DNase I to remove genomic DNA contamination. This is a protocol for preparation of total RNA from cultured human fibroblast cell lines grown in 25- or 75-cm^2 flasks, which has been adapted from the TRIzol Reagent protocol. During RNA isolation and analysis, it is essential to maintain an RNase-free environment. All reagents, tubes, and pipets should be RNase free.

1. Aspirate culture medium from cells grown in monolayer that have reached 70 to 100% confluence, and wash cultures twice with sterile phosphate-buffered saline.
2. Add 1 mL TRIzol reagent per 10 cm^2 of cells (i.e., 1 mL for 1×10^6 cells), and lyse cells in TRIzol by pipetting up and down in a 21-gage needle and syringe until solid matter disappears, then incubate at room temperature for 5 min.
3. Transfer lysate to 1.5-mL polypropylene microcentrifuge tubes (maximum volume of 1 mL into a 1.5-mL tube).
4. Add 0.2 mL of chloroform per 1 mL of RNA reagent, shake vigorously for 15 s, then incubate at room temperature for 2 to 3 min.
5. Centrifuge the homogenate at 12,000g for 15 min at 4°C. The homogenate will form two phases: DNA and protein reside in the lower organic phase and in the interface, with RNA in the upper aqueous phase.
6. Transfer the colorless aqueous phase, which contains the RNA, to a fresh microcentrifuge tube. Only recover approx 95% to avoid carrying over contaminants from the organic/aqueous interface.
7. Precipitate the RNA by adding an equal volume of isopropanol. Leave for 10 min at 4°C, then centrifuge at 12,000g (4°C) for 10 min.
8. Discard the supernatant and wash the RNA pellet twice with 75% ethanol (1 mL of 75% ethanol per 1 mL of initial solution used) by shaking, then centrifuging for 5 min at 7500g (4°C). Air-dry the pellet for 5–10 min (do not over dry, because it will be more difficult to dissolve), then dissolve in 50–100 µL of DEPC-treated water.
9. The yield and purity of the RNA preparation can be determined by measuring the optical density on a spectrophotometer. Take an aliquot of RNA (1–2 µL), dilute in RNase-free TE, and measure the spectrophotometric absorbance at 260 and 280 nm. The OD A260:A280 ratio should be approx 1.8 to 2.0. Total RNA yields fall in the range of 5 to 15 µg from 1×10^6 mammalian cells and can be calculated using the formula: RNA isolated (µg/mL) = OD^{260nm} × dilution factor × 40 µg/mL. Samples can be stored at –70°C.
10. Treating RNA samples with DNase I, add:
    a. 1 µg RNA preparation in 8 µL DEPC-treated water.
    b. 1 µL 10X DNase I buffer (100 m*M* Tris-HCl pH 7.5; 25 m*M* MgCl$_2$; and 5 m*M* CaCl$_2$).

c. 1 μL DNase I (1 U).
Incubate for 15 min at room temperature. Add 1 μL stop solution (50 mM EDTA) and inactivate by heating at 70°C for 5 min. Cool on ice. Heating also denatures hairpins in the RNA, so the RNA can be used directly in reverse transcription. Alternatively, samples can be stored at –70°C.

3.5.6. RT-PCR of Complementary DNA

SuperScript III RT may be used to synthesize first-strand complementary DNA (cDNA) from a total RNA preparation. The first-strand cDNA synthesis reaction can be primed using random hexamers, oligo(dT), or gene-specific primers. We use oligo(dT)$_{20}$ as a more specific priming method. This hybridizes to 3' poly(A) tails, which are found in most eukaryotic mRNAs. First-strand synthesis can also be specifically primed with a 3'-terminus gene-specific primer PCR primer; however, oligo(dT) produces an RT-PCR product more consistently and is our method of choice. In the second step, PCR is performed in a separate tube using primers specific for *ELN*. The primers are designed so that they span exon–intron boundaries to allow specific PCR amplification only from the cDNA template and not from any residual contaminating genomic DNA. Some of primer sequences designed from the *ELN* cDNA sequence that we have used successfully are included in **Table 1** (*see* **Note 2**).

3.5.7. First-Strand cDNA Synthesis

1. The following procedure can to convert 1 pg to 5 μg of total RNA into first-strand cDNA. In a 0.5-mL sterile tube add:
   a. x μL of total RNA (maximum 5 μg).
   b. 1 μL of 50 μM oligo(dT)20 primer, or 2 μM gene-specific primer.
   c. 1 μL of 10 mM dNTP mix.
   d. DEPC-treated water to 10 μL.
   Incubate at 65°C for 5 min, then place on ice for at least 1 min.
2. Prepare the following cDNA synthesis reaction mix:
   a. 2 μL of 10X RT buffer.
   b. 4 μL of 25 mM MgCl$_2$.
   c. 2 μL of 0.1 M dithiothreitol.
   d. 1 μL of 40 U/μL RNase Inhibitor (RNaseOUT).
   e. 1 μL of 200 U/μL SuperScript III RT.
   Recombinant RNase Inhibitor (RNaseOUT) is included to prevent degradation of target RNA caused by ribonuclease contamination of the RNA preparation.
3. Add 10 μL of cDNA Synthesis Mix to each RNA plus primer mixture, mix, and collect by brief centrifugation. Incubate for 50 min at 50°C.
4. Inacivate the enzyme by heating at 85°C for 5 min. Cool the tubes on ice.
5. Add 1 μL of RNase H and incubate for 20 min at 37°C. Removing the RNA template from the cDNA:RNA hybrid molecule by digestion with RNase H after first-strand synthesis increases the sensitivity of the PCR step (especially for long templates). The cDNA synthesis reaction can be stored at –20°C or used directly for PCR.

3.5.8. Amplification of Target ELN cDNA

The cDNA prepared may be amplified directly using PCR. Two microliters of cDNA can be used for PCR, however, for some targets, adding more template may be required to increase the product yield. cDNA prepared from a normal control individual should be tested alongside the SVAS sample to aid the identification of aberrantly spliced cDNA or differences in levels of *ELN* gene expression. A ubiquitously expressed housekeeping gene, such as human β-*ACTIN* can be included as an internal control to allow semiquantitative analysis of the *ELN* transcript. Using the β-*ACTIN* gene primers (*see* **Table 1**), a 353-bp RT-PCR product is produced, which can be used as an internal indicator of normal transcript levels in the tissue tested.

1. Prepare a PCR mixture for each control reaction. For each control reaction, add the following to a 0.2-mL tube on ice:
   a. DEPC-treated water   38.1 μL
   b. 10X PCR buffer without Mg^{2+} 5 μL
   c. 50 m*M* $MgCl_2$ 1.5 μL
   d. 10 m*M* dNTP mix   1 μL
   e. 10 μ*M* sense primer   1 μL
   f. 10 μ*M* antisense primer   1 μL
   g. cDNA   2 μL
   h. 5 U/μL *Taq* DNA polymerase   0.4 μL
   i. Final volume   50 μL
2. Mix the contents of the tube. Centrifuge briefly to collect the reaction components.
3. Place reaction mixture in preheated (94°C) thermal cycler. Perform an initial denaturation step: 94°C for 2 min followed by 35 cycles of:
   a. 94°C for 15 s.
   b. 55°C for 30 s.
   c. 72°C for 1 min (increase for larger product, 1 min/1 kb of sequence).
   d. Final extension at 72°C for 10 min.
   After completion, maintain reactions at 4°C.
4. Analyze 10 μL of each sample with a DNA ladder on a 2% agarose gel using ethidium bromide staining to visualize the RT-PCR products. Aberrant *ELN* splicing or exon deletions or insertions will be observed as DNA bands that migrate differently compared with the normal control. Reduced *ELN* expression can be measured semiquantitatively with radioactively labeled probes, using protocols described elsewhere (*9,10*).
5. RT-PCR products can also be analyzed by direct sequencing with the BigDye cycle sequencing kit, using the RT-PCR primers.

4. Notes

1. If desired, the quality of the PCR products may be assessed by agarose gel electrophoresis before DHPLC analysis. In our experience, such quality control, fol-

lowed by reamplification of weak or failed PCR products, may significantly reduce the instrument time needed for complete mutation analysis.
2. *ELN* cDNA Genbank accession number: NM_000501. All nucleotide sequences cited here can be accessed from the Entrez Nucleotide database available at the following web address: http://www.ncbi.nlm.nih.gov/entrez/query.fcgi?db=Nucleotide&cmd=search&term=Z24075+.

Acknowledgments

We thank Marc W. Crepeau for technical assistance. This work was supported by The Wellcome Foundation (MT) and, in part, by grant HL073703 (ZU) from the National Heart Lung and Blood Institute, the National Institutes of Health.

References

1. Mecham, R. P. and Davis, E. C. (1994) Elastic fibre structure and assembly, in *Extracellular Matrix Assembly and Structure* (Yurchenko, P. D., Birk, D. E, and Mecham, R. P., eds.), Academic, San Diego, CA, pp. 281–314.
2. Indik, Z., Yeh, H., Ornstein-Goldstein, N., et al. (1989) Structure of the elastin gene and alternative splicing of elastin mRNA: implications for human disease. *Am. J. Med. Genet.* **34,** 81–90.
3. Tassabehji, M., Metcalfe, K., Donnai, D., et al. (1997) Elastin: genomic structure and point mutations in patients with supravalvular aortic stenosis. *Hum. Mol. Genet.* **6,** 1029–1036.
4. Williams, J. C., Barratt-Boyes, B. G., and Lowe, J. B. (1961) Supravalvular aortic stenosis. *Circulation* **24,** 1311–1318.
5. Eisenberg, R., Young, D., Jacobson, B., and Boito, A. (1964) Familial supravalvular aortic stenosis. *Am. J. Dis. Child.* **108,** 341–347.
6. Li, D. Y., Toland, A. E., Boak, B. B., et al. (1997) Elastin point mutations cause an obstructive vascular disease, supravalvular aortic stenosis. *Hum. Mol. Genet.* **6,** 1021–1028.
7. Metcalfe, K., Rucka, A. K., Smoot, L., et al. (2000) Elastin: mutational spectrum in supravalvular aortic stenosis. *Eur. J. Hum. Genet.* **8,** 955–963.
8. Urban, Z., Michels, V. V., Thibodeau, S. N., Donis-Keller, H., Csiszar, K., and Boyd, C. D. (1999) Supravalvular aortic stenosis: a splice site mutation within the elastin gene results in reduced expression of two aberrantly spliced transcripts. *Hum. Genet.* **104,** 135–142.
9. Urban, Z., Michels, V. V., Thibodeau, S. N., et al. (2000) Isolated supravalvular aortic stenosis: functional haploinsufficiency of the elastin gene as a result of nonsense-mediated decay. *Hum. Genet.* **106,** 577–588.
10. Urban, Z., Zhang, J., Davis, E. C., et al. (2001) Supravalvular aortic stenosis: genetic and molecular dissection of a complex mutation in the elastin gene. *Hum. Genet.* **109,** 512–520.

11. Urban, Z., Riazi, S., Seidl, T. L., et al. (2002) Connection between elastin haploinsufficiency and increased cell proliferation in patients with supravalvular aortic stenosis and Williams-Beuren syndrome. *Am. J. Hum. Genet.* **71,** 30–44.

12. Curran, M. E., Atkinson, D. L., Ewart, A. K., Morris, C. A., Leppert, M. F., and Keating, M. T. (1993) The elastin gene is disrupted by a translocation associated with supravalvular aortic stenosis. *Cell* **73,** 159–168.

13. Ewart, A. K., Jin, W., Atkinson, D., Morris, C. A., and Keating, M. T. (1994) Supravalvular aortic stenosis associated with a deletion disrupting the elastin gene. *J. Clin. Invest.* **93,** 1071–1077.

14. Olson, T. M., Michels, V. V., Urban, Z., et al. (1995) A 30 kb deletion within the elastin gene results in familial supravalvular aortic stenosis. *Hum. Mol. Genet.* **4,** 1677–1679.

15. Tassabehji, M., Metcalfe, K., Karmiloff-Smith, A., et al. (1999) Williams syndrome: use of chromosomal microdeletions as a tool to dissect cognitive and physical phenotypes. *Am. J. Hum. Genet.* **64,** 118–125.

16. Tassabehji, M., Metcalfe, K., Hurst, J., et al. (1998) An elastin gene mutation producing abnormal tropoelastin and abnormal elastic fibres in a patient with autosomal dominant cutis laxa. *Hum. Mol. Genet.* 7, 1021–1028.

17. Zhang, M. C., He, L., Giro, M., Yong, S. L., Tiller, G. E., and Davidson, J. M. (1999) Cutis laxa arising from frameshift mutations in exon 30 of the elastin gene (ELN). *J. Biol. Chem.* **274,** 981–986.

18. Rodriguez-Revenga, L., Iranzo, P., Badenas, C., Puig, S., Carrio, A., and Mila, M. (2004) A novel elastin gene mutation resulting in an autosomal dominant form of cutis laxa. *Arch. Dermatol.* **140,** 1135–1139.

19. Urban, Z., Gao, J., Pope, F. M., and Davis, E. C. (2005) Autosomal dominant cutis laxa with severe lung disease: sythesis and matrix deposition of mutant tropoelastin. *J. Invest. Dermatol.* **124,** 1193–1199.

20. Onda, H., Kasuya, H., Yoneyama, T., et al. (2001) Genomewide-linkage and haplotype-association studies map intracranial aneurysm to chromosome 7q11. *Am. J. Hum. Genet.* **69,** 804–819.

21. Suggs, S. V., Wallace, R. B., Hirose, T., Kawashima, E. H., and Itakura, K. (1981) Use of synthetic oligonucleotides as hybridization probes: isolation of cloned cDNA sequences for human beta 2-microglobulin. *Proc. Natl. Acad. Sci. USA* **78,** 6613–6617.

22. Bassam, B. J., Caetano-Anolles, G., and Gresshoff, P. M. (1991) Fast and sensitive silver staining of DNA in polyacrylamide gels. *Anal. Biochem.* **196,** 80–83.

23. Foster, K., Ferrell, R., King-Underwood, L., et al. (1993) Description of a dinucleotide repeat polymorphism in the human elastin gene and its use to confirm assignment of the gene to chromosome 7. *Ann. Hum. Genet.* **57(Pt 2),** 87–96.

24. Urban, Z., Csiszar, K., Fekete, G., and Boyd, C. D. (1997) A tetranucleotide repeat polymorphism within the human elastin gene (ELNi1). *Clin. Genet.* **51,** 133–134.

9

"Chip"ping Away at Heart Failure

J. David Barrans and Choong-Chin Liew

Summary

Studies in the field of microarray technology have exploded onto the scene to delve into the unknown underlying mechanisms and pathways in molecular disease. Diseases of the cardiovascular system, particularly those with unexplained molecular etiologies, such as heart failure, have more recently been investigated using array technology. Our laboratory has sought to examine gene expression profiles of human heart failure using a 10,000+ element cardiovascular-based complementary DNA microarray constructed in-house, termed the "CardioChip." Our studies have identified panels of genes, such as those encoding sarcomeric and cytoskeletal proteins, stress proteins, and Ca^{2+} regulators, that are differentially expressed in disease conditions as compared with samples from nonfailing hearts. Microarrays are effective tools for examining molecular portraits of the cardiovascular disease condition.

Key Words: Microarray; heart failure; cardiomyopathy; genomics; cardiovascular disease.

1. Introduction

Heart failure resulting from cardiomyopathy is a major cause of morbidity and mortality in North America. Typically, cardiomyopathy is diagnosed in at least four forms, including dilated (DCM), hypertrophic (HCM), restrictive, and arrythmogenic cardiomyopathy. DCM, the most common form of cardiomyopathy, is characterized by a dilated left atrium and ventricle and thin ventricular walls, as compared with a normal heart *(1)*. By contrast, HCM predominantly involves myocyte hypertrophy, leading to a thickening of the posterior wall of the left ventricle to meet metabolic demands of the body. In both cases, cardiac output and efficiency are compromised, leading to a gradual and eventual demise of the cardiac tissue.

Although DCM and HCM share common clinical endpoints, the same cannot be said about the molecular mechanisms involved in each condition (reviewed in **ref. 2**). The study of the molecular mechanisms underlying the development and progression of this syndrome has been rather challenging.

From: *Methods in Molecular Medicine, vol. 126: Congenital Heart Disease: Molecular Diagnostics*
Edited by: M. Kearns-Jonker © Humana Press Inc., Totowa, NJ

Much of the difficulty arises from the sometimes indistinct boundaries between primary, causative events or processes and more secondary phenomena resulting from appropriate or inappropriate physiological adaptations to primary events.

The early 21st century has seen the rise of genomic technologies that examine the entire genome of an organism. Although techniques such as positional cloning (whereby genes are characterized according to their chromosomal locations) had been earlier used to a limited extent, genomics truly came into widespread use during the long and arduous Human Genome Project and similar projects in other organisms. Although these projects have looked at the collection of genes present in respective organisms, they typically do not offer insight into gene expression at first blush; thus, other studies making use of expressed sequence tags sought to examine which genetic transcripts were turned on and turned off in various conditions, leading to or preventing disease manifestation. The investigation of gene expression has become particularly important in the cardiovascular sciences, either alone or in combination with environmental stimuli. The concept of cardiovascular genomics began in earnest in the late 1980s and early 1990s, with the construction and sequencing of a fetal heart complementary DNA (cDNA) library in our laboratory *(3–8)*. However, large-scale endeavors of this type have been time-consuming, laborious, and prohibitively expensive to most laboratory establishments.

Since the mid-1990s, studies in genomics have turned to microarray technology *(9)*. Although simple in their theory and design—essentially a high-throughput Southern blot on a very small scale—microarrays have revolutionized the examination of global gene expression. The excitement in the scientific community regarding the prospects of microarrays spawned an exponential increase in the number of articles in the literature dealing with microarrays, because this technology represents a reductive method, whereby complex gene expression patterns can be distilled to identify specific genes or chromosomal locations involved in a given disease state. Initial studies in yeast revealed unique gene expression profiles between different chromosomes, using a glass slide spotted with clones derived from yeast genomic DNA *(10)*. Since then, the use of microarrays to examine global gene expression has seen an exponential increase, most profoundly in cancer, e.g., melanoma *(11)*; hepatocellular carcinoma *(12)*; osteosarcoma *(13)*; breast cancer *(14)*; gastric carcinoma *(15,16)*; and lymphoma *(16–19)*. DNA microarrays are a highly sensitive (detection limit is 1 in 100,000 for cDNA microarrays and 1 in 300,000 for oligonucleotide arrays, relative to messenger RNA (mRNA) abundance *[20,21]*) and high-throughput approach for expression profiling. As with other technology, microarrays (and microarray science, in general) have been evolving at a rapid pace. Early versions used nylon membranes as a solid base, mimicking those used by traditional blotting strategies *(20,22)*. Today, the most widely used DNA microarrays come in two main platforms, although with slight variations. One uses the photolithographic synthesis of oligodeoxynucleotides directly onto silicon chips, more commonly manifested in the Affymetrix GeneChip®. The other uses a robotic or ink-jet printer style system to spot cDNA (polymerase chain reaction [PCR] products or plasmids) onto coated (usually poly-L-lysine or γ-amino polysilane) standard glass microscope slides *(23–26)*. In both cases, individual or duplicate spots on the array represent individual genes. Photolithography, a technology borrowed from the semiconductor industry, was implemented with DNA synthesis into the microarray field by Fodor and colleagues at Affymetrix. In this process of cyclic coupling and deprotection, a photomask is used to reveal a defined region on a glass wafer. Photoprotected DNA bases are sequentially added to the chip, enabling the preparation of a first-order oligonucleotide microarray directly on the chip. The reduction of sample handling and the use of synthetic reagents are important advantages for ensuring high chip-to-chip fidelity. Eleven probe sets on the GeneChip are assigned to each gene, represented by at least a 25-base oligomer derived from strategic sections of the gene. With the ability to represent more than 38,000 distinct transcripts on a single chip, this microarray attempts to give an extremely robust genetic platform for global expression profiling from genes all across the genome, especially for humans and mouse species.

On a cDNA array, DNA spots from unique genes are placed in a grid-like fashion directly onto the surface of the slide. Current technologies allow for the placement of several picoliters each of more than 10,000 full-length elements in an area of less than 1 cm^2. Fluid can be deposited in one of three or more methods. Schena and Brown pioneered the addition of yeast genes using a "quill pen" *(23,27)*. In this approach, a prepared DNA sample (e.g., a PCR product) is loaded into a spotting nib by capillary action, and a small volume is transferred to a solid surface by physical contact between the pin and the solid substrate. After the first spotting cycle, the nib (or set of nibs) is washed and a second sample is loaded and deposited. Another technique (used in our laboratory) incorporates the principles of surface tension by suspending a portion of liquid into a ring. A conjoining pin mechanism pokes into, but does not disrupt, the ring of liquid and touches the slide at a precise location. A variation on the drop system of microarrays is the use of a modified ink-jet printer, designed at a critical point in the infancy of spotted-array technology, when overzealous investigators turned to less expensive and more practical methods to participate in large-scale gene expression endeavors. In this approach, a DNA sample is loaded into a miniature nozzle equipped with a piezoelectric fitting (or other form of propulsion), which is used to expel a precise amount of liquid from the jet onto the slide.

Regardless of the system, comparisons of gene expression between any two samples can be performed. Typically, the two mRNA pools of interest are oligo-dT primed and labeled with fluorescent tags (e.g., Cy3 or Cy5) and hybridized independently (oligo array) or simultaneously to a single array (cDNA on glass slides). A fluorescent scanner then reads the chip or slide (after appropriate washing and so on) to generate a visual image representing the signals obtained from the two fluorescent tags. The ratio between the two signals for each spot is calculated, and differences in signal intensity are representative of differences in expression levels between the two transcript populations for each gene. Each type of microarray has its advantage, but there are also several downsides. Despite coming down in price, commercial oligonucleotide-based arrays have been hampered by prohibitive initial set up costs and the fact that two nonreusable chips are typically required for each experiment. cDNA microarrays are less costly to produce only if the required number of cDNA clones are readily available; there is also the issue of sample cross-contamination if appropriate wash steps are not addressed. The Affymetrix GeneChip is currently a popular platform of choice for the oligo-array consumer considering the vast number of genes on the array, but its closed reagent system and strict patent-related issues restrict its usefulness in novel gene discovery. Greater flexibility with chip designs and clones on hand benefit cDNA array use; however, the current method for labeling, hybridization, and image analysis is a veritable hodgepodge of protocols provided in the literature and through on-line user groups. This lack of standardization has hampered the progress of acceptance by more cautious members of the scientific community, as witnessed by an apparent overflow of review articles on microarrays and the relatively few manuscripts contributing original data.

Although microarray use has been successfully applied to conditions such as cancer *(18)*, its penetration into the cardiovascular sciences was not as vigorous at the outset. Initial studies with the GeneChip and cDNA arrays have examined gene expression after myocardial infarction *(28)* and in DCM *(29,30)*. In the first study, approx 7000 clones from a rat left ventricle cDNA library were spotted and hybridized with labeled heart RNA samples from different times after myocardial infarction. In the second study, two human left ventricle free-wall samples from patients with DCM were compared with normal hearts and analyzed using the Affymetrix Hu6800® GeneChip. In both cases, the gene for atrial natriuretic peptide (among other genes) was significantly upregulated in diseased hearts, confirming previous evidence *(31–34)*. Both of these studies provided an important initial basis for subsequent microarray studies in cardiovascular disease, which had been lacking in the field. This has led to subsequent gene expression studies of diverse cardiac conditions, including cardiac hypertrophy *(35–37)*, DCM *(38)*, end-stage heart failure *(39)*, fibrosis *(40)*, and response to left ventricular assist device implantation *(41)*.

Our laboratory has taken advantage of our vast previously acquired resources and has constructed what we think is the first ever custom-made cardiovascular-based cDNA microarray, which we term the CardioChip *(42,43)*. Its practicality and flexibility has allowed us to conceptualize the molecular events surrounding end-stage heart failure. We have used our CardioChip to explore gene expression in end-stage DCM and HCM relative to normal heart function *(42,43)*. RNA was extracted from the left ventricular free wall of seven patients undergoing transplantation, and from five samples from nonfailing hearts. More than 100 transcripts were consistently differentially expressed in DCM more than 1.5-fold. Not surprisingly, the gene for atrial natriuretic peptide was found to be upregulated in DCM (19-fold compared with samples from nonfailing hearts; $p < 0.05$). In addition, we found differences in transcripts encoding numerous sarcomeric and cytoskeletal proteins, stress response proteins, and transcription/translation regulators. Downregulation was most prominently observed with cell-signaling channels and mediators, particularly those involved in Ca^{2+} pathways. We also observed a selection of genes that were differentially expressed between HCM and DCM (including *calsequestrin*, *lipocortin*, and *lumican*), indicating that, despite similar clinical endpoints, heart failure resulting from HCM and DCM occurs through different molecular pathways *(44)*. Among both upregulated and downregulated transcripts, were novel, uncharacterized cDNAs, which serve as the basis for further investigation. Complementing our microarray analysis was verification of expression using quantitative real-time reverse transcriptase PCR (RT-PCR). Our studies provided preliminary molecular profiles of DCM and HCM using the largest human heart-specific cDNA microarray of the day. In recent years, we have developed molecular portraits to predict pathways and etiology of such diseases as heart failure and Chagas' cardiomyopathy *(45–47)*.

The protocol outlined in this chapter illustrates one embodiment of methods for determining gene expression using cDNA microarrays typical of the methods used in our laboratory. Although other methods exist, and may prove beneficial to the individual user, we have found that this regimen has offered the most consistent results.

2. Materials
1. TRIzol® buffer.
2. Diethylpyrocarbonate (DEPC)-treated water.
3. Oligo-dT.
4. 200 m*M* dNTP.
5. First-strand buffer.

 6. Cy3- and Cy5-dUTP.
 7. Reverse transcriptase (SuperScript®).
 8. 0.5 *M* NaOH.
 9. 10 m*M* EDTA.
10. 0.5 *M* Tris-HCl, pH 7.0.
11. Gel exclusion chromatography column.
12. DIG EasyHyb® hybridization solution (Roche).
13. Yeast tRNA (10 mg/mL).
14. Human Cot1 DNA.
15. Poly-dA.
16. Salmon sperm DNA (10 mg/mL).
17. HybriSlips® (Sigma-Aldrich, St. Louis, MO).
18. 1X sodium chloride-sodium citrate (SSC), 0.1% sodium dodecyl sulphate (SDS).
19. 50-mL conical tubes.

3. Methods

3.1. PCR Products

In the process of our large-scale sequencing project, PCR products were generated from human fetal and adult heart, familial hypertrophic cardiomyopathy heart, and vascular phage cDNA libraries, as described previously *(5–7,48)*. After sequence-similarity searching using BLAST *(49)* in the non-redundant database and database of ESTs, an annotated database of clones was compiled. **Table 1** illustrates the categorical distribution of the PCR products used on the CardioChip.

3.2. PCR Product Purification and Construction of 10,368-Element cDNA Microarray

Rescue individual clones from phage (λ ZAP) into phagemid vector (for 3'-end sequencing and further experimental analysis, e.g., protein expression).

1. Amplify phagemids by PCR (T3 and T7 forward and reverse primers, respectively), in 96-well microplates (Corning).
2. Visualize inserts on a 1% agarose minigel.
3. Randomly assign clones to individual wells of a 96-well microplate (Corning).
4. Purify 50 µL of each PCR product with 5 µL of 3 *M* ammonium acetate and 125 µL of 95% ethanol at −20°C overnight.
5. The next day, centrifuge the plates at 4000 rpm for 30 min at 4°C.
6. Decant the supernatant. After two washes with 50 µL of 70% ethanol, air-dry the resulting DNA pellets.
7. Resuspend pellets in 20 µL of 3X SSC.

To construct the CardioChip, spot 108 of the microplates (containing 10,368 nonredundant PCR products) onto CMT-UltraGAPS® amino-silane-coated

Table 1
Categorical Distribution of the 10,368 Expressed Sequence Tags (ESTs)
on the CardioChip

Category of EST	Number of clones on array (% of total)
Known, matched gene[a]	4002 (38.6)
Matched other EST in dbEST[b]	1818 (17.5)
Unmatched, putative novel EST[c]	4356 (42.0)
Bacterial clones (negative controls)	192 (1.8)

[a]Includes matches to full-length hypothetical proteins in the non-redundant database of GenBank.
[b]Includes matches to human genome sequences in the non-redundant database of GenBank.
[c]Includes matches to sequences in the unfinished high-throughput genomic sequences database of GenBank.

glass microarray slides (Corning) using a GMS 417 arrayer (Affymetrix, Santa Clara, CA), and postprocess the arrays, as previously described *(11)*.

3.3. Fluorescent Probe Labeling and Hybridization

Extract total RNA from tissue samples using TRIzol reagent (Gibco BRL-Life Technologies), according to the manufacturer's protocol (*see* **Note 1**). We used samples of unique normal human adult heart (left ventricular free wall of five nonfailing human adult hearts, rejected as donors because of infection) and of DCM heart (explanted hearts from patients undergoing transplantation).

3.3.1. Label Probes and Hybridize to Microarray Slides (see **Notes 2–4**)

1. Suspend 10 µg of each total RNA species in 8 µL DEPC-treated water.
2. Add 2 µL oligo-dT$_{15-18}$, incubate at 65°C for 2 min.
3. Add reaction mixture to each sample:
   a. 4 µL first-strand buffer.
   b. 1 µL dNTP (total concentration = 200 µ*M*).
   c. 4 µL Cy3- or Cy5-dUTP stock (Amersham).
   d. 1 µL SuperScript RT.
4. Incubate at 42°C for 2 h, adding an additional 1 µL RT to each sample after 1 h.
5. Stop reaction with 5 µL of 0.5 *M* NaOH and 5 µL of 10 m*M* EDTA for 5 min, then neutralize with 0.5 *M* Tris-HCl.
6. Remove excess label by gel exclusion chromatography (ProbeQuant G-50®, Amersham), according to the manufacturer's protocol.
7. Mix the two probes of interest (one with Cy3 and one with Cy5).
8. Reduce to a volume of 10 µL using a speed vacuum.
9. Combine with 30 µL of hybridization solution (stock solution containing the following as blocking agents):

    a. 100 µL DIG EasyHyb hybridization solution (Roche).
    b. 5 µL of 10 mg/mL yeast tRNA.
    c. 5 µL human Cot1 DNA.
    d. 5 µL poly-dA.
    e. 5 µL of 10 mg/mL salmon sperm DNA.
10. Add probe mixture to microarray slide and cover with cover slip.
11. Hybridize slide in a sealed dry chamber in a 37°C water bath overnight.

3.3.2. Slide Scanning (see **Notes 5** and **6**)

1. The next day, wash the slides in a slide-washing basin, first with 1X SSC to remove the cover slip (HybriSlips; Sigma), then with three successive washes of 1X SSC/0.1% SDS for 15 min each at 50°C, followed by a rinse with 1X SSC.
2. Remove excess fluid on the slides by placing them into individual 50-mL conical tubes and centrifuging at 500 rpm for approx 2 min.
3. Scan the slides using an appropriate microarray scanner, first at 635 nm (for Cy5), then at 532 nm (for Cy3).

3.4. Data Processing (see **Notes 7–11**)

1. Superimpose the Cy3 and Cy5 scans for each slide. Turn the gain to the maximum value.
2. Place a grid on the superimposed image, ensuring that the grid locators completely cover the illuminated spots.
3. Obtain values corresponding to the level of fluorescent intensity for each spot and import to an Excel® spreadsheet.
4. Subtract the local background from the fluorescent value of each spot to obtain a net value.
5. Determine median ratio for each spot (calculated as the ratio of the median fluorescence from each pixel, minus the background, of Cy5 to Cy3). Submit this expression data to hierarchical clustering analysis.

3.5. Verification of Candidate Gene Expression Using Quantitative Real-Time RT-PCR (see **Notes 12** and **13**)

1. Design forward and reverse primers for the selected genes, including an internal control.
2. Take 100 ng of total RNA per reaction and prepare the quantitative RT-PCR solution:
    a. 50 µL total volume containing 1X SYBR® Green PCR Master Mix.
    b. 0.25 U/µL Multiscribe® RT (Applied BioSystems, Foster City, CA).
    c. 0.4 U/µL RNase inhibitor.
    d. 10 pmoles of each forward and reverse primer.
3. Perform the reactions in a 96-well format, with the following cycling parameters: 30 min at 48°C, and 40 cycles of 30 s at 94°C and 1 min at 60°C.

4. Notes

1. RNA quality is an important limiting factor in conducting a microarray experiment. Always run the sample on a formaldehyde gel to check the integrity of the RNA; clear 28S, 18S, and 5S bands should be visible with no genomic DNA contamination. Check the optical density of the sample at 260 nm/280 nm to ensure a ratio of at least 1.8.

2. Labeling, overnight hybridization, washing, and scanning MUST be performed in reduced light, i.e., as close to dark conditions as possible. Increased light exposure will bleach the dyes and impair proper signal generation from the spots on the array.

3. One method for verifying the integrity of the hybridization method is by reverse labeling. Take the same samples and reverse the fluorescent dye used in the first experiment (i.e., if the DCM heart samples were labeled with Cy3 and samples from nonfailing hearts with Cy5 in the first experiment; for the second experiment, label samples from DCM hearts with Cy5 and samples from nonfailing hearts with Cy3). Ideally, the ratios of each spot should be inverse—e.g., spot A with a DCM to nonfailing ratio of 2.5 in the first experiment should have a nonfailing to DCM ratio of 0.4 in the second experiment. However, we noted that this phenomenon typically occurs with genes that are more vastly expressed in one sample than in the other, and when each set of hybridizations is performed at least three times, preferably more.

4. To assess the intersample variation, a parallel labeling against each of the samples can be performed with human universal reference RNA, and hybridized together. The universal RNA acts as a common reference to which any future sample can be compared.

5. To ensure that uniform spotting on the array has occurred, one slide out of the lot was tested by staining with a 1:10,000 dilution of SYBR Green I (Applied Biosystems), which detects double-stranded DNA. The slide was scanned in the Cy3 channel (532 nm) and visualized using ScanAlyze (M. Eisen, Stanford University, CA) and PhotoShop (Adobe, San Jose, CA). Aberrant spots or regions of inconsistencies on the slide were flagged, and, as necessary, the spotting process was repeated.

6. Scanning of Cy5 and Cy3 channels was performed using the GMS 418 Array Scanner (Affymetrix). Cy5 is more sensitive, so it should be scanned first.

7. Raw scanned images were processed using ScanAlyze 2.44 microarray image analysis software (M. Eisen, available at: http://rana.lbl.gov, Stanford University, CA).

8. To account for incomplete hybridization on each spot, in our analysis, we only included those spots in which at least 50% of the pixels (within the defined area of the spot) displayed a fluorescence at least 1.5 times higher than background in all experiments. Spots whose net fluorescent value did not exceed the mean value obtained from the 192 bacterial negative-control spots were excluded.

9. Another, older method for normalizing spot intensity is to use a scatterplot. The level of normalization required is based on the deviation of signal from the mean Cy3 signal. The factor by which the Cy3 fluorescence signal is reduced can be determined by plotting the raw net signals from each channel on a scatterplot. The slope of the resulting trend line is used as a multiplying factor against the Cy3 fluorescence value of each spot. The resulting slope has a value of 1.0 and, thus, proper ratios can be calculated.

10. To assess the reproducibility of hybridization results and assess intraassay variation, one can examine the correlation of the median ratio values for each filtered spot on the array from at least three replicate experiments (i.e., using the same RNA sample divided into three separate aliquots).

11. Hierarchical cluster analysis and/or intensity filtering was also performed, using commercially available software, such as GeneSpring v6.1 (Silicon Genetics, Redwood City, CA).

12. In 96-well format, for each gene of interest, single quantitative RT-PCR reactions were performed on each individual DCM heart mRNA sample ($n = 7$) and each nonfailing adult heart mRNA sample ($n = 5$). As an internal control, primers for glycerol phosphate dehydrogenase were also designed and amplified in parallel with the genes of interest.

13. Primers were designed online (http://alces.med.umn.edu/rawprimer.html), verified for complementarity (http://www.basic.northwestern.edu/biotools/oligocalc.html), and searched against the public database to confirm unique amplification products (http://www.ncbi.nlm.nih.gov).

References

1. Towbin, J. A. and Bowles, N. E. (2000) Genetic abnormalities responsible for dilated cardiomyopathy. *Curr. Cardiol. Rep.* **2,** 475–480.
2. Hwang, J. J., Dzau, V. J., and Liew, C. C. (2001) Genomics and the pathophysiology of heart failure. *Current Cardiol. Rep.* **3,** 198–207.
3. Jandreski, M. A. and Liew, C. C. (1987) Construction of a human ventricular cDNA library and characterization of a beta myosin heavy chain cDNA clone. *Hum. Genet.* **76,** 47–53.
4. Liew, C.C. (1993) A human heart cDNA library—the development of an efficient and simple method for automated DNA sequencing. *J. Mol. Cell. Cardiol.* **25,** 891–894.
5. Hwang, D. M., Hwang, W. S., and Liew, C. C. (1994) Single pass sequencing of a unidirectional human fetal heart cDNA library to discover novel genes of the cardiovascular system. *J. Mol. Cell. Cardiol.* **26,** 1329–1333.
6. Hwang, D. M., Dempsey, A. A., Wang, R. X., et al. (1997) A genome-based resource for molecular cardiovascular medicine: toward a compendium of cardiovascular genes. *Circulation* **96,** 4146–4203.
7. Liew, C. C., Hwang, D. M., Fung, Y. W., et al. (1994) A catalogue of genes in the cardiovascular system as identified by expressed sequence tags. *Proc. Natl. Acad. Sci. USA* **91,** 10,645–10,649.

8. Barrans, J. D. (2002) *Genomic Exploration of Cardiovascular-Based Gene Expression*, PhD Thesis, University of Toronto, Department of Laboratory Medicine and Pathobiology.
9. Liew, C. C., Hwang, D. M., Wang, R. X., et al. (1997) Construction of a human heart cDNA library and identification of cardiovascular based genes (CVBest). *Mol. Cell. Biochem.* **172,** 81–87.
10. Shalon, D., Smith, S. J., and Brown, P. O. (1996) A DNA microarray system for analyzing complex DNA samples using two-color fluorescent probe hybridization. *Genome Res.* **6,** 639–645.
11. DeRisi, J., Penland, L., Brown, P. O., et al. (1996) Use of a cDNA microarray to analyse gene expression patterns in human cancer. *Nat. Genet.* **14,** 457–460.
12. Lau, W. Y., Lai, P. B., Leung, M. F., et al. (2000) Differential gene expression of hepatocellular carcinoma using cDNA microarray analysis. *Oncol. Res.* **12,** 59–69.
13. Wolf, M., El-Rifai, W., Tarkkanen, M., et al. (2000) Novel findings in gene expression detected in human osteosarcoma by cDNA microarray. *Cancer Genet. Cytogenet.* **123,** 128–132.
14. van 't Veer, L. J., Dai, H., van de Vijver, M. J., et al. (2002) Gene expression profiling predicts clinical outcome of breast cancer. *Nature* **415,** 530–536.
15. Mori, M., Mimori, K., Yoshikawa, Y., et al. (2002) Analysis of the gene-expression profile regarding the progression of human gastric carcinoma. *Surgery* **131(1 Suppl),** S39–47.
16. Hippo, Y., Taniguchi, H., Tsutsumi, S., et al. (2002) Global gene expression analysis of gastric cancer by oligonucleotide microarrays. *Cancer Res.* **62,** 233–240.
17. Alizadeh, A., Eisen, M., Davis, R. E., et al. (1999) The lymphochip: a specialized cDNA microarray for the genomic-scale analysis of gene expression in normal and malignant lymphocytes. *Cold Spring Harb. Symp. Quant. Biol.* **64,** 71–78.
18. Alizadeh, A. A., Eisen, M. B., Davis, R. E., et al (2000) Distinct types of diffuse large B-cell lymphoma identified by gene expression profiling. *Nature* **403,** 503–511.
19. Shipp, M. A., Ross, K. N., Tamayo, P., et al. (2002) Diffuse large B-cell lymphoma outcome prediction by gene-expression profiling and supervised machine learning. *Nat. Med.* **8,** 68–74.
20. Granjeaud, S., Nguyen,C., Rocha, D., Luton, R., and Jordan, B.R. (1996) From hybridization image to numerical values: a practical, high throughput quantification system for high density filter hybridizations. *Genet. Anal.* **12,** 151–162.
21. Bertucci, F., Bernard, K., Loriod, B., et al. (1999) Sensitivity issues in DNA array-based expression measurements and performance of nylon microarrays for small samples. *Hum. Mol. Genet.* **8,** 1715–1722.
22. Nguyen, C., Rocha, D., Granjeaud, S., et al. (1995) Differential gene expression in the murine thymus assayed by quantitative hybridization of arrayed cDNA clones. *Genomics* **29,** 207–216.
23. Schena, M., Shalon, D., Davis, R. W., and Brown, P. O. (1995) Quantitative monitoring of gene expression patterns with a complementary DNA microarray. *Science* **270,** 467–470.

24. Lockhart, D. J. and Winzeler, E. A. (2000) Genomics, gene expression and DNA arrays. *Nature* **405,** 827–836.
25. Bowtell, D. D. (1999) Options available—from start to finish—for obtaining expression data by microarray. *Nat. Genet.* **21(1 Suppl),** 25–32.
26. Lipshutz, R. J., Fodor, S. P., Gingeras, T. R., and Lockhart, D. J. (1999) High density synthetic oligonucleotide arrays. *Nat. Genet.* **21(1 Suppl),** 20–24.
27. Schena, M., Shalon, D., Heller, R., Chai, A., Brown, P. O., and Davis, R. W. (1996) Parallel human genome analysis: microarray-based expression monitoring of 1000 genes. *Proc. Natl. Acad. Sci. USA* **93,** 10,614–10,619.
28. Stanton, L. W., Garrard, L. J., Damm, D., et al. (2000) Altered patterns of gene expression in response to myocardial infarction. *Circ. Res.* **86,** 939–945.
29. Yang, J., Moravec, C. S., Sussman, M. A., et al. (2000) Decreased SLIM1 expression and increased gelsolin expression in failing human hearts measured by high-density oligonucleotide arrays. *Circulation* **102,** 3046–3052.
30. Yang, J., Moravec, C. S., Sussman, M. A., et al. (2000) Expression profiling reveals distinct sets of genes altered during induction and regression of cardiac hypertrophy. *Proc. Natl. Acad. Sci. USA* **97,** 6745–6750.
31. Hanatani, A., Yoshiyama, M., Kim, S., et al. (1998) Assessment of cardiac function and gene expression at an early phase after myocardial infarction. *Jpn. Heart J.* **39,** 375–388.
32. Mittmann, C., Munstermann, U., Weil, J., et al. (1998) Analysis of gene expression patterns in small amounts of human ventricular myocardium by a multiplex RNase protection assay. *J. Mol. Med.* **76,** 133–140.
33. Lowes, B. D., Minobe, W., and Abraham, W. T. (1997) Changes in gene expression in the intact human heart: downregulation of alpha-myosin heavy chain in hypertrophied, failing ventricular myocardium. *J. Clin. Invest.* **100,** 2315–2324.
34. Mendez, R. E., Pfeffer, J. M., Ortola, F. V., et al. (1987) Atrial natriuretic peptide transcription, storage, and release in rats with myocardial infarction. *Am. J. Physiol.* **253,** H1449–1455.
35. Friddle, C. J., Koga, T., Rubin, E. M., et al. (2000) Expression profiling reveals distinct sets of genes altered during induction and regression of cardiac hypertrophy. *Proc. Natl. Acad. Sci. USA* **97,** 6745–6750.
36. Haase, D., Lehmann, M. H., Korner, M. M., et al. (2002) Identification and validation of selective upregulation of ventricular myosin light chain type 2 mRNA in idiopathic dilated cardiomyopathy. *Eur. J. Heart Fail.* **4,** 23–31.
37. Napoli, C., Lerman, L.O., Sica, V., Lerman, A., Tajana, G., and de Nigris, F. (2003) Microarray analysis: a novel research tool for cardiovascular scientists and physicians. *Heart* **89,** 597–604.
38. Grzeskowiak, R., Witt, H., Drungowski, M., et al. (2003) Expression profiling of human idiopathic dilated cardiomyopathy. *Cardiovasc. Res.* **59,** 400–411.
39. Steenbergen, C., Afshari, C. A., Petrank, J. G., et al. Alterations in apoptotic signaling in human idiopathic cardiomyopathic hearts in failure. *Am. J. Physiol. Heart. Circ. Physiol.* **284,** H268–H276.

40. Kapoun, A. M., Liang, F., O'Young, G., et al. B-type natriuretic peptide exerts broad functional opposition to transforming growth factor-β in primary human cardiac fibroblasts. Fibrosis, myofibroblast conversion, proliferation, and inflammation. *Circ. Res.* **94,** 453–461.

41. Chen, M. M., Ashley, E. A., Deng, D. X., et al. (2003) Novel role for the potent endogenous inotrope apelin in human cardiac dysfunction. *Circulation* **108,** 1432–1439.

42. Barrans, J. D., Stamatiou, D., and Liew, C. C. (2001) Construction of a human cardiovascular cDNA microarray: portrait of the failing heart. *Biochem. Biophys. Res. Comm.* **280,** 964–969.

43. Barrans, J. D., Allen, P. D., Stamatiou, D., Dzau, V. J., and Liew, C. C. (2002) Global gene expression profiling of end-stage dilated cardiomyopathy using a human cardiovascular-based cDNA microarray. *Am. J. Path.* **160,** 2035–2043.

44. Hwang, J. J., Allen, P. D., Tsseng, G. C., et al. (2002) Microarray gene expression profiles in dilated and hypertrophic cardiomyopathic end-stage heart failure. *Physiol. Genomics* **10,** 31–44.

45. Liew, C. C. and Dzau, V. (2004) Molecular genetics and genomics of heart failure. *Nat. Rev. Genet.* **5,** 811–825.

46. Liew, C. C. (2005) Expressed genome molecular signatures of heart failure. *Clin. Chem. Lab. Med.* **43,** 462–469.

47. Cunha-Neto, E., Dzau, V. J., Allen, P. D., et al. (2005) Cardiac gene expression profiling provides evidence for cytokinopathy as a molecular mechanism in Chagas disease cardiomyopathy. *Am. J. Path.* **167,** 305–313.

48. Hwang, D. M., Dempsey, A. A., Lee, C. Y., and Liew, C. C. (2000) Identification of differentially expressed genes in cardiac hypertrophy by analysis of expressed sequence tags. *Genomics* **66,** 1–14.

49. Altschul, S. F., Gish, W., Miller, W., Myers, E. W., and Lipman, D. (1990) Basic local alignment search tool. *J. Mol. Biol.* **215,** 403–410.

10

Molecular Diagnostics of Catecholaminergic Polymorphic Ventricular Tachycardia Using Denaturing High-Performance Liquid Chromatography and Sequencing

Alex V. Postma, Zahurul A. Bhuiyan, and Hennie Bikker

Summary

Catecholaminergic polymorphic ventricular tachycardia (CPVT) is an arrhythmogenic disease characterized by adrenergic-induced arrhythmias in the form of bidirectional and PVT. CPVT is a distinct clinical entity associated with a high mortality rate of up to 50% by the age of 30 yr. Recently, the molecular diagnostics of this disease have become increasingly important because underlying mutations can be found in more than 60% of the identified CPVT patients. Along with the fact that treatment with β-blockers has a favorable outcome in CPVT patients, and given the risk of sudden death, the identification of causative mutations in CPVT is important because it can greatly augment early diagnosis and subsequent preventive strategies. In this chapter, we describe the molecular diagnostics, as performed in our lab, of the three genes known to be involved in CPVT, the cardiac ryanodine receptor gene, the cardiac calsequestrin gene, and the inwardly rectifying potassium channel *KCNJ2*.

Key Words: CPVT; RYR2; CASQ2; *KCNJ2*; DHPLC; sequencing.

1. Introduction

Catecholaminergic polymorphic ventricular tachycardia (CPVT) is a rare arrhythmogenic disease characterized by syncopal events and sudden cardiac death at a young age *(1)*. CPVT is a distinct clinical entity associated with a high mortality rate of up to 50% by the age of 30 yr. Its key features include childhood onset of syncope and collapse triggered by exercise and other stressful scenarios, with reproducible polymorphic and/or bidirectional ventricular tachycardia demonstrated during exercise testing and catecholamine infusion. Cardiac investigations show no evidence of structural heart disease, and the resting 12-lead electrocardiogram is unremarkable, including the QT interval.

From: *Methods in Molecular Medicine, vol. 126: Congenital Heart Disease: Molecular Diagnostics*
Edited by: M. Kearns-Jonker © Humana Press Inc., Totowa, NJ

Cases have been reported throughout the world, and both sexes seem to be susceptible. Recently, the molecular diagnostics of CPVT has become increasingly important because underlying mutations can be found in more than 60% of the identified CPVT patients *(2,3)*. Along with the fact that treatment with β-blockers has a favorable outcome in CPVT patients, and given the risk of sudden death, the identification of causative mutations in CPVT is important because it can greatly augment early diagnosis and subsequent preventive strategies. In this chapter, we describe the molecular diagnostics, as performed in our lab, of the three genes currently known to be involved in CPVT.

1.1. Autosomal-Dominant CPVT, the Cardiac Ryanodine Receptor

Many cases of CPVT are familial, and the first extensive report with a definite linkage analysis was published by Swan et al., and showed linkage of CPVT with chromosome 1q42-43 *(4)*. This report was followed by publications that associated mutations in a gene from the 1q42-43 region, the cardiac-specific ryanodine receptor type 2 *(RYR2)*, with CPVT *(1,5,6)*. Ryanodine receptor channels are intracellular Ca^{2+}-release channels that form a homotetrameric membrane-spanning calcium channel on the sarcoplasmic reticulum. The *RyR2* gene is located on chromosome 1q42 and consists of 105 exons, which translate into 15 kb of complementary DNA. *RYR2* encodes a protein of 4967 amino acids, making it the largest known ion channel to date. At present, approx 50 mutations have been reported in more than 52 families *(1,2,5–8)*. The various mutations cluster within four regions in the RyR2 protein: the N-terminal side; around the binding site of FKBP12.6, a protein that stabilizes the RyR2 channel *(9)*; the calcium binding site; and the channel-forming transmembrane domains.

1.2. Autosomal-Recessive CPVT, the Cardiac Calsequestrin Gene

In contrast to the majority of CPVT patients, who have an autosomal-dominant mode of inheritance *(RYR2)*, two studies have recently demonstrated a recessive form of CPVT *(3,10)*. The affected patients of these four families all shared an area on chromosome 1p13-21. Subsequently, homozygous mutations in the cardiac calsequestrin gene *(CASQ2)* located in that region were found to underlie this recessive form of CPVT. Strikingly, the heterozygous carriers of the mutations were devoid of any clinical symptoms or electrocardiographic anomalies. The phenotypes of the recessive *CASQ2* CPVT patients seem more severe compared with the *RyR2* CPVT patients. The *CASQ2* gene consists of 11 exons and encodes a protein that serves as the major Ca^{2+} reservoir within the sarcoplasmic reticulum lumen of cardiac myocytes. However, although *CASQ2* mutations are often autosomal recessive, some reports indicate that autosomal-dominant inheritance with reduced penetrance can be part of the clinical spectrum of *CASQ2* CPVT *(3)*.

1.3. Overlapping Diseases: Andersen and CPVT, the KCNJ2 Gene

Mutations of the *KCNJ2* gene are known to be causative in Andersen syndrome (AS), a disease characterized by potassium-sensitive periodic paralysis, dysmorphic features, and PVT *(11)*. However, mutations in *KCNJ2* result in a pleiotropy of phenotypic AS variations, including all, some, or a single characteristic of AS. Moreover, there is evidence that *KCNJ2* only produces CPVT characteristics with a very low penetrance of prominent dysmorphic features, suggesting that some AS patients may present as CPVT patients *(12,13)*. These "overlap" patients have syncope, exercise-induced PVT, and a normal QTc interval. However, in contrast to CPVT, they can also exhibit polymorphic ventricular beats in the resting electrocardiogram. The *KCNJ2* gene is a background ion channel involved in maintaining the membrane potential of cardiomyocytes during diastole. It is located on chromosome 17q23.1-q24.2 and consists of a single coding exon.

1.4. Molecular Diagnostics of CPVT

It is clear that there is a strong genetic component in CPVT, and, currently, underlying mutations are found in approx 60% of patients with CPVT. Depending on the clinical presentation of the disease and the family history, the appropriate genes can be screened for in CPVT patients. Because the causative genes differ so much in size, the diagnostics for CPVT are challenging. The main gene involved in CPVT, *RYR2*, has 105 exons, *CASQ2* has 11 exons, and *KCNJ2* has 1 exon. Thus, the strategies for the genetic screening of patients with CPVT depend on the size of the genes involved, the equipment available, and the cost effectiveness. Our lab currently uses denaturing high-performance liquid chromatography (DHPLC) analysis for the *RYR2* and the *CASQ2* genes, and sequence analysis for the *KCNJ2* gene. In **Subheading 3.**, we outline the various techniques we use to screen CPVT patients for the genes of interest. In our laboratory, patients with a CPVT diagnosis are screened first for *RYR2*, subsequently for *CASQ2*, and finally for *KCNJ2*, this order is based on the prevalence of mutations.

2. Materials

2.1. Polymerase Chain Reaction

1. 10X polymerase chain reaction (PCR) buffer (Roche).
2. 5X PCR buffer. For 1 mL:
   a. 250 µL of 1 *M* Tris-HCl, pH 9.0.

b. 140 µL of 0.5 *M* (NH$_4$)SO$_4$.
c. 100 µL dimethylsulfoxide.
d. 75 µL Tween-20.
e. 435 µL ddH$_2$O.
3. 25 m*M* MgCl$_2$ (Applied Biosystems [ABI]).
4. dNTPs, 1.25 m*M* for each NTP (Amersham Pharmacia).
5. 20 pmol/µL primers (*see* **Note 1**).
6. Super Taq (HT Biotechnology).
7. 5 m*M* betaine (Sigma).
8. Strip tubes/caps (VWR).
9. 96-well plate (Biozym).

2.2. Sequencing

1. BigDye Terminator v3.0 (ABI).
2. 5X sequencing buffer (supplied with BigDye Terminator v3.0) (ABI).
3. 5 m*M* betaine (Sigma).
4. Strip tubes/caps (VWR).

2.3. Gel Electrophoresis Analysis

1. Agarose.
2. 1X Tris-acetate-EDTA (TAE):
   a. 0.04 *M* Tris-acetate.
   b. 0.001 *M* EDTA, pH 8.0.
3. Ethidium bromide (10 mg/mL).
4. 10X loading buffer (25 mL):
   a. 6.25 g Ficoll 400.
   b. 0.5 mL of 0.5 m*M* EDTA.
   c. 0.25 mL of 10% sodium dodecyl sulphate.
   d. 0.0625 g Orange G (Merck).
   e. Add ddH$_2$O to bring up to 25 mL.

2.4. Denaturing High-Performance Liquid Chromatography

1. 0.1 *M* triethylamine acetate (pH 7.0) (Transgenomic).
2. Acetonitrile (Transgenomic) (*see* **Note 2**).

2.5. Equipment

1. Thermocycler.
2. Gel electrophoresis device.
3. Gel image-capture device, Eagle-eye II (Stratagene).
4. ABI PRISM® DNA Analyzer (ABI).
5. Computer with sequence analysis software (ABI) and WAVE Maker™ software (Transgenomic).
6. DHPLC-WAVE™ system (Transgenomic).

3. Methods

3.1. Direct Sequence

3.1.1. PCR Reaction

1. Amplify genomic DNA for sequence analysis in 20 µL reaction mixtures containing:
   a. 3.0 µL of 25 ng/µL genomic DNA.
   b. 4.0 µL of 5X PCR buffer.
   c. 1.2 µL of 25 mM MgCl$_2$.
   d. 2.25 µL of 1.25 mM dNTPs.
   e. 0.4 µL of each 20 pmol/µL primer.
   f. 0.1 µL Super Taq (HT Biotechnology).
   g. 4.0 µL of 5 mM Betaine.
   h. 4.65 µL ddH$_2$O (*see* **Note 3**).
2. Perform PCR using an initial denaturing step of 94°C for 3 min, followed by 35 cycles of the following touch-down PCR protocol: denaturation at 94°C for 45 s, annealing at 66 to 52°C (*see* **Note 4**) for 45 s, and extension at 72°C for 1 min.
3. Store the product mixture at 4°C until further use.

3.1.2. Gel Electrophoresis Analysis

1. The PCR products are tested on an agarose gel to determine the outcome and specificity of the reaction. Single, crisp bands indicate a successful PCR product that can be used for subsequent sequence analysis.
2. Prepare a 1.5% (w/v) agarose gel with 1X TAE, with 5 µL of 10 mg/mL ethidium bromide added to each 100 mL of gel solution. Run the electrophoresis in a 1X TAE buffer.
3. Add 1 µL of 10X loading buffer to a sample of 5 µL of each PCR product, and load the reaction mixture onto the agarose gel. Use a stock ladder (100-bp ladder) to determine the size of the products.
4. Perform electrophoresis at 100 V/100 mA; running time depends on product size and gel length.
5. Capture the gel image (photograph or computer) under long-wave UV to determine the result of the PCR. If the PCR was successful, sequence the sample.

3.1.3. Sequencing Reaction

1. Assemble the sequencing reaction (10 µL total volume) by adding 3.0 µL of PCR product diluted 1:5 to a strip tube containing:
   a. 1.0 µL BigDye Terminator v3.0.
   b. 1.0 µL of sequencing primer (2 pmol/µL).
   c. 2.0 µL 5X sequencing buffer.
   d. 2.0 µL 5 mM betaine.
   e. 1.0 µL ddH$_2$O (*see* **Notes 3** and **5**).
2. Denature the DNA initially by incubating the reaction mixture at 94°C for 2 min.

3. Perform cycle sequencing with 24 cycles of denaturation at 96°C for 10 s, primer annealing at 50°C for 5 s, and primer extension at 60°C for 4 min; and with a single, final extension step at 60°C for 10 min (*see* **Note 6**).
4. Store the product mixture at 4°C until loading onto the capillary DNA sequencer.

3.2. Denaturing High-Performance Liquid Chromatography

3.2.1. PCR Reaction

1. Amplify genomic DNA for DHPLC analysis in 50-μL reaction mixtures containing:
   a. 2.0 μL of 25 ng/μL genomic DNA.
   b. 5.0 μL of 10X DHPLC-PCR buffer (Roche).
   c. 3.0 μL of 25 mM MgCl$_2$.
   d. 8.0 μL of 1.25 mM dNTPs.
   e. 1.0 μL of each 20 pmol/μL primer.
   f. 0.1 μL Super Taq (HT Biotechnology).
   g. 30 μL ddH$_2$O (*see* **Note 7**).
2. Perform PCR using an initial denaturing step of 94°C for 3 min, followed by 35 cycles of the following touch-down PCR protocol: denaturation at 94°C for 45 s, annealing at 66 to 52°C for 45 s, and extension at 72°C for 1 min (*see* **Note 4**).
3. Store the product mixture at 4°C until further use.

3.2.2. Gel Analysis of PCR Products

1. PCR products for subsequent DHPLC analysis are checked using agarose gels in the manner described in **Subheading 3.1.3.** Only PCR products with single, crisp bands are to be used in the DHPLC analysis (*see* **Note 8**).

3.2.3. DHPLC Analysis

1. For each amplicon, the PCR product of wild-type DNA (healthy control) has to be mixed with the patient's product at equimolar ratios (*see* **Note 9**); subsequently, the resulting mix is subjected to a 5 min, 95°C denaturing step in a PCR machine, followed by a gradual reannealing from 95°C to room temperature during 1 h. This ensures the formation of equimolar ratios of homoduplex and heteroduplex species. The mixed products can be stored at 4°C for several weeks, or used immediately.
2. The temperatures needed for successful resolution of heteroduplex molecules are determined by running amplicon-specific melting curves and by using the DHPLC melting algorithm WAVE Maker of the WAVE instrument. Melting curves are determined as follows: the elution time of a specific fragment under standard conditions is determined. This specific gradient is then tested for the same PCR product for temperatures ranging from 48 to 70°C, and retention time vs temperature are graphed to yield a fragment-specific melting curve. The optimal analysis temperature is defined by a maximal decrease of retention time in a minimal temperature range. However, the complexity of the melting curve may

need between one and four different temperatures for fragment analysis. On average, three different temperatures to cover the entire DNA fragment of interest are necessary (*see* **Note 10**). The chosen temperatures are stored by the software and can be reused for subsequent samples for the same amplicon.

3. The (mixed) samples are loaded into the DHPLC machine and covered with a (96-well) rubber mat to avoid evaporation of the products. It is advisable to also use a negative control (water control of the PCR) and a positive control (a known aberration in the amplicon examined) during each DHPLC run. Enter whether you are using strips or plates into the DHPLC software and use an injection volume of 8 μL per (mixed) DNA sample per temperature.

4. The (mixed) samples are separated at a flow rate of 0.9 mL/min by means of a linear acetonitrile gradient. Generally, analysis takes approx 4 min/sample, including column regeneration and re-equilibration to starting conditions. The column mobile phase consists of a mixture of 0.1 M triethylamine acetate (pH 7.0) (buffer B) with 25% acetonitrile (buffer A).

5. Subsequently, the DHPLC is run with the optimal temperatures and gradients, and the results are stored for analysis.

3.3. Sequence Variation Identification by DNA Analysis

Whether sequence variations of aberrant DHPLC samples will be determined or variation in a patient's sequence will be directly identified, the methods for finding sequence variations remain the same. Always sequence samples from at least two different individuals, i.e., a confirmed healthy control DNA sample sequenced together with DNA samples of the patient(s) of interest. After the sequencing run on the ABI PRISM 310 DNA Analyzer (or similar machine), trim and reanalyze the sequence traces of all of the sequences with the ABI Sequence Analysis software. In this way, poor quality bases can be removed and the sequencing signal can be boosted. Subsequently, the ABI Factura program is used to mark and annotate sequence variations and areas of low signal quality. The final step is to align the cleaned-up sequences. For this, we use the ABI Sequence Navigator program. After importing eight sequences into the program (including a healthy control), "Clustal alignment" with the default settings will provide the best alignment. If necessary, sequences performed with a reverse primer can also be imported and converted to inversed complementary sequences to complete the alignment (*see* **Note 11**). After the alignment, we let the program mark all of the differences in a given position using the option "create shadow/compute ambiguity sequences." This marks all of the places in the alignment with possible differences, including homozygous mutations or polymorphisms (**Fig. 1**). Similar options for marking ambiguity in sequences are available in the ABI Auto Assembler program. We subsequently display the alignments at the points of interest (places with ambiguity) and determine the source of the ambiguity (**Fig. 1**). In case of a possible

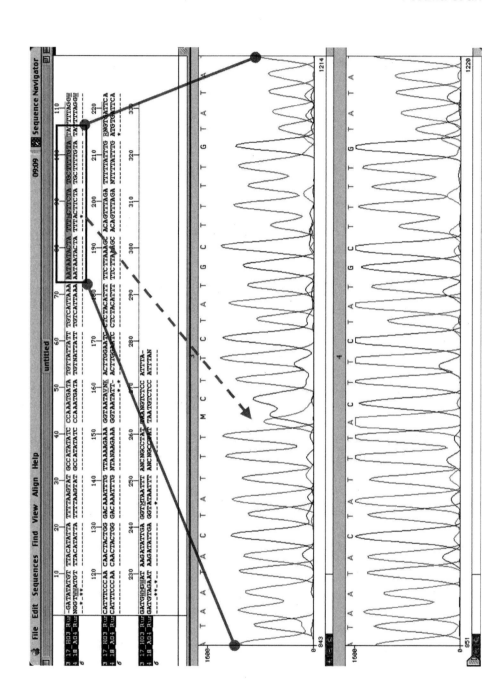

mutation, polymorphism, or disruption of the reading frame, screenshots are taken for archiving, and the sequence of interest can be printed. It is important to understand that sequence variations can always arise from the PCR technique itself and, therefore, aberrant sequences need to be validated by amplifying control DNA and patient DNA in a additional subsequent PCR reaction. Moreover, it is important to check whether the aberrant sequence is truly a mutation, or a (rare) polymorphism. In general, an aberration is labeled as a mutation if it is absent from more than 200 control alleles. However, the causality of any given mutation depends on DNA analysis in family members, coupled to the clinical history and expression analysis. This approach and good-quality sequences provide a balance between speed of analysis and accuracy. We use the sequencing techniques for various exons of *CASQ2* (*see* **Note 12**) and all of the *KCNJ2* samples. After identifying a possible mutation, it is imperative to finish screening the remaining exons as well.

3.4. Sequence Variation Identification by DHPLC Analysis

The main reason to perform DHPLC analysis is that it is a fast and accurate method for screening for mutations. Samples resulting in aberrant patterns always have to be sequenced to determine the nature of the sequence variation. Even if the DHPLC pattern resembles a pattern of a known polymorphism for the amplicon examined, sequencing is still necessary, because this does not exclude the possibility that a mutation close to the polymorphism is masked, or that an unknown mutation causes a similar pattern. DHPLC is used to filter out the wild-type sequences to decrease the amount of patient samples to be sequenced. It is important to analyze the patient's samples at each temperature indicated by the WAVE maker software, because some sequence aberrations can only be seen at one specific temperature. To obtain a reliable analysis, a second researcher should always check the DHPLC results. DHPLC samples are compared at each temperature, and any aberrant patterns are marked and printed for archiving purposes (**Fig. 2**). Subsequently, the sequence analysis on the aberrant samples can be performed directly from the PCR product loaded in the DHPLC machine using the methods described in **Subheading 3.2.3.** It is important to understand that amplicons with numerous sequence variations will severely hamper a reliable DHPLC analysis. Therefore, DHPLC analysis is only performed on amplicons that do not contain frequent polymorphisms (*see*

Fig. 1. (*opposite page*) Example of a clustal alignment of sequences in which any ambiguity between sequences is marked with an asterisk; in the lower panel, a close-up view of the ambiguity is displayed. Note that up to eight sequences can be aligned and analyzed at the same time.

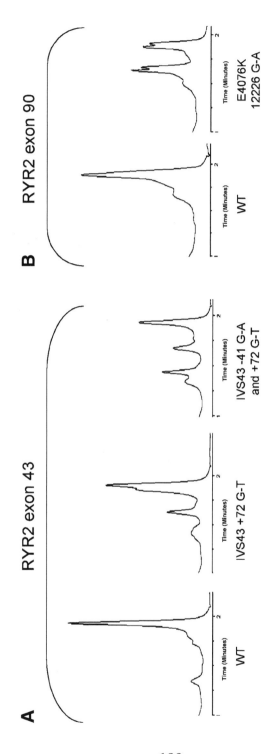

Fig. 2. Examples of aberrant DHPLC profiles caused by the presence of (**A**) no, one, or two polymorphisms in exon 43 of *RYR2*, and (**B**) a known mutation, E4076K, in exon 90 of *RYR2*.

Note 12). We use DHPLC analysis for the majority of the *CASQ2* samples and all of the *RYR2* samples. After identifying a possible mutation, it is imperative to finish screening the remaining exons as well.

4. Notes

1. Primers were designed with a target melting temperature of 60°C. It is important to design the forward and reverse primer in introns as far upstream or downstream as necessary, because this will ensure that any sequence variations around the splice sites and branch sites are included in the analysis. Make sure that the chosen primers do not overlap with single-nucleotide polymorphisms. Moreover, it is important to keep in mind that accurate DHPLC analysis is only possible ±50 bp downstream or upstream from any given primer. Primers for *RYR2* are available from Tiso et al. *(5)*; primers for *CASQ2* and *KCNJ2* are available from the authors on request.

2. Acetonitrile is a hazardous chemical and can penetrate the skin, therefore, caution is warranted when replacing the containers; always use gloves. Moreover, the waste product of the DHPLC machine also contains acetonitrile and it is, therefore, recommended to place a fume hood above the waste container to capture any hazardous fumes.

3. Betaine is used in the PCR and sequencing steps to reduce self-coiling of GC-rich areas and to lower melting temperatures; in our experience betaine has substantial beneficial effects on all PCR/sequence reactions.

4. In a PCR touch-down protocol, the annealing temperature is lowered (proportionally) for each successive cycle; the first cycle is performed at the first temperature indicated in the protocol and is subsequently lowered each cycle until the last temperature mentioned is reached at the end of the final cycle.

5. Sequence reactions can be purified using spin columns or gel filtration, however, in our experience, a dilution of 1:5 of the PCR product works equally well, and saves time and costs. If the dilution of a PCR product produces unusable results during sequencing, one can always revert to other methods of purification.

6. If the product is GC rich, it might help if the temperature of the annealing step of the sequencing reaction is raised, for instance from 50°C to 55°C or even 58°C.

7. When using DHPLC in patient analysis, it is crucial to use PCR reaction buffers that do not contain solvent or detergents (found in most PCR buffers), such as dimethylsulfoxide, glycerol, Tween-20, or betaine. These products can damage the columns of the DHPLC machine; therefore, PCR buffers without such products should be used. However, if these products are necessary for a specific PCR, the PCR products can be filtered by column purification and subsequently used in the DHPLC.

8. PCR products for subsequent DHPLC analysis need to be specific; any double bands or smears on gel analysis point to a PCR with side products. These side products will interfere with the DHPLC analysis by producing incorrect patterns and might even mask real polymorphisms or mutations.

9. Homozygous mutations are difficult to detect in a DHPLC because aberrant homozygous patterns might differ only slightly, or even not at all, compared with homozygous normal alleles. Mixing of wild-type DNA with patient DNA results in heteroduplexes that are easier to detect. However, in case of a clear family history with autosomal-dominant inheritance (most of the CPVT cases) one could take the risk to analyze patient DNA without mixing with wild-type DNA to speed analysis.

10. A set of random samples plus a positive control is to be used for the initial optimization of the PCR amplicons of interest. The DHPLC conditions are adjusted so that the elution profile of the positive control is different from the wild-type sample. When no positive control is available, conditions are considered to be optimal at the temperature and corresponding gradient immediately before a significant decrease in the retention time of the amplicon and/or an excessive broadening of the peak, indicating excess denaturation. Useful temperatures are typically located in the range of 50 to 75% of the helical fraction for the amplicons analyzed.

11. Initially unidirectional sequencing per patient is used (i.e., only a forward primer). If aberrant sequences are found, a new PCR is performed, and, in the subsequent sequence reaction, both the forward and reverse primers are used.

12. Direct sequencing is warranted for *CASQ2* exons 1, 7 (contains a poly T tail in the 5' intron; therefore, a reverse primer is recommended), 8, 9, and 10 because they contain numerous polymorphisms.

References

1. Priori, S. G., Napolitano, C., Tiso, N., et al. (2001) Mutations in the cardiac ryanodine receptor gene (hRyR2) underlie catecholaminergic polymorphic ventricular tachycardia. *Circulation* **103(2)**, 196–200.
2. Priori, S. G., Napolitano, C., Memmi, M., et al. (2002) Clinical and molecular characterization of patients with catecholaminergic polymorphic ventricular tachycardia. *Circulation* **106(1)**, 69–74.
3. Postma, A. V., Denjoy, I., Hoorntje, T. M., et al. (2002) Absence of calsequestrin 2 causes severe forms of catecholaminergic polymorphic ventricular tachycardia. *Circ. Res.* **91(8)**, e21–26.
4. Swan, H., Piippo, K., Viitasalo, M., et al. (1999) Arrhythmic disorder mapped to chromosome 1q42-q43 causes malignant polymorphic ventricular tachycardia in structurally normal hearts. *J. Am. Coll. Cardiol.* **34(7)**, 2035–2042.
5. Tiso, N., Stephan, D. A., Nava, A., et al. (2001) Identification of mutations in the cardiac ryanodine receptor gene in families affected with arrhythmogenic right ventricular cardiomyopathy type 2 (ARVD2). *Hum. Mol. Genet.* **10(3)**, 189–194.
6. Laitinen, P. J., Brown, K. M., Piippo, K., et al. (2001) Mutations of the cardiac ryanodine receptor (RyR2) gene in familial polymorphic ventricular tachycardia. *Circulation* **103(4)**, 485–490.

7. Bauce, B., Rampazzo, A., Basso, C., et al. (2002) Screening for ryanodine receptor type 2 mutations in families with effort-induced polymorphic ventricular arrhythmias and sudden death: early diagnosis of asymptomatic carriers. *J. Am. Coll. Cardiol.* **40(2),** 341–349.

8. Postma, A. V., Denjoy, I., Kamblock, J., et al. (2005) Catecholaminergic polymorphic ventricular tachycardia: RYR2 mutations, bradycardia, and follow-up of the patients. *J. Med. Gen.* **42,** 863–870.

9. Meissner, G. (2002) Regulation of mammalian ryanodine receptors. *Front. Biosci.* **7,** d2072–2080.

10. Lahat, H., Pras, E., Olender, T., et al. (2001) A missense mutation in a highly conserved region of CASQ2 is associated with autosomal recessive catecholamine-induced polymorphic ventricular tachycardia in Bedouin families from Israel. *Am. J. Hum. Genet.* **69(6),** 1378–1384.

11. Plaster, N. M., Tawil, R., Tristani-Firouzi, M., et al. (2001) Mutations in Kir2.1 cause the developmental and episodic electrical phenotypes of Andersen's syndrome. *Cell* **105(4),** 511–519.

12. Andelfinger, G., Tapper, A. R., Welch, R. C., et al. (2002) KCNJ2 mutation results in Andersen syndrome with sex-specific cardiac and skeletal muscle phenotypes. *Am. J. Hum. Genet.* **71(3),** 663–668.

13. Donaldson, M. R., Jensen, J. L., Tristani-Firouzi, M., et al. (2003) PIP2 binding residues of Kir2.1 are common targets of mutations causing Andersen syndrome. *Neurology* **60(11),** 1811–1816.

11

Mutation Detection in Tumor Suppressor Genes Using Archival Tissue Specimens

Aristotelis Astrinidis and Elizabeth Petri Henske

Summary

Tuberous sclerosis complex (TSC) is a neurocutaneous syndrome characterized by seizures, mental retardation, and benign tumors of many organs, including the brain, kidneys, skin, retina, and heart. TSC is caused by mutations in the *TSC1* and *TSC2* tumor suppressor genes. The genes follow the two-hit model for tumorigenesis, with germline mutations inactivating one allele and somatic mutations inactivating the remaining wild-type allele. Allelic loss (also called loss of heterozygosity [LOH]) in the 9q34 and 16p13 regions has been found in many tumor types from TSC patients. Cardiac rhabdomyomas are frequently found in infants with TSC. Because rhabdomyomas often spontaneously regress, access to fresh tissue is limited. In this chapter, we present methodology for detection of genetic inactivation of *TSC1* and *TSC2* in paraffin-embedded archival tissues. The template DNA is obtained either by direct scraping of tissue or after laser capture microdissection. LOH analysis is performed after polymerase chain reaction amplification of microsatellite markers in the 9q34 and 16p13 regions and denaturing polyacrylamide gel electrophoresis. Mutation detection is performed using single-strand conformation polymorphisms on mutation detection enhancement gels. Finally, variant bands are amplified and analyzed by direct sequencing.

Key Words: Tuberous sclerosis complex (TSC); *TSC1*; *TSC2*; tumor suppressor genes; rhabdomyomas; laser capture microdissection (LCM); loss of heterozygosity (LOH); single-strand conformation polymorphisms (SSCP); direct sequencing; variant bands.

1. Introduction

Rhabdomyomas, which are the most common pediatric cardiac neoplasm, are frequently associated with tuberous sclerosis complex (TSC) *(1)*. TSC is an autosomal-dominant syndrome characterized by seizures, mental retardation, autism, and benign tumors of the brain, heart, kidney, and skin *(2,3)*. Mutations in the *TSC1* or *TSC2* tumor suppressor genes cause TSC *(4,5)* and pulmonary lymphangioleiomyomatosis *(6,7)*. According to Knudson's two-hit hypothesis for tumorigenesis, two mutational events are necessary for tumor

From: *Methods in Molecular Medicine, vol. 126: Congenital Heart Disease: Molecular Diagnostics*
Edited by: M. Kearns-Jonker © Humana Press Inc., Totowa, NJ

initiation; the first is a germline or somatic mutation, in familial or sporadic cases, respectively *(8)*. The second event affects the remaining wild-type allele of the tumor suppressor gene and is usually a deletion of a chromosomal region, which is termed allelic loss or loss of heterozygosity (LOH). However, it is not unusual for the second hit to be a smaller mutation, such as a nonsense or missense mutation.

Rhabdomyomas arise during fetal development, and usually spontaneously regress during early childhood *(9)*. Therefore, surgical resection is usually avoided, access to tissue (particularly fresh tissue) is very limited, and relatively little is known about their pathogenesis. This chapter focuses on the methods for genetic analysis of the *TSC1* and *TSC2* genes using archival, paraffin-embedded tissue specimens. Template DNA can be obtained either by direct scraping from tissue sections or after laser capture microdissection (LCM). Two types of genetic analyses are described: LOH using microsatellite markers, and mutational analysis using single-strand conformation polymorphisms (SSCP) followed by direct sequencing. Although the methodology refers to the *TSC1* and *TSC2* genes, it can be applied in any tumor suppressor gene.

The complexity of the *TSC1* and *TSC2* genes, with 21 and 41 coding exons, respectively, and the absence of obvious mutational hot spots in either gene, make screening for mutations challenging. All mutations in *TSC1* cause premature protein termination (nonsense or frameshift mutations), whereas, in *TSC2*, there are also missense mutations *(10–13)*. LOH has been found in 60% of renal angiomyolipomas *(14,15)*, and in pulmonary lymphangioleiomyomatosis *(6,16,17)*. LOH in TSC tumors is more frequent in the *TSC2* gene region of chromosome 16p13 *(18)*, than in the *TSC1* region (9q34).

2. Materials

1. Xylene.
2. Harry's modified hematoxylin solution.
3. Eosin Y solution.
4. Histology slide extraction buffer: 50 mM KCl, 10 mM Tris-HCl, pH 8.3, 1.5 mM MgCl$_2$, 100 µg/mL bovine serum albumin, 0.45% v/v Tween-20, 0.45% v/v Nonidet P-40.
   Sterilize by filtering, aliquot, and store at –20°C. Before using, add proteinase K at a final concentration of 1 mg/mL.
5. PixCell II LCM microscope, and CapSure transfer caps (Arcturus Biosciences, Mountain View, CA).
6. 10X TK buffer: 500 mM Tris-HCl, pH 8.9, 10 mM NaCl, 20 mM EDTA, 5% v/v Tween-20.
   Sterilize by filtering, aliquot, and store at –20°C. Before using, add proteinase K at a final concentration of 2 mg/mL.

7. Taq DNA polymerase, 10X polymerase buffer, and 50 mM MgCl$_2$.
8. dNTP mix: 10 mM of each dATP, dCTP, dGTP and dTTP.
9. α[^{32}P]-dCTP, 3000 Ci/mmol, 10 mCi/mL.
10. 10 μM oligonucleotide primers for the microsatellite markers (Invitrogen, Carlsbad, CA), and for each of the exons of *TSC1* and *TSC2*.
11. Mineral oil.
12. Vertical polyacrylamide gel unit (30-cm height, 38-cm width) with 0.4-mm spacers and shark tooth-type comb.
13. Siliconizing solution (i.e., Sigmacoat; Sigma, St. Louis, MO).
14. 10X Tris-borate-EDTA (TBE) buffer: 0.89 M Tris-borate, pH 8.3, 0.02 M EDTA.
15. 40% acrylamide gel solution: 38% w/v acrylamide, 2% w/v *bis*-acrylamide (N,N'-methylene*bis*acrylamide).
    Filter and store at 4°C in tinted bottle.
16. Urea.
17. 10% w/v ammonium persulfate. Store in aliquots at –20°C.
18. TEMED.
19. 2X denaturing loading buffer. Store in aliquots at –20°C: 50% formamide, 0.1% bromophenol blue, 0.1% xylene cyanol.
20. 3MM Whatman chromatography paper.
21. 2X mutation detection enhancement (MDE) gel solution (Cambrex, East Rutherford, NJ).
22. Agarose gel electrophoresis unit.
23. Polymerase chain reaction (PCR) purification kit (i.e., Qiagen, Valencia, CA).
24. Gel extraction kit (i.e., Qiagen).
25. Tris-HCl-EDTA (TE) buffer: 10 mM Tris-HCl, pH 8.0, 1 mM EDTA.
26. Self-stick fluorescent labels.

3. Methods

The methods below describe in detail:

1. The extraction of DNA either directly from the histology slide, or from LCM material.
2. LOH analysis using microsatellite markers.
3. SSCP to detect variant bands.
4. Direct sequencing of variant bands to detect mutations or polymorphisms.
5. Analysis of LOH and SSCP/direct sequencing results.

3.1. Extraction of DNA From Archival Tissue Specimens

Archival, paraffin-embedded tissue can be used for the extraction and amplification of DNA (*see* **Note 1**). If the tissue under investigation is homogenous and clearly defined, direct scraping and extraction can be used. If the tissue of interest is small or the cells of interest are mixed with normal cells, a microdissection procedure can be used. From the several microdissection methods available, we use the LCM, which was developed by the National Institutes of Health (*19*) and marketed by Arcturus Biosciences Inc.

3.1.1. Preparation of Hematoxylin and Eosin-Stained Slides

1. Cut 5- to 7-μm-thick sections and mount on microscopy slides. Use uncoated slides for LCM.
2. Remove paraffin by dipping slides twice in xylene for 2 min.
3. Rehydrate tissue by dipping for 2 min in decreasing ethanol concentrations: twice in 100% ethanol, once in 95% ethanol, and once in 70% ethanol. Rehydrate completely twice in dH_2O for 2 min.
4. Dip slide in hematoxylin solution for 10 s.
5. Rinse slide twice in dH_2O (three dips).
6. Dip slide for 2 min in 70 and 95% ethanol, consecutively.
7. Dip slide in eosin Y (five dips).
8. Wash slide twice in 95% ethanol for 2 min.
9. Dehydrate slide in 100% ethanol for 2 min.
10. Air-dry slide. Do not allow excessive drying if slides are to be used for LCM.

3.1.2. Scraping of Tissue Directly Into DNA Histology Slide Extraction Buffer

1. Use a hematoxylin and eosin-stained section to identify the area to be used for DNA extraction. Mark the area of interest on an adjacent *unstained* slide with a fine-tip permanent marker.
2. Using a clean razor blade, remove all excess paraffin from the unstained slide.
3. Scrape the tissue from the area of interest, avoiding normal tissue.
4. Using a sterile microbiological loop, transfer the tissue into histology slide extraction buffer (~150 μL/cm^2 of tissue, *see* **Note 2**).
5. Vortex briefly and incubate at 65°C overnight.
6. Heat inactivate proteinase K at 95°C for 10 min.
7. Spin briefly, aliquot extracted DNA, and store at –20°C.

3.1.3. Use of LCM to Obtain Tissue

In LCM, a microscope is used to facilitate the visualization of lightly stained tissue sections. A transparent cap with a polymer (capturing film) rests on top of the tissue section under the objective lens. The user can fire a laser beam, which melts and attaches the polymer to the underlying tissue. The precision of LCM has allowed researchers to capture single cells from tissue sections (*see* **Note 3**).

1. Prepare 1X TK buffer by a 1:10 dilution of 10X TK buffer in dH_2O.
2. Perform LCM on a lightly hematoxylin and eosin-stained uncoated slide.
3. If capturing more than 100 cells, add 50 μL of 1X TK buffer on top of the CapSure cap. Cap a 0.5-mL microcentrifuge tube using the tool provided by the manufacturer. Invert the tube so that the extraction solution is always in contact with the captured cells. Incubate at 55°C overnight.
4. If capturing less than 100 cells, use a sterile scalpel to excise the area of transfer film containing the captured cells. Using sterile forceps, transfer the film into a

0.2-mL PCR tube, add 10 to 20 μL of 1X TK buffer, and incubate at 55°C overnight.
5. Spin tubes briefly. Heat inactivate proteinase K at 95°C for 10 min.
6. Store extracted DNA at –20°C.

3.2. PCR Amplification for LOH and SSCP Analysis

Because the fixatives used in archival tissue damage nucleic acids, it is difficult to amplify targets larger than 300 bp, and it is advisable to choose or design primers that will amplify DNA fragments smaller than 200 bp. For the *TSC1* genomic region (chromosomal location 9q34), we use the D9S1198 and D9S1199 microsatellite markers. For the *TSC2* genomic region (16p13), we use D16S291, D16S418, D16S475, D16S663, and Kg8. The primer information for the *TSC1* and *TSC2* exons has been previously published *(20,21)*. Normal DNA adjacent to the tumor analyzed must always be included in the study to provide positive controls for the presence of heterozygosity and/or the normal SSCP pattern. The PCR products are radiolabeled by direct incorporation of ^{32}P-dCTP in the reaction, resolved in polyacrylamide gels, and visualized after autoradiography (*see* **Note 4**).

1. Dilute DNA samples extracted directly from pathology slides 1:10 to 1:100 in dH$_2$O. DNA after LCM must *not* be diluted. Use 2 μL of DNA sample per reaction.
2. In a 0.2-mL PCR tube (or 96-well PCR plate for multiple samples), set up a 10-μL PCR reaction according to **Table 1**.
3. Overlay PCR reactions with 10 μL mineral oil.
4. Perform the amplification using the following cycling conditions: 95°C for 5 min, 30 cycles of (95°C for 30 s; 55°C for 30 s; and 72°C for 30 s), 72°C for 5 min (*see* **Note 5**).
5. Store the samples at –20°C until analyzed.

3.3. LOH Analysis Using Microsatellite Markers

LOH analysis is performed after PCR amplification of highly polymorphic microsatellite markers that are close to the gene of interest. Microsatellite markers in unrelated chromosomal locations are used as negative controls. The PCR products are resolved in denaturing polyacrylamide gels.

3.3.1. Preparation of Denaturing Polyacrylamide Gel

1. Wash the glass plates of the vertical electrophoresis unit thoroughly and dry.
2. Under a fume hood, apply 0.5 to 1 mL of siliconizing solution onto a small piece of tissue paper and smear on the inner surface of the back glass plate. Remove traces of siliconizing solution by washing the glass plate with dH$_2$O. Wipe and allow to air-dry (*see* **Note 6**).
3. Wash the inner surface of the front glass plate with 70% ethanol. Wipe and allow to air-dry.

Table 1
PCR Reaction for LOH and SSCP Analysis

	Final concentration	Volume (mL)
10X PCR buffer	1X	1.0
50 mM MgCl$_2$	1.5 mM	0.3
10 mM dNTP mix	0.2 mM	0.2
10 μM forward primer	1.5 μM	1.5
10 μM reverse primer	1.5 μM	1.5
DNA		2.0
10 μCi/μL of α[^{32}P]-dCTP	0.1 μCi/μL	0.1
dH$_2$O		3.0
5 U/μL of *Taq* polymerase	0.2 U/μL	0.4
Total		10.0

4. Assemble the unit and lay flat, back plate facing up. Clean the comb with ethanol, and dry.
5. Prepare gel solution by mixing 5 mL of 10X TBE, 7.5 mL of 40% acrylamide gel solution, and 21 g of urea, in a final volume of 50 mL (*see* **Note 7**).
6. Add 350 μL of 10% ammonium persulfate and mix.
7. Add 20 μL TEMED and mix.
8. Using a 50-mL syringe, pour the acrylamide gel solution between the two glass plates. Gently tap the top glass plate to avoid formation of air bubbles. Fill the unit with gel solution to the top.
9. Insert the straight edge of the comb between the two glass plates, approx 5 mm from the edge of the glass plate. Clamp the two glass plates together using three large paper clamps (*see* **Note 8**).
10. Let gel polymerize for 1 h.
11. Remove the clamps. Remove the comb and clean it.

3.3.2. Electrophoresis and Autoradiography

1. Use 1X TBE as the running buffer. Prerun the gel at 65W for 15 min, until the gel temperature is 55°C (*see* **Note 9**).
2. Add an equal volume of 2X denaturing loading buffer into each PCR reaction.
3. Denature DNA by heating at 99°C for 5 min. Immediately put in ice for 2 min.
4. Stop the prerun and flush the gel surface with running buffer. Insert the comb between the two glass plates, so that the shark teeth are buried 1 mm in the polyacrylamide gel.
5. Load 4 μL of the denatured samples.
6. Perform the electrophoresis at 55W, maintaining the gel temperature at 55°C, until the bromophenol blue front reaches the bottom of the gel.

7. Stop the electrophoresis and disassemble the unit. Lay the glass plates flat, back plate on top. *Gently* separate the glass plates by inserting a spatula between them. Place a 3MM Whatman paper on top of the gel. Allow the 3MM Whatman paper to stick for a few minutes, and slowly lift one end of the filter paper. Cover the gel with plastic wrap, place in gel drier, and dry under vacuum at 80°C for 1 h.
8. Perform autoradiography at –80°C, using intensifying screens.

3.4. Mutational Analysis Using SSCP

SSCP is based on the ability of single-stranded DNA molecules to migrate in nondenaturing polyacrylamide gels. The mobility of those molecules depends on the DNA sequence; single nucleotide changes can greatly affect the mobility, resulting in mobility shifts between the test and wild-type DNA. Although SSCP is not a very sensitive mutation detection method (70–80% detection rate of mutant DNA species), it is simple and fairly cost effective when analyzing large number of samples.

3.4.1. Preparation of SSCP Gel

1. Follow **steps 1–4** of **Subheading 3.3.1.**
2. Prepare gel solution by mixing 3 mL of 10X TBE and 12.5 mL of 2X MDE gel solution, in a final volume of 50 mL.
3. Add 200 µL of 10% ammonium persulfate and mix.
4. Add 20 µL of TEMED and mix.
5. Follow **steps 8–11** of **Subheading 3.3.1.**

3.4.2. Electrophoresis

1. Add an equal volume of 2X denaturing loading buffer in each PCR reaction.
2. Heat at 99°C for 5 min, then snap-chill on ice for 5 min.
3. Flush the surface of the SSCP gel with running buffer (1X TBE). Insert the comb so that the shark teeth are buried 1 mm in the polyacrylamide gel.
4. Load 4 µL of sample in each well.
5. Perform electrophoresis at 100 to 160V for 16 to 24 h (*see* **Note 10**). Follow **Subheading 3.3.2., steps 7** and **8.**

3.5. Direct DNA Sequencing

SSCP analysis is indicative of the presence of a nucleotide change in the test DNA. In many instances, false-positive results and complex banding patterns arise from DNA molecules that have more than one stable three-dimensional conformation. To exclude the possibility that the variant band is caused by an error during DNA amplification, a second, independent, confirmation of the SSCP result is needed. Finally, direct sequencing is used to identify the exact nucleotide change. Direct sequencing can be performed after PCR amplification of DNA extracted from tissue sections or LCM material, or from variant bands.

3.5.1. Extraction of DNA From Variant Bands

1. Line up the autoradiography with the dried SSCP gel over a light box (*see* **Note 11**).
2. Mark the region of the gel corresponding to a variant band with a fine-tipped marker.
3. Cut the filter paper and gel containing the variant band, allowing a 2-mm margin on each side.
4. Immerse the cutout filter paper/gel in 100 μL dH$_2$O for 1 h.
5. Aspirate as much liquid as possible, and store gel at –20°C.

3.5.2. Amplification and Purification of DNA for Direct Sequencing

1. Use DNA from scraped paraffin-embedded tissue, LCM, or from a variant band.
2. Set up a 50-μL PCR reaction according to **Table 2**.
3. Overlay the reaction with 20 μL mineral oil.
4. Use the optimized cycling conditions for the specific exon.
5. Resolve one-tenth (5 μL) of the PCR reaction in an 1% agarose/0.5X TBE vertical gel.
6. If PCR product *does not* have nonspecific bands, use a PCR purification kit to purify DNA from buffer, dNTPs, primers, and enzyme. Elute in the smallest possible amount of TE buffer or dH$_2$O.
7. If PCR product *has* nonspecific bands, resolve the remaining PCR reaction on an agarose gel, excise the appropriate gel slice, and purify using a gel purification kit. Elute in the smallest possible amount of TE buffer or dH$_2$O.
8. Perform direct sequencing in the purified PCR product with the primers used for amplification.

3.6. Analysis of LOH and SSCP/Direct Sequencing Results

3.6.1. Reading an LOH Gel

LOH is observed as an absence of an allelic band in the tumor sample, compared with the presence of both allelic bands in the normal sample for heterozygous markers. In some instances, normal DNA can contaminate the tumor sample. In this case, the observed LOH is not complete. Because smaller DNA fragments are favored during a PCR amplification reaction, LOH is harder to demonstrate for the smaller of the two alleles of a heterozygous marker.

3.6.2. Distinguishing Mutations From Polymorphisms After DNA Sequencing

Some of the variations observed in the *TSC1* or *TSC2* genes are caused by common polymorphisms. These are easy to identify because they occur in high frequencies (>0.05) in the general population. Frameshifting and nonsense mutations are considered disease-causing mutations, because they both result in premature termination of protein synthesis. Missense mutations are harder to classify as disease-causing or rare polymorphisms. If the mutation is identi-

Table 2
PCR Reaction for Direct Sequencing Analysis

	Final concentration	Volume (mL)
10X PCR buffer	1X	5.0
50 mM MgCl$_2$	1.5 mM	1.5
10 mM dNTP mix	0.2 mM	1.0
10 μM forward primer	1.5 μM	7.5
10 μM reverse primer	1.5 μM	7.5
DNA		5.0
dH$_2$O		20.5
5 U/μL of Taq polymerase	0.2 U/μL	2.0
Total		50.0

fied in normal DNA, the researcher can test normal DNA from other members of the family. A disease-causing mutation will segregate with the affected individuals of a large pedigree. Parental DNA can be particularly informative in patients with TSC whose parents are unaffected. Approximately 60% of TSC patients represent new germline mutations. In these cases, the disease-causing mutation will not be present in parental DNA. However, in complex disorders, such as TSC, extensive clinical evaluation may be needed to exclude a diagnosis in the parents.

4. Notes

1. In addition to the tissue of interest, DNA from normal cells must also be obtained. The normal DNA is essential for LOH, and may be needed for SSCP studies to distinguish between germline and somatic mutations. Peripheral blood lymphocytes are a good source of high quality normal DNA, although any normal tissue can be used, including microdissected normal cells adjacent to the tumor.
2. This amount of buffer is critical. Using too much or too little buffer will impair the DNA amplification.
3. Slide preparation and staining will greatly affect the conditions (pulse duration and power of laser beam) for successful capture. It is preferable to stain the slide and perform the capture the same day. If LCM is to be performed on another day, the slides can be stored in a desiccator. However, storing for long periods is not indicated, because the tissue tends to adhere more strongly to the glass slide. If the cells are resistant to capture, try increasing the power and duration of the laser pulse. If the cells of interest are morphologically indistinguishable from the surrounding cells, immunohistochemically stained slides with a marker specific to the cells of interest can be used.
4. We regularly use 1 to 2.5 μL of extracted DNA in a standard 10-μL PCR reaction. It is advisable to optimize PCR conditions, using as low as 0.5 ng of high-

quality template (i.e., genomic DNA from peripheral blood or cultured cells). Because the amount of template DNA per reaction is very small (especially for LCM-extracted DNA), take additional precautions to prevent cross contamination. Always include a dH_2O control PCR reaction. When setting up PCR reactions, use aerosol-barrier tips and a designated set of automatic pipettors.

5. The annealing temperature (55°C) must be optimized for each oligonucleotide pair. PCR conditions that are optimal for other sources of high-quality DNA may need reoptimization when amplifying archival DNA. In some instances, the annealing temperature is significantly lower (5–10°C) for archival DNA. If nonspecific DNA fragments are present that cannot be removed after optimization, a "hot-start" technique should be used. It is best to amplify and analyze multiple patients at the same time, so that it is easier to identify the alleles and banding patterns during LOH and SSCP analyses, respectively.

6. Siliconizing solutions are volatile and toxic. They should be applied in a fume hood. After siliconization, *do not* wash this plate with ethanol. It is best if the same glass plate is siliconized each time. Some researchers use bonding solutions for the opposite (front) glass plate, but we find that unnecessary.

7. Urea dissolves better in warm solution. However, the acrylamide solution must be allowed to cool at room temperature before adding ammonium persulfate and TEMED, otherwise, rapid polymerization will occur.

8. Clamping the two glass plates together is necessary for appropriate and uniform gel thickness, and eliminates cross contamination of samples during loading. The acrylamide solution polymerizes within 30 to 45 min, but the gel should not be used for an additional 2 h. The gel can be stored at 4°C overnight, but it must be equilibrated at room temperature for at least 2 h before use.

9. The wattage of the electrophoresis depends on the gel surface. The wattages suggested are for 30 × 38-cm gels. Gel temperature should be maintained at 50°C to 60°C during the electrophoresis of samples.

10. Single-stranded DNAs are better resolved in low-voltage runs. Increasing the voltage excessively will increase the temperature of the gel and destroy the three-dimensional conformations of the single-stranded DNA. Several conditions can affect the mobility of single-stranded DNAs and the ability of SSCP to distinguish between wild-type and mutant molecules. Two of the conditions commonly used are: the addition of 10% glycerol in the nondenaturing gels, and electrophoresis at 4°C. In the latter case, equilibrate the gel and running buffer temperature at 4°C for at least 2 h before loading.

11. Use fluorescent labels during autoradiography for easy orientation.

References

1. Webb, D., Thomas, R. D., and Osborne, J. (1993) Cardiac rhabdomyomas and their association with tuberous sclerosis. *Arch. Dis. Child.* **68,** 367–370.

2. Roach, E. S., Gomez, M. R., and Northrup, H. (1998) Tuberous sclerosis complex consensus conference: revised clinical diagnostic criteria. *J. Child. Neurol.* **13,** 624–628.

3. Gomez, M., Sampson, J. R., and Whittemore, V. H. (1999) *Tuberous Sclerosis Complex*, 3rd ed, Oxford University Press, New York.

4. The European Chromosome 16 Tuberous Sclerosis Consortium. (1993) Identification and characterization of the tuberous sclerosis gene on chromosome 16. *Cell* **75**, 1305–1315.
5. van Slegtenhorst, M., de Hoogt, R., Hermans, C., et al. (1997) Identification of the tuberous sclerosis gene TSC1 on chromosome 9q34. *Science* **277**, 805–808.
6. Carsillo, T., Astrinidis, A., and Henske, E. P. (2000) Mutations in the tuberous sclerosis complex gene TSC2 are a cause of sporadic pulmonary lymphangioleiomyomatosis. *Proc. Natl. Acad. Sci. USA* **97**, 6085–6090.
7. Sato, T., Seyama, K., Fujii, H., et al. (2002) Mutation analysis of the TSC1 and TSC2 genes in Japanese patients with pulmonary lymphangioleiomyomatosis. *J. Hum. Genet.* **47**, 20–28.
8. Knudson, A. (1971) Mutation and cancer: statistical study of retinoblastoma. *Proc. Natl. Acad. Sci. USA* **68**, 820–823.
9. Bosi, G., Lintermans, J. P., Pellegrino, P. A., Svaluto-Moreolo, G., and Vliers, A. (1996) The natural history of cardiac rhabdomyoma with and without tuberous sclerosis. *Acta. Paediatr.* **85**, 928–931.
10. Jones, A. C., Shyamsundar, M. M., Thomas, M. W., et al. (1999) Comprehensive mutation analysis of TSC1 and TSC2-and phenotypic correlations in 150 families with tuberous sclerosis. *Am. J. Hum. Genet.* **64**, 1305–1315.
11. Niida, Y., Lawrence-Smith, N., Banwell, A., et al. (1999) Analysis of both TSC1 and TSC2 for germline mutations in 126 unrelated patients with tuberous sclerosis. *Hum. Mutat.* **14**, 412–422.
12. van Slegtenhorst, M., Verhoef, S., Tempelaars, A., et al. (1999) Mutational spectrum of the TSC1 gene in a cohort of 225 tuberous sclerosis complex patients: no evidence for genotype-phenotype correlation. *J. Med. Genet.* **36**, 285–289.
13. Dabora, S. L., Jozwiak, S., Franz, D. N., et al. (2001) Mutational analysis in a cohort of 224 tuberous sclerosis patients indicates increased severity of TSC2, compared with TSC1, disease in multiple organs. *Am. J. Hum. Genet.* **68**, 64–80.
14. Carbonara, C., Longa, L., Grosso, E., et al. (1994) 9q34 loss of heterozygosity in a tuberous sclerosis astrocytoma suggests a growth suppressor-like activity also for the TSC1 gene. *Hum. Mol. Genet.* **3**, 1829–1832.
15. Henske, E. P., Neumann, H. P., Scheithauer, B. W., Herbst, E. W., Short, M. P., and Kwiatkowski, D. J. (1995) Loss of heterozygosity in the tuberous sclerosis (TSC2) region of chromosome band 16p13 occurs in sporadic as well as TSC-associated renal angiomyolipomas. *Genes Chromosomes Cancer* **13**, 295–298.
16. Smolarek, T. A., Wessner, L. L., McCormack, F. X., Mylet, J. C., Menon, A. G., and Henske, E. P. (1998) Evidence that lymphangiomyomatosis is caused by TSC2 mutations: chromosome 16p13 loss of heterozygosity in angiomyolipomas and lymph nodes from women with lymphangiomyomatosis. *Am. J. Hum. Genet.* **62**, 810–815.
17. Yu, J., Astrinidis, A., and Henske, E. P. (2001) Chromosome 16 loss of heterozygosity in tuberous sclerosis and sporadic lymphangiomyomatosis. *Am. J. Respir. Crit. Care. Med.* **164**, 1537–1540.
18. Carbonara, C., Longa, L., Grosso, E., et al. (1996) Apparent preferential loss of heterozygosity at TSC2 over TSC1 chromosomal region in tuberous sclerosis hamartomas. *Genes Chromosomes Cancer* **15**, 18–25.

19. Emmert-Buck, M. R., Bonner, R. F., Smith, P. D., et al. (1996) Laser capture microdissection. *Science* **274,** 998–1001.

20. Hornigold, N., Devlin, J., Davies, A., Aveyard, J., Habuchi, T., and Knowles, M. (1999) Mutation of the 9q34 gene TSC1 in sporadic bladder cancer. *Oncogene* **18,** 2657–2661.

21. Au, K.-S., Rodriguez, J., Finch, J., et al. (1997) Germ-line mutational analysis of the TSC2 gene in 90 tuberous sclerosis patients. *Am. J. Hum. Genet.* **62,** 286–294.

12

Friedreich Ataxia

Detection of GAA Repeat Expansions and Frataxin Point Mutations

Massimo Pandolfo

Summary

Friedreich ataxia (FA) is an autosomal-recessive disease primarily characterized by progressive neurological disability. A significant proportion of patients also present with a hypertrophic cardiomyopathy, which may, in some cases, cause premature death. FA is caused by insufficient levels of the protein, frataxin, which is involved in mitochondrial iron metabolism. All patients carry at least one copy of an intronic GAA triplet-repeat expansion that interferes with frataxin transcription. Normal chromosomes contain up to 35 to 40 GAA triplets in an Alu sequence localized in the first intron of the frataxin gene; FA chromosomes carry from approx 70 to more than 1000 GAA triplets. The molecular diagnosis of FA is, therefore, based on the detection of this expansion, which is present in homozygosity in more than 95% of the cases. The remaining patients are heterozygous for the GAA expansion and carry a frataxin point mutation as the other pathogenic allele. The expanded GAA triplet repeat may be detected by polymerase chain reaction (PCR) amplification followed by agarose gel electrophoresis analysis. In our hands, carefully performed PCR testing, in particular, if fragment detection is enhanced by hybridization with a GAA oligonucleotide probe, is as effective in identifying patients and carriers as is Southern blot analysis of genomic DNA, and allows a more accurate sizing of the repeat. Furthermore, in the case of smaller expansions, the amplified fragment may be directly sequenced to identify very rare nonpathogenic variant repeats, such as GAAGGA. Sequence analysis of the five coding exons of the frataxin gene should be performed in clinically affected individuals who are heterozygous for an expanded GAA repeat to identify point mutations.

Key Words: Ataxia; neurodegenerative diseases; cardiomyopathies; expanded triplet repeats; mutation analysis; polymerase chain reaction; Southern blot; DNA sequencing.

From: *Methods in Molecular Medicine, vol. 126: Congenital Heart Disease: Molecular Diagnostics*
Edited by: M. Kearns-Jonker © Humana Press Inc., Totowa, NJ

1. Introduction

Friedreich ataxia (FA) is an autosomal-recessive disease characterized by progressive neurological disability, cardiomyopathy, and increased risk of diabetes mellitus. The disease, which currently has no treatment, affects roughly 2 to 3 in 100,000 people. Because of a founder effect of the main responsible mutation, the disease only affects individuals of European, North African, Middle Eastern, and Indian origins. In most cases, the neurological symptoms dominate the clinical picture, however, a significant proportion of patients have their life shortened because of heart disease. In addition, rare patients have disease onset with symptoms and signs of cardiomyopathy.

1.1. Clinical Presentation

The typical onset of FA is around puberty *(1–6)*, but it may be earlier *(7,8)*. After the gene was mapped and identified, it became clear that late-onset cases exist, even in late adult life (late-onset FA) *(9,10)*. The typical presentation at onset is with gait instability or generalized clumsiness. Among nonneurological manifestations, scoliosis, often considered to be idiopathic, may precede the onset of ataxia. Rare patients (5%) are diagnosed with idiopathic hypertrophic cardiomyopathy and treated as such for up to 2 to 3 yr before neurological symptoms appear *(1–4)*.

1.2. Neurological Signs and Symptoms

Mixed cerebellar and sensory ataxia characterizes the disease. It begins as truncal ataxia causing swaying, imbalance, and falls. Subsequently, the ataxic nature of gait becomes evident, with irregular steps, veering, and difficulty in turning. With further progression, gait becomes broad based, with frequent losses of balance, requiring intermittent support. A cane, and then a walker, becomes necessary. Finally, on average, 10 to 15 yr after onset, patients lose the ability to walk, stand, and sit without support. Evolution is variable; however, with mild cases patients are still ambulatory decades after onset. Limb ataxia appears after truncal ataxia, impairing writing, dressing, and handling utensils. Ataxia is progressive and unremitting, although periods of stability are frequent at the beginning of the illness. Dysarthria appears within 5 yr of clinical onset *(1–4)*, and has a cerebellar character *(11,12)*. Dysphagia, particularly for liquids, appears with advancing disease. Cognitive functions are generally well-preserved.

Findings at the neurological examination indicate the underlying pathology. Involvement of the central and peripheral sensory system results in deep sensory loss and abolished reflexes *(1,2)*. Pyramidal tract degeneration causes extensor plantar responses and progressive muscular weakness, which become severe only late in the progression of the disease. Ataxia and not weakness is the primary cause for loss of ambulation, even when patients become wheelchair-bound, they still maintain, on average, 70% of their normal strength in the lower limbs *(13)*. The relative impact of sensory neuropathy and of pyramidal tract degeneration varies from patient to patient, resulting most often in the described picture of areflexia associated with extensor plantar responses. However, sometimes, one component prevails, thus, some patients have retained reflexes or flexor plantar responses. These are usually milder cases of the disease. Some involvement of lower motor neurons is common and is revealed by distal amyotrophy in the four limbs *(2)*. When patients are wheelchair-bound, disuse atrophy occurs. The typical oculomotor abnormality is fixation instability with square-wave jerks *(14)*. Various combinations of cerebellar, vestibular, and brainstem oculomotor signs may be observed, but gaze-evoked nystagmus is uncommon and ophthalmoparesis does not occur. Approximately 30% of patients with FA develop optic atrophy, with or without visual impairment *(1,2,4,15–17)*, and 20% have sensorineural hearing loss *(18,19)*. Optic atrophy and sensorineural hearing loss tend to be associated with each other and with diabetes *(1,20)*.

1.3. Heart Disease

The cardiomyopathy of FA is most commonly asymptomatic; however, in a significant minority of patients it may contribute to disability and cause premature death, particularly in those with earlier age of onset *(1–4,21–28)*. Shortness of breath (40%) and palpitations (11%) are the most common first symptoms *(1)*. As the disease evolves, patients may develop arrhythmias, which may be fatal, and congestive heart failure. At end-stage disease, the cardiomyopathy becomes dilative, with progression of heart failure and eventually cardiogenic shock and death.

1.4. Other Signs and Symptoms

Approximately 10% of patients with FA develop diabetes mellitus, and 20% have carbohydrate intolerance. The mechanisms are complex, with β-cell dysfunction *(29)* and atrophy *(30)*, as well as peripheral insulin resistance *(31)*. Oral hypoglycemic drugs may initially give adequate control, but insulin eventually becomes necessary.

Skeletal abnormalities are common. Kyphoscoliosis may cause pain and cardiorespiratory problems. *Pes cavus* and *pes equinovarus* may further affect ambulation.

Autonomic disturbances, most commonly cold and cyanotic legs and feet, become increasingly frequent as the disease advances *(32)*. Parasympathetic abnormalities, such as decreased heart rate variability parameters have been reported *(33)*. Urinary problems, usually urgency, are rare.

1.5. Laboratory Investigations

FA causes typical neurophysiological abnormalities. Sensory nerve action potentials are severely reduced or, most often, lost *(34–36)*. Motor and sensory (when measurable) nerve conduction velocities are, instead, within or just below the normal range. These findings clearly distinguish an early case of FA from a case of hereditary demyelinating sensorimotor neuropathy.

Central nervous system magnetic resonance imaging shows a thinned spinal cord, but no major atrophy of brain structures. Even the cerebellum is apparently normal or only mildly atrophic in more advanced cases *(37)*.

The electrocardiogram shows inverted T waves in essentially all patients with FA, ventricular hypertrophy in most patients, conduction disturbances in approx 10% of patients, and, occasionally, supraventricular ectopic beats and atrial fibrillation *(3,4,26,27)*. The electrocardiogram may vary in time with occasional normal recordings, however, repeated recordings remain the most-sensitive test for the FA cardiomyopathy. Echocardiography and Doppler–echocardiography demonstrate concentric hypertrophy of the ventricles (62%) or asymmetric septal hypertrophy (29%), with diastolic function abnormalities *(2,38)*.

Recently, abnormalities in heart and skeletal muscle metabolism have been detected by phosphorus magnetic resonance spectroscopy, in particular, a reduced rate of adenosine triphosphate (ATP) synthesis. These abnormalities are a direct consequence of the primary genetic defect that affects mitochondrial function.

1.6. Prognosis

Patients with FA become wheelchair-bound, on average, 15 yr after onset of symptoms, but the variability is very large *(2,8)*. Early onset and left ventricular hypertrophy predict a faster rate of progression *(8,19)*. The burden of neurological impairment, cardiomyopathy, and, occasionally, diabetes, shortens life expectancy *(8)*. Survival may be significantly prolonged with treatment of cardiac symptoms (particularly arrhythmias), with antidiabetic treatment, and with preventing and controlling complications resulting from prolonged neurological disability.

1.7. Molecular Genetics

The FA gene (*FRDA*) *(39,40)* encodes a small mitochondrial matrix protein, frataxin, that is highly conserved in evolution. A single frataxin gene is found in all eukaryotes, including fungi and plants. A homolog, CyaY, is present in

Gram-negative bacteria and in other prokaryotes, such as *Rickettsia prowazeckii*, thought to be related to the hypothetical mitochondrial precursor. *FRDA* is expressed in all cells, but at variable levels in different tissues and during development *(41,42)*. In adult humans, *frataxin* messenger RNA is most abundant in the heart, brain, and spinal cord; followed by liver, skeletal muscle, and pancreas.

Patients with FA have a profound but not complete frataxin deficiency, with a small residual amount of normal protein. FA is caused by a so-far, unique mutation mechanism: the expansion of an intronic GAA triplet-repeat sequence (TRS), for which most patients are homozygous. Smaller expansions allow a higher residual gene expression *(43)*. Accordingly, the severity and age of onset of the disease are, in part, determined by the size of the expanded GAA TRS, in particular, of the smaller allele *(20,44)*. Lengths of the GAA TRS corresponding to pathological *FRDA* alleles can adopt a triple-helical structure in physiological conditions and can inhibit transcription in vitro and in vivo *(45–47)*. Approximately 2% of FA chromosomes carrying GAA repeats of normal lengths have missense, nonsense, or splice-site mutations ultimately affecting the frataxin coding sequence (**Fig. 1**) *(48)*.

1.8. Pathogenesis

Structural studies have been carried out on frataxin *(49,50)* and its bacterial homolog, CyaY *(51)*, by nuclear magnetic resonance and by crystallography. These investigations revealed a novel structural motif, called the frataxin fold, unique to frataxin and CyaY proteins. The structure is compact, overall globular, containing an N-terminal α-helix, a middle β-sheet region composed of seven β-strands, a second α-helix, and a C-terminal coil. The α-helices are folded on the β-sheet, with the C-terminal coil filling a groove between the two α-helices. On the outside, a ridge of negatively charged residues and a patch of hydrophobic residues are highly conserved, suggesting that they interact with a large ligand, probably a protein.

Knockout of the yeast frataxin homologous gene (*YFH1*) has provided the first information on frataxin function. Most YFH1 knockout yeast strains, called Δ*yfh1*, lose the ability to carry out oxidative phosphorylation, cannot grow on nonfermentable substrates, and lose mitochondrial DNA *(52,53)*. In Δ*YFH1*, iron accumulates in mitochondria, more than 10-fold in excess of wild-type yeast, at the expense of cytosolic iron. Loss of respiratory competence requires the presence of iron in the culture medium, and occurs more rapidly as iron concentration in the medium is increased, suggesting that permanent mitochondrial damage is the consequence of iron toxicity *(54)*. Iron in mitochondria can react with reactive oxygen species that form in these organelles and generate the highly toxic hydroxyl radical through the Fenton reaction with

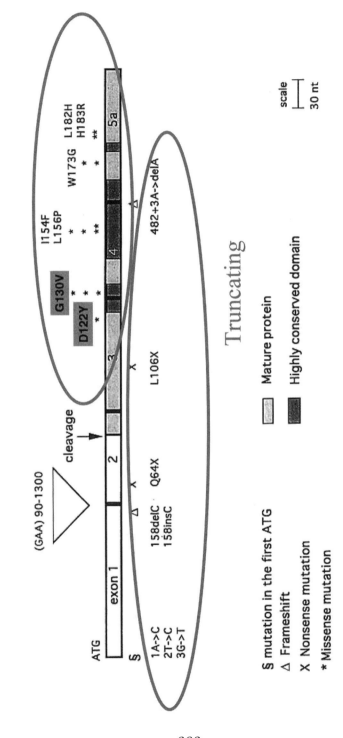

Fig. 1. Examples of mutation affecting the frataxin coding sequence. The two highlighted missense mutations are associated with a mild phenotype. Notice that the missense mutations are clustered after the cleavage site that removes the mitochondrial targeting N-terminal peptide.

H_2O_2. The hydroxyl radical causes lipid peroxidation, and protein and nucleic acid damage. Occurrence of the Fenton reaction in $\Delta YFH1$ yeast cells is suggested by their highly enhanced sensitivity to H_2O_2 (52).

In $\Delta yfh1$ yeast, iron is trapped in mitochondria, and there is a deficit in cytosolic iron, causing a marked induction (10- to 50-fold) of the high-affinity iron transport system on the cell membrane, normally not expressed in yeast cells that are iron replete (52). Consequently, iron crosses the plasma membrane in large amounts and further accumulates in mitochondria, engaging the cell in a vicious cycle. Experimental evidence suggests that frataxin stimulates a flux of nonheme iron out of mitochondria (54).

Respiratory chain complexes I, II, and III, and aconitase are impaired in $\Delta yfh1$ yeast (55). These enzymes contain iron–sulfur clusters (ISCs) in their active sites. ISCs are synthesized in mitochondria and are highly sensitive to free radicals (56). Remarkably, all yeast mutants defective in ISC synthesis have mitochondrial iron accumulation, apparently caused by defective iron export out of mitochondria, because it occurs in $\Delta yfh1$. Recent data point to a direct involvement of frataxin in an early step of ISC synthesis (57), through an interaction with the scaffold protein Isu1, in which the first ISC assembly takes place, probably facilitating iron incorporation (58). This finding suggests that frataxin may be a mitochondrial iron chaperone, protecting the iron from reactive oxygen species and making it bioavailable. Recent data support this view, suggesting that frataxin also acts as an iron chaperone in heme synthesis (59) and in the modulation of aconitase activity (60). A much higher affinity of frataxin for the heme synthesis enzyme, ferrochelatase, than for Isu1 (59) would explain why heme synthesis is resistant to low frataxin levels and is essentially unaffected in patients with FA (61). To act as an iron chaperone, frataxin must have iron-binding properties. Adamec et al. (62) first reported the ability of yfh1p, when exposed to a high iron concentration (iron to protein ratio of 40:1), to form a high molecular weight complex containing approx 60 frataxin molecules and 3000 Fe^{3+} atoms in a ferritin-like structure; however, the in vivo relevance of this finding has been controversial. Subsequent studies by the same group suggested that frataxin has an intrinsic ferroxidase activity and that it may bind and chaperone Fe^{2+} at lower iron to protein ratios (63).

Altered iron metabolism, free radical damage, and mitochondrial dysfunction all occur in patients with FA. Iron deposits are found in myocardial cells from patients with FA (64). Oxidative stress is revealed by increased plasma levels of malondialdehyde, a lipid peroxidation product (65), and increased urinary 8-hydroxy-2'-deoxyguanosine, a marker of oxidative DNA damage (66). We directly showed increased free-radical production in cultured cells engineered to produce reduced levels of frataxin (67). In addition, patients' fibroblasts are sensitive to low doses of H_2O_2, doses that induce apoptosis at lower doses than in control fibroblasts *(68)*, suggesting that even nonaffected cells are in an at-risk status for oxidative stress as a consequence of the primary genetic defect. FA fibroblasts also show abnormal antioxidant responses, in particular, a blunted increase in mitochondrial superoxide dismutase triggered by iron and by oxidants in control cells *(69)*. Mitochondrial dysfunction has been proven to occur in vivo in patients with FA. Phosphorus magnetic resonance spectroscopy analysis of skeletal muscle and heart shows a reduced rate of ATP synthesis *(70)*. Finally, and most importantly, the same multiple iron–sulfur protein enzyme dysfunctions found in Δ*YFH1* yeast are found in affected tissues from patients with FA *(55)*.

1.9. Animal Models

The generation of a frataxin knockout mouse *(71)* has revealed that homozygous knockout mice die as early as embryonic day 7. To date, viable mouse models have been obtained through a conditional gene-targeting approach. A heart and striated muscle frataxin-deficient line and a line with more generalized, including neural, frataxin deficiency have been generated *(72)*. These mice reproduce important progressive pathophysiological and biochemical features of the human disease: cardiac hypertrophy without skeletal muscle involvement in the heart and striated muscle frataxin-deficient line, large sensory neuron dysfunction without alteration of the small sensory and motor neurons in the more generalized frataxin-deficient line, and deficient activities of complexes I to III of the respiratory chain and of the aconitases in both lines. Time-dependent intramitochondrial iron accumulation occurs in the heart of the heart and striated muscle frataxin-deficient line. These animals provide an important resource for pathophysiological studies and for testing of new treatments. However, they still do not mimic the situation occurring in the human disease, because conditional gene targeting leads to complete loss of frataxin in some cells at a specific time in development, whereas FA is characterized by partial frataxin deficiency in all cells and throughout life. An attempt to closely mimic the human disease by inserting a GAA TRS into the mouse gene by homologous recombination has succeeded in generating mice with a partial reduction in frataxin, but this was not sufficient to induce a pathological phenotype *(73)*. Recently, a mouse model recreating the neurological features of the human disease was obtained using a tamoxifen-inducible Cre recombinase under the control of a neuron-specific prion protein promoter *(74)*. These mice present a general locomotor deficit without a defect in muscle strength, beginning at approx 10 wk, and, further, develop a clear progressive ataxia leading to loss of spontaneous ambulation at approx 1 yr of age. In addition, electromyographic studies show a significant decrease in sensorimotor reflexes after sciatic nerve stimulation, indicating that the large myelinated proprioceptive sensory neurons are functionally defective, causing sensory and spinocer-ebellar ataxia, a distinctive pathological characteristic of FRDA.

1.10. Perspectives for Treatment

The findings presented in **Subheading 1.8.** paved the way for the develop-ment of pharmacological treatments. Because of their ability to stimulate oxi-dative phosphorylation and to act as potent free-radical scavengers, coenzyme Q derivatives have been considered a promising treatment for FA. Coenzyme Q10 and its short chain analog, idebenone, have both been clinically tested. Despite a short-term (3 mo) study showing no effect on heart size or function *(75)*, several small open-label trials and a single double-blind, placebo-con-trolled trial concluded that idebenone is able to reduce cardiac hypertrophy in patients with FA *(76–78)*. Only one study, however, showed some functional improvement along with heart-size reduction *(78)*. Studies in mouse models of FA cardiomyopathy also confirmed a positive effect of idebenone on cardiac size and function and on survival *(79)*. In addition, a positive effect on cardiac and calf muscle energy metabolism of a cocktail of 400 mg/d of coenzyme Q10 and 2100 IU/d of vitamin E could be demonstrated by ^{31}P-magnetic resonance spectroscopy in 10 FRDA patients *(80)*. Conversely, thus far, it has not been possible to document any significant effect of these drugs on neurological symptoms. Although detection of a modest effect could not be possible with the design limitations of the clinical trials that have been conducted, pharma-cokinetic factors may also be involved, because one study indicates that idebenone levels in the cerebrospinal fluid are very low when the drug is given at the dosage used in most trials *(81)*.

Newer pharmacological approaches, still at the experimental or preclinical stages, include modified coenzyme Q derivatives that are targeted to mitochon-dria *(82)*; other antioxidants; glutathione peroxidase mimetics *(83)*; and a very promising group of new iron chelators that can reach the mitochondrial com-partment and possibly act more like iron chaperones (frataxin-like) in remov-ing iron than traditional chelators do.

Finally, approaches that are being explored in the laboratory and may hold some promise include gene replacement therapy, protein replacement, and sub-stances that are able to boost frataxin gene expression, either through a direct effect or by interfering with the structure adopted by the GAA expansion.

1.11. Molecular Methods for Diagnosing FA

The diagnostic molecular test for FA is aimed to detect the unstable hyperexpansion of the GAA triplet repeat in the first intron of the FRDA gene, that is found in 98% of FA chromosomes. Normal alleles contain between 6 and 36 GAA triplets. In whites, two groups of normal alleles are found: short normal (SN) alleles of less than 12 repeats and long normal (LN) alleles of more than 12 triplets. SN alleles are present on approx 80% of the chromosomes, most contain nine triplets. LN alleles have a broad distribution, with a median of approx 16 to 18 triplets. Stable LN alleles with more than 27 triplets are usually interrupted by GAGGAA or GAAGGA hexanucleotide units, whereas uninterrupted alleles with 34 or more triplets can hyperexpand and should be considered "premutation" alleles. Alleles found in individuals with FA are called expanded (E) and have 66 to more than 1500 triplets. E alleles show meiotic and mitotic instability. Occasionally, alleles in the E range are stable and nonpathogenic. These are usually less than 150 triplets in size and contain variant sequences, e.g., GAAGGA repeats. As detailed in **Subheading 3.3.**, sequencing of alleles in this size range, as well as some very long LN alleles, may be indicated in particular circumstances.

Polymerase chain reaction (PCR) or Southern blot can be used to detect the expansion (**Fig. 2**). PCR requires only a small amount of DNA, but high-quality DNA is extremely important. Ambiguous results, particularly in heterozygote detection, can be resolved by subsequent hybridization of PCR products with an oligonucleotide probe containing a GAA or CTT repeat. Southern blot requires more DNA and is less accurate for determining the number of repeats; however, it has full sensitivity in detecting E alleles at the heterozygous state.

2. Materials

1. Agarose and DNA sequencing gel equipment.
2. Thermocycler for PCR.
3. Oligonucleotide primers.
4. rTth DNA polymerase.
5. dNTP mix, 2 mM each.
6. 10X PCR buffer.
7. ^{32}P-ATP for end labeling of oligonucleotides.
8. ^{32}P end-labeling kit for oligonucleotides.
9. Restriction enzymes.
10. ^{32}P-dCTP for probe labeling.
11. DNA probe-labeling kit.
12. HybondN+ membranes.
13. Whatman filter paper no. 1.
14. 10X saline sodium citrate (SSC): 1.5 M sodium chloride and 0.15 M sodium citrate.
15. 1% sodium dodecyl sulfate.
16. Film, intensifying screens, and cassettes for autoradiography.
17. Dimethylsulfoxide.
18. DNA sequencing kit, including dNTPs, ddNTPs, DNA polymerase, and buffer; for manual or automated sequencing.

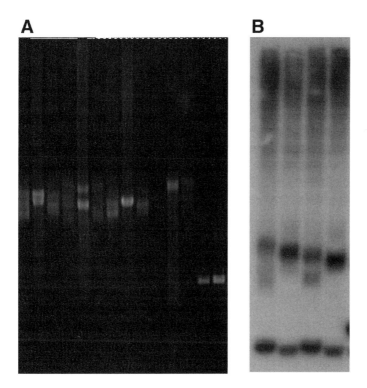

Fig. 2. (A) PCR analysis of the GAA triplet repeat in the frataxin gene. The two lanes on the extreme right correspond to normal individuals, all other lanes to Patients with FA. Notice how several samples generate multiple bands, a sign of somatic instability of the expanded repeats. **(B)** PCR analysis of FA carriers. Amplified fragments were blotted and hybridized with a $(CTT)_{10}$ oligonucleotide probe to enhance sensitivity.

3. Methods

3.1. PCR Analysis

When testing for *FRDA* carrier status, we routinely perform two different PCR reactions. The first is a long-range PCR that generates fragments of 1350 + 3n bp (n being the number of GAA triplets), using the primers 2500F *(40)* and 104FGAA *(8)*. This reaction is performed in a final volume of 50 µL, using 200 ng of genomic DNA, 20 pmoles of each primer, a final concentration of each dNTP of 0.2 mM, 1 U of rTth polymerase, and 5 µL of 10X buffer (as provided by the polymerase manufacturer). Temperature cycling is: 94°C for 1 h; followed by 10 cycles of 15 min at 94°C and 3.5 h at 67°C; then by 20 cycles of 15 min at 94°C, 30 min at 66°C, and 3 h at 68°C, with a 20 min increase at each cycle. In our experience, these PCR conditions are optimal for the detection of expanded repeats, both in the homozygous and heterozygous state (*see* **Note 1**). The second reaction is optimal for the detection and sizing of repeats in the normal range. It generates fragments of 451 + 3n bp (n = number of GAA triplets) using the GAA-F/GAA-R primers (as described in **ref. 40**). Analysis of GAA-F/GAA-R PCR products on 2% agarose gels clearly resolves SN from LN alleles. To maximize sensitivity, we routinely transfer the amplified fragments obtained by 2500F/104FGAA and by GAAF/GAAR PCR to a nylon membrane (Hybond N+), and hybridize them with an ^{32}P end-labeled $(CTT)_{10}$ oligonucleotide. Hybridization is for 3 h at 42°C, followed by two 5 h washes at room temperature, first with 2X SSC, then with 0.1X SSC.

3.2. Southern Blot Analysis

The Southern blot method **(44)** involves digestion of genomic DNA with the *Bsi*HKAI enzyme, which yields a 2.4-kb target DNA fragment (*see* **Note 2**). Ten micrograms of genomic DNA are digested by *Bsi*HKAI (New England Biolabs), electrophoresis is performed in 0.9% agarose gel, the gels are blotted on HybondN+ membranes (Amersham), and the samples are hybridized with a ^{32}P-radiolabeled 463-bp genomic fragment containing exon 1 of the frataxin gene. This fragment can be obtained by PCR amplification from genomic DNA using the forward primer, CAAGTTCCTCCTGTTTAG, and the reverse primer, CCGCGGCTGTTCCCGG. Blots are washed in 0.2X SSC and 0.1% sodium dodecyl sulfate twice at room temperature and twice at 60°C, and exposed for autoradiography at –80°C with an intensifying screen.

3.3. Sequencing of the Frataxin Intronic Repeat

Sequencing of the frataxin intronic repeat may be useful whenever it is important to differentiate small pathogenic E alleles from very long, nonpathogenic variant repeats or potentially unstable from stable LN alleles (*see* **Note 3**). Most cases involve diagnosis of carrier status; occasionally, for the small E alleles, diagnosis of FA may be involved. Pathogenic alleles contain uninterrupted stretches of more than 66 GAA triplets, unstable LN alleles have uninterrupted stretches of more than 34 GAA triplets.

GAA-F/GAA-R amplification products are purified from NuSieve gels using the QIAquick Gel Extraction Kit (Qiagen), and directly sequenced using the Sequenase PCR Product Sequencing Kit (USB). Because of the presence of a poly-A stretch preceding the GAA repeat, which interferes with the sequencing reaction, samples are sequenced on the opposite (CTT) strand, using the GAA-R primer.

3.4. Detection of Frataxin Point Mutations

Frataxin point mutations should be searched in ataxic individuals who are heterozygous for an E and a normal allele at the GAA repeat (**Fig. 2**). No patient with point mutations in both frataxin alleles has been found thus far, probably because the complete or quasi-complete loss of frataxin function that would follow is incompatible with life, as indicated by the knockout mouse model *(71)*.

No mutation in the frataxin coding sequence could be identified in up to 40% of heterozygous patients with a GAA expansion in some series *(48)*. Some of these cases may be *bona fide* FA cases and have mutations deep into introns or in regulatory sequences. Some, however, may have a different disease and carry a GAA expansion by chance, given its high frequency (1 in 90 people) in whites.

Carrier testing by point mutation analysis is currently limited to family members of individuals with known point mutations. The frequency of frataxin point mutations is approx 1 in 40 GAA expansions *(48)*, thus, exclusion of the expansion leaves a 1 in 4000 risk of being a carrier. This risk may vary in different populations, for example, it is close to 0 in French Canadians, because all FRDA patients with this ancestry have two expanded GAA repeats, and higher in individuals from the Naples, Italy region, where the I154F mutation is relatively frequent *(40,48)*. Testing for a locally prevalent point mutation may, in this case, be added to expansion analysis when determining carrier status.

The following intronic primers are used to amplify the five frataxin exons from genomic DNA (50–100 ng) (**Note 4 *[40,48]***):

Exon 1 (240 bp): forward, AGCACCCAGCGCTGGAGG; reverse, CCG CGGCTGTTCCCGG

Exon 2 (168 bp): forward, AGTAACGTACTTCTTAACTTTGGC; reverse, AGAGGAAGATACCTATCACGTG

Exon 3 (227 bp): forward, AAAATGGAAGCATTTGGTAATCA; reverse, AGTGAACTAAAATTCTTAGAGGG

Exon 4 (250 bp): forward, AAGCAATGATGACAAAGTGCTAAC; reverse, TGGTCCACAATGTCACATTTCGG

Exon 5a (223 bp): forward, CTGAAGGGCTGTGCTGTGGA; reverse, TGTCCTTACAAACGGGGCT

Amplifications for exons 2, 3, 4, and 5a consist of 30 cycles of: 1 min at 94°C, 1 min at 55°C, and 1 min at 72°C. To amplify the highly GC-rich exon 1, the annealing temperature is raised to 68°C and 10% dimethylsulfoxide is added to the reaction.

Amplified fragments are gel purified and directly sequenced on both strands using the same forward and reverse primers.

Some mutations can be confirmed by restriction enzyme-based assays *(48)* . Mutations affecting the ATG initiation codon and the H183 codon disrupt an NlaIII restriction site (CATG/). D122Y and the L156P changes create new restriction sites for RsaI (GT/AC) and for HaeIII (GG/CC), respectively. 158delC and 158insC mutations in exon 1 are resolved on sequencing gels of

TaqI digestion products of exon 1 PCR fragments, yielding 54- and 56-bp labeled fragments, respectively *(48)*. Other mutations can be detected using allele-specific oligonucleotide hybridization or allele specific amplification *(48)* (**Note 5**).

4. Notes

1. PCR detection of GAA expansions is fast, sensitive, effective, and requires little genomic DNA. We used this method in approx 800 molecular tests for FA or for carrier status. One possible source of error when interpreting the results of a PCR test comes from the observation that some individuals seem to be carriers of a large expansion along with either a small and a large normal allele, or an allele in the normal range and a small expansion (up to 120–150 triplets). In some cases, several apparently fully expanded bands are visible, particularly when the gel is overloaded. These larger bands represent heteroduplex molecules formed during the PCR coamplification of repeats of different length. This phenomenon must be taken into account when performing the molecular test to detect FRDA carriers to avoid false-positive results. We recommend always performing the two PCR reactions when testing for the FRDA GAA expansion, and to add Southern blot analysis of genomic DNA if any uncertainty is left by the PCR results.

2. Southern blot analysis is used by many diagnostic labs because it allows a clear, usually unquestionable detection of expanded repeats in affected subjects as well as in heterozygous carriers. Disadvantages are mainly related to the need for larger amounts of genomic DNA, and the time consuming and more complex protocol, particularly at a time when genomic Southern blotting is performed less frequently and technical personnel may not be familiar with this technique. Another disadvantage is the difficulty of accurately sizing expanded bands, particularly when they are close to the normal range.

3. Sequencing the expanded repeat is technically challenging. The best results are obtained by sequencing the CTT strand, in which DNA polymerase slippages are less likely to occur. The occurrence of interruptions in the GAA repeated sequence, such as GAAGGA, GGGA, GAAA, and similar variants, is particularly important to distinguish shorter pathogenic repeats, mostly or entirely composed of uninterrupted GAA, from similar-size nonpathogenic repeats, mostly composed of variant repeats, e.g., GAAGGA hexanucleotides. Fortunately, such variant sequences are less likely to cause DNA polymerase slippages, and, therefore, easier to sequence.

4. The sequencing of frataxin exons and the neighboring intronic sequence offers no special difficulty except for exon 1, which is highly GC rich. Some laboratories perform preliminary analyses to select exons to sequence, such as single-strand conformation polymorphism or denaturing high-performance liquid chromatography. In our experience, given the small number of fragments to analyze and the limited number of tests to perform for this rare disorder, there is no clear advantage compared with directly sequencing all fragments, which is what we routinely do. In addition, single-strand conformation polymorphism and

denaturing high-performance liquid chromatography are less sensitive for the GC-rich exon 1, therefore, this exon must be sequenced anyway.

5. There have been reported cases of genomic deletions involving the frataxin gene. Affected subjects carrying this type of mutation are always compound heterozygotes for the GAA expanded repeat. Separate PCR amplification of each exon in these cases may give a normal result, because the frataxin coding sequence is complete and normal on the chromosome with the GAA expansion. If such a case is suspected, as in a clinically affected individual who is heterozygous for the GAA expanded repeat and has a normal frataxin coding sequence, either quantitative PCR or genomic Southern blot analysis should be performed on each exon. This is usually done in specialized research laboratories.

References

1. Geoffroy, G., Barbeau, A., Breton, G., et al. (1976) Clinical description and roentgenologic evaluation of patients with Friedreich ataxia. *Can. J. Neurol. Sci.* **3,** 279–286.
2. Harding, A. E. (1981) Friedreich ataxia: a clinical and genetic study of 90 families with an analysis of early diagnosis criteria and intrafamilial clustering of clinical features. *Brain* **104,** 589–620.
3. Filla, A., De Michele, G., Caruso, G., Marconi, R., and Campanella, G. (1990) Genetic data and natural history of Friedreich disease: a study of 80 Italian patients. *J. Neurol.* **237,** 345–351.
4. Muller-Felber, W., Rossmanith, T., Spes, C., Chamberlain, S., Pongratz, D., and Deufel, T. (1993) The clinical spectrum of Friedreich ataxia in German families showing linkage to the FRDA locus on chromosome 9. *Clin. Investig.* **71,** 109–114.
5. Campanella, G., Filla, A., De Falco, F., Mansi, D., Durivage, A., and Barbeau A. (1980) Friedreich ataxia in the south of Italy: A clinical and biochemical survey of 23 patients. *Can. J. Neurol. Sci.* **7,** 351–357.
6. D'Angelo, A., Di Donato, S., Negri, G., Beulche, F., Uziel, G. and Boeri, R. (1980) Friedreich ataxia in northern Italy: I. Clinical, neurophysiological and in vivo biochemical studies. *Can. J. Neurol. Sci.* **7,** 359–365.
7. Ulku, A., Arac, N., and Ozeren, A. (1988) Friedreich ataxia: a clinical review of 20 childhood cases. *Acta Neurol. Scand.* **77,** 493–497.
8. De Michele, G., Di Maio, L., Filla, A., et al. (1996) Childhood onset of Friedreich ataxia: a clinical and genetic study of 36 cases. *Neuropediatrics* **27,** 3–7.
9. Klockgether, T., Chamberlain, S., Wullner, U., et al. (1993) Late-onset Friedreich ataxia. Molecular genetics, clinical neurophysiology, and magnetic resonance imaging. *Arch. Neurol.* **50,** 803–806.
10. De Michele, G., Filla, A., Cavalcanti, F., et al. (1994) Late onset Friedreich disease: clinical features and mapping of mutation to the FRDA locus. *J. Neurol. Neurosurg. Psychiatry* **57,** 977–979.
11. Gentil, M. (1990) Dysarthria in Friedreich disease. *Brain Lang.* **38,** 438–448.
12. Cisneros, E. and Braun, C. M. (1995) Vocal and respiratory diadochokinesia in Friedreich ataxia. Neuropathological correlations. *Rev. Neurol. (Paris)* **151,** 113–123.

13. Beauchamp, M., Labelle, H., Duhaime, M., and Joncas, J. (1995) Natural history of muscle weakness in Friedreich's Ataxia and its relation to loss of ambulation. *Clin. Orthop.* **311,** 270–275.

14. Spieker, S., Schulz, J. B., Petersen, D., Fetter, M., Klockgether, T., and Dichgans, J. (1995) Fixation instability and oculomotor abnormalities in Friedreich ataxia. *J. Neurol.* **242,** 517–521.

15. Kirkham, T. H. and Coupland, S. G. (1981) An electroretinal and visual evoked potential study in Friedreich ataxia. *Can. J. Neurol. Sci.* **8,** 289–294.

16. Livingstone, I. R., Mastaglia, F. L., Edis, R., and Howe, J. W. (1981) Visual involvement in Friedreich ataxia and hereditary spastic ataxia. A clinical and visual evoked response study. *Arch. Neurol.* **38,** 75–79.

17. Rabiah, P. K., Bateman, J. B., Demer, J. L., and Perlman, S. (1997) Ophthalmologic findings in patients with ataxia. *Am. J. Ophthalmol.* **123,** 108–117.

18. Ell, J., Prasher, D., and Rudge, P. (1984) Neuro-otological abnormalities in Friedreich ataxia. *J. Neurol. Neurosurg. Psychiatry* **47,** 26–32.

19. Cassandro, E., Mosca, F., Sequino, L., De Falco, F. A., and Campanella, G. (1986) Otoneurological findings in Friedreich ataxia and other inherited neuropathies. *Audiol.* **25,** 84–91.

20. Montermini, L., Richter, A., Morgan, K., et al. (1997) Phenotypic variability in Friedreich ataxia: role of the associated GAA triplet repeat expansion. *Ann. Neurol.* **41,** 675–682.

21. Leone, M., Rocca, W. A., Rosso, M.G., Mantel, N., Schoenberg, B. S., and Schiffer, D. (1988) Friedreich disease: survival analysis in an Italian population. *Neurology* **38,** 1433–1438.

22. Hartman, J. M. and Booth, R. W. (1960) Friedreich ataxia: a neurocardiac disease. *Am. Heart J.* **60,** 716–720.

23. Boyer, S. H., Chisholm, A. W., and McKusick, V. A. (1962) Cardiac aspects of Friedreich ataxia. *Circulation* **25,** 493–505.

24. Harding, A. E. and Hewer, R. L. (1983) The heart disease of Friedreich ataxia. A clinical and electrocardiographic changes in 30 cases. *Q. J. Med.* **52,** 489–502.

25. Pentland, B. and Fox, K. A. (1983) The heart in Friedreich ataxia. *J. Neurol. Neurosurg. Psychiatry* **46,** 1138–1142.

26. Child, J. S., Perloff, J. K., Bach, P. M., Wolfe, A. D., Perlman, S., and Kark, R. A. (1986) Cardiac involvement in Friedreich ataxia: a clinical study of 75 patients. *J. Am. Coll. Cardiol.* **7,** 1370–1378.

27. Alboliras, E. T., Shub, C., Gomez, M. R., et al. (1986) Spectrum of cardiac involvement in Friedreich ataxia: clinical, electrocardiographic and echocardiographic observations. *Am. J. Cardiol.* **58,** 518–524.

28. Maione, S., Giunta, A., Filla, A., et al. (1997) May age onset be relevant in the occurrence of left ventricular hypertrophy in Friedreich ataxia? *Clin. Cardiol.* **20,** 141–145.

29. Finocchiaro, G., Baio, G., Micossi, P., Pozza, G., and Di Donato, S. (1988) Glucose metabolism alterations in Friedreich ataxia. *Neurology* **38,** 1292–1296.

30. Schoenle, E. J., Boltshauser, E. J., Baekkeskov, S., Landin Olsson, M., Torresani, T., and von Felten, A. (1989) Preclinical and manifest diabetes mellitus in young

patients with Friedreich ataxia: no evidence of immune process behind the islet cell destruction. *Diabetologia* **32,** 378–381.

31. Fantus, I. G., Seni, M. H., and Andermann, E. (1993) Evidence for abnormal regulation of insulin receptors in Friedreich ataxia. *J. Clin. Endocrinol. Metab.* **76,** 60–63.
32. Margalith, D., Dunn, H. G., Carter, J. E., and Wright, J. M. (1984) Friedreich ataxia with dysautonomia and labile hypertension. *Can. J. Neurol. Sci.* **11,** 73–77.
33. Pousset, F., Kalotka, H., Durr, A., et al. (1996) Parasympathetic activity in Friedrich's ataxia. *Am. J. Cardiol.* **78,** 847–850.
34. McLeod, J. G. (1971) An electrophysiological and pathological study of peripheral nerves in Friedreich ataxia. *J. Neurol. Sci.* **12,** 333–349.
35. Peyronnard, J. M., Bouchard, J. P., and Lapointe, M. (1976) Nerve conduction studies and electromyography in Friedreich ataxia. *Can. J. Neurol. Sci.* **3,** 313–317.
36. Ackroyd, R.S., Finnegan, J.A., and Green, S.H. (1984) Friedreich ataxia. A clinical review with neurophysiological and echocardiographic findings. *Arch. Dis. Child.* **59,** 217–221.
37. Wullner, U., Klockgether, T., Petersen, D., Naegele, T., and Dichgans, J. (1993) Magnetic resonance imaging in hereditary and idiopathic ataxia [see comments]. *Neurology* **43,** 318–325.
38. Morvan, D., Komajda, M., Doan, L. D., et al. (1992) Cardiomyopathy in Friedreich ataxia: a Doppler-echocardiographic study. *Eur. Heart J.* **13,** 1393–1398.
39. Chamberlain, S., Shaw, J., and Rowland, A. (1998) Mapping of mutation causing Friedreich's ataxia to human chromosome 9. *Nature* **334,** 248–250.
40. Campuzano, V., Montermini, L., Moltó, M. D., et al. (1996) Friedreich ataxia: autosomal recessive disease caused by an intronic GAA triplet repeat expansion. *Science* **271,** 1423–1427.
41. Koutnikova, H., Campuzano, V., Foury, F., Dollé, P., Cazzalini, O., and Koenig, M. (1997) Studies of human, mouse and yeast homologues indicate a mitochondrial function for frataxin. *Nat. Genet.* **16,** 345–351.
42. Jiralerspong, S., Liu, Y., Montermini, L., Stifani, S., and Pandolfo, M. (1997) Frataxin shows developmentally regulated tissue-specific expression in the mouse embryo. *Neurobiol. Dis.* **4,** 103–113.
43. Campuzano, V., Montermini, L., Lutz, Y., et al. (1997) Frataxin is reduced in Friedreich ataxia patients and is associated with mitochondrial membranes. *Hum. Mol. Genet.* **6,** 1771–1780.
44. Dürr, A., Cossée, M., Agid, Y., et al. (1996) Clinical and genetic abnormalities in patients with Friedreich ataxia. *N. Engl. J. Med.* **335,** 1169–1175.
45. Ohshima, K., Montermini, L., Wells, R. D., and Pandolfo, M. (1998) Inhibitory effects of expanded GAA•TTC triplet repeats from intron I of the Friedreich ataxia gene on transcription and replication in vivo. *J. Biol. Chem.* **273,** 14,588–15,595.
46. Sakamoto, N. K., Ohshima, K. L., Montermini, L. M., Pandolfo, M., and Wells, R. D. (2001) Sticky DNA, a self-associated complex formed at long GAA•TTC re-

peats in intron 1 of the Frataxin gene, inhibits transcription. *J. Biol. Chem.* **276,** 27,171–27,177.

47. Sakamoto, N., Chastain, P. D., Parniewski, P., et al. (1999) Sticky DNA: self-association properties of long GAA•TTC repeats in R•R•Y triplex structures from Friedreich ataxia. *Mol. Cell* **3,** 465–475.

48. Cossée, M., Dürr, A., Schmitt, M., et al. (1999) Frataxin point mutations and clinical presentation of compound heterozygous Friedreich ataxia patients. *Ann. Neurol.* **45,** 200–206.

49. Dhe-Paganon, S., Shigeta, R., Chi, Y. I., Ristow, M., and Shoelson, S. E. (2000) Crystal structure of human frataxin. *J. Biol. Chem.* **275,** 30,753–30,756.

50. Musco, G., Stier, G., Kolmerer, B., et al. (2000) Towards a structural understanding of Friedreich ataxia: the solution structure of frataxin. *Structure Fold. Des.* **8,** 695–707.

51. Cho, S. J., Lee, M. G., Yang, J. K., Lee, J. Y., Song, H. K., and Suh, S. W. (2000) Crystal structure of Escherichia coli CyaY protein reveals a previously unidentified fold for the evolutionarily conserved frataxin family. *Proc. Natl. Acad. Sci. USA* **97,** 8932–8937.

52. Babcock, M., de Silva, D., Oaks, R., et al. (1997) Regulation of mitochondrial iron accumulation by Yfh1, a putative homolog of frataxin. *Science* **276,** 1709–1712.

53. Wilson, R. B. and Roof, D. M. (1997) Respiratory deficiency due to loss of mitochondrial DNA in yeast lacking the frataxin homologue. *Nat. Genet.* **16,** 352–357.

54. Radisky, D. C., Babcock, M. C., and Kaplan, J. (1999) The yeast frataxin homologue mediates mitochondrial iron efflux. Evidence for a mitochondrial iron cycle. *J. Biol. Chem.* **274,** 4497–4499.

55. Rötig, A., deLonlay, P., Chretien, D., et al. (1997) Frataxin gene expansion causes aconitase and mitochondrial iron–sulfur protein deficiency in Friedreich ataxia. *Nat. Genet.* **17,** 215–217.

56. Gardner, P. R., Rainieri, I., Epstein, L. B., and White, C. W. (1995) Superoxide radical and iron modulate aconitase activity in mammalian cells. *J. Biol. Chem.* **270,** 13,399–13,405.

57. Muhlenhoff, U., Gerber, J., Richhardt, N., and Lill, R. (2003) Components involved in assembly and dislocation of iron–sulfur clusters on the scaffold protein Isu1p. *EMBO J.* **22,** 4815–4825.

58. Yoon, T. and Cowan, J. A. (2003) Iron–sulfur cluster biosynthesis. Characterization of frataxin as an iron donor for assembly of [2Fe-2S] clusters in ISU-type proteins. *J. Am. Chem. Soc.* **125,** 6078–6084.

59. Yoon, T. and Cowan, J. A. (2004) Frataxin-mediated iron delivery to ferrochelatase in the final step of heme biosynthesis. *J. Biol. Chem.* **279,** 25,943–25,946.

60. Bulteau, A. L., O'Neill, H. A., Kennedy, M. C., Ikeda-Saito, M., Isaya, G., and Szweda, L. I. (2004) Frataxin acts as an iron chaperone protein to modulate mitochondrial aconitase activity. *Science* **305,** 242–245.

61. Pandolfo, M. (2002) Iron metabolism and mitochondrial abnormalities in Friedreich ataxia. *Bl. Cells Mol. Dis.* **29,** 536–547.

62. Adamec, J., Rusnak, F., Owen, W. G., et al. (2000) Iron-dependent self-assembly

of recombinant yeast frataxin: implications for Friedreich ataxia. *Am. J. Hum. Genet.* **67,** 549–562.

63. Park, S., Gakh, O., O'Neill, H. A., et al. (2003) Yeast frataxin sequentially chaperones and stores iron by coupling protein assembly with iron oxidation. *J. Biol. Chem.* **278** , 31,340–31,345.

64. Lamarche, J. B., Côté, M., and Lemieux, B. (1980) The cardiomyopathy of Friedreich ataxia morphological observations in 3 cases. *Can. J. Neurol. Sci.* **7,** 389–396.

65. Emond, M., Lepage, G., Vanasse, M., and Pandolfo, M. (2000) Increased levels of plasma malondialdehyde in Friedreich ataxia. *Neurology* **55,** 1752–1753.

66. Schulz, J. B., Dehmer, T., Schols, L., et al. (2000) Oxidative stress in patients with Friedreich ataxia. *Neurology* **55,** 1719–1721.

67. Santos, M., Ohshima, K., and Pandolfo, M. (2001) Frataxin deficiency enhances apoptosis in cells differentiating into neuroectoderm. *Hum. Mol. Genet.* **10,** 1935–1944.

68. Wong, A., Yang, J., Cavadini, P., et al. (1999) The Friedreich ataxia mutation confers cellular sensitivity to oxidant stress which is rescued by chelators of iron and calcium and inhibitors of apoptosis. *Hum. Mol. Genet.* **8,** 425–430.

69. Jiralerspong, S., Ge, B., Hudson, T. J., and Pandolfo, M. (2001) Manganese superoxide dismutase induction by iron is impaired in Friedreich ataxia cells. *FEBS Lett.* **509,** 101–105.

70. Lodi, R., Cooper, J. M., Bradley, J. L., et al. (1999) Deficit of in vivo mitochondrial ATP production in patients with Friedreich ataxia. *Proc. Natl. Acad. Sci. USA* **96,** 11,492–11,495.

71. Cossée, M., Puccio, H., Gansmuller, A., et al. (2000) Inactivation of the Friedreich ataxia mouse gene leads to early embryonic lethality without iron accumulation. *Hum. Mol. Genet.* **9,** 1219–1226.

72. Puccio, H., Simon, D., Cossee, M., et al. (2001) Mouse models for Friedreich ataxia exhibit cardiomyopathy, sensory nerve defect and Fe-S enzyme deficiency followed by intramitochondrial iron deposits. Nat. Genet. **27,** 181–186.

73. Miranda, C. J., Santos, M. M., Ohshima, K., et al. (2002) Frataxin knockin mouse. *FEBS Lett.* **512,** 291–297.

74. Simon, D., Seznec, H., and Gansmuller, A. (2004) Friedreich ataxia mouse models with progressive cerebellar and sensory ataxia reveal autophagic neurodegeneration in dorsal root ganglia. *J. Neurosci.* **24,** 1987–1995.

75. Schols, L., Vorgerd, M., Schillings, M., Skipka, G., and Zange, J. (2001) Idebenone in patients with Friedreich ataxia. *Neurosci. Lett.* **306(3),** 169–172.

76. Hausse, A. O., Aggoun, Y., Bonnet, D., et al. (2002) Idebenone and reduced cardiac hypertrophy in Friedreich's ataxia. *Heart* **87(4),** 346–349.

77. Mariotti, C., Solari, A., Torta, D., Marano, L., Fiorentini, C., and Di Donato, S. (2003) Idebenone treatment in Friedreich patients: one-year-long randomized placebo-controlled trial. *Neurol.* **60(10),** 1676–1679.

78. Buyse, G., Mertens, L., Di Salvo, G., et al. (2003) Idebenone treatment in

Friedreich's ataxia: neurological, cardiac, and biochemical monitoring. *Neurol.* **60(10),** 1679–1681.

79. Seznec, H., Simon, D., Monassier, L., et al. (2004) Idebenone delays the onset of cardiac functional alteration without correction of Fe-S enzymes deficit in a mouse model for Friedreich ataxia. *Hum. Mol. Genet.* **13(10),** 1017–1024.

80. Lodi, R., Hart, P. E., Rajagopalan, B., et al. (2001) Antioxidant treatment improves in vivo cardiac and skeletal muscle bioenergetics in patients with Friedreich's ataxia. *Ann. Neurol.* **49,** 590–596.

81. Schols, L., Vorgerd, M., Schillings, M., Skipka, G., and Zange, J. (2001) Idebenone in patients with Friedreich ataxia. *Neurosci. Lett.* **306,** 169–172.

82. Hausse, A.O., Aggoun, Y., Bonnet, D., et al. (2002) Idebenone and reduced cardiac hypertrophy in Friedreich's ataxia. *Heart* **87,** 346–349.

83. Mariotti, C., Solari, A., Torta, D., Marano, L., Fiorentini, C., and Di Donato, S. (2003) Idebenone treatment in Friedreich patients: one-year-long randomized placebo-controlled trial. *Neurol.* **60,** 1676–1679.

13

The Cardiovascular Manifestations of Alagille Syndrome and *JAG1* Mutations

Elizabeth Goldmuntz, Elizabeth Moore, and Nancy B. Spinner

Summary

Alagille syndrome is an autosomal-dominant disorder characterized by hepatic, cardiac, ocular, skeletal, and facial abnormalities. The disease gene, Jagged1 (*JAG1*), was identified by molecular analyses of chromosomal alterations involving chromosome 20p. Total gene deletions (3–7%) and intragenic mutations (70%) of *JAG1* have been identified in Alagille patients. Identifying *JAG1* mutations is challenging, given its size of 26 exons. Methods to identify both whole-gene deletions and intragenic mutations of *JAG1* are described in detail, including fluorescence *in situ* hybridization (FISH), conformation-sensitive gel electrophoresis (CSGE), and complementary DNA (cDNA) sequencing.

Key Words: Alagille syndrome; congenital heart disease; *JAG1*; fluorescence *in situ* hybridization; mutation detection; conformation-sensitive gel electrophoresis; peripheral pulmonary stenosis; tetralogy of Fallot.

1. Introduction

Alagille, or arteriohepatic dysplasia, syndrome is a multisystem, autosomal-dominant disorder independently described by two investigators more than 30 yr ago *(1,2)*. The original clinical diagnostic criteria required the demonstration of bile duct paucity on liver biopsy in addition to three of the five following characteristics: cholestatic liver disease, cardiac anomalies, skeletal anomalies, ocular abnormalities, and characteristic facies. Typical skeletal anomalies included butterfly vertebrae, and typical eye anomalies included posterior embryotoxon. Renal anomalies were also commonly reported. Approximately 5 to 10% of patients were found to have abnormal karyotypes involving the short arm of chromosome 20, thereby defining a probable disease locus. Additional molecular analyses identified the smallest region of overlap, and candidate gene analyses identified mutations in affected patients

From: *Methods in Molecular Medicine, vol. 126: Congenital Heart Disease: Molecular Diagnostics*
Edited by: M. Kearns-Jonker © Humana Press Inc., Totowa, NJ

in a gene mapping to the disease locus, called *JAG1* *(3,4)*. Therefore, the disease gene for Alagille syndrome is now known to be *JAG1*.

1.1. Cardiovascular Manifestations of Alagille Syndrome

As noted, Alagille syndrome is characterized in part by cardiac anomalies. Earlier reports had demonstrated that the right side of the heart, including the pulmonary arterial bed, was most commonly affected. We recently reviewed a large cohort of patients with Alagille syndrome who were tested for *JAG1* mutations in our center to better define the cardiovascular phenotype of this disorder and to identify any genotype–phenotype correlations *(5)*. This study demonstrated that 93% of patients with Alagille syndrome had some cardiovascular anomaly, ranging from a murmur consistent with peripheral pulmonary stenosis (PPS; mild changes) to tetralogy of Fallot with pulmonary atresia (severe defects). Overall, 76% of the cohort had PPS; 35% of the cohort had PPS in isolation, whereas the rest (41%) had PPS in conjunction with other cardiac anomalies. Right-sided cardiac defects were most common (55% of entire cohort), but left-sided cardiac abnormalities were also seen (7%). Multiple other anomalies (14%), including septal defects (10%), were identified as well. In this study, there was no correlation between the type and location of *JAG1* mutation and cardiac phenotype.

1.2. JAG1 Mutations in Congenital Heart Disease

Because a cardiovascular phenotype seems to be so highly penetrant in Alagille syndrome, many questioned whether patients with cardiac defects in the absence of hepatic disease could have *JAG1* mutations. Inspection of pedigrees and individuals harboring a *JAG1* mutation demonstrated marked clinical variability. In these families, some individuals carrying a *JAG1* mutation had very mild features or a "microform" of Alagille syndrome, whereas others with the same mutation manifested all of the features of Alagille syndrome *(3,6)*. Moreover, some patients predominantly manifested a cardiac phenotype with no overt hepatic involvement.

Subsequent reports highlight the potential contribution of *JAG1* mutations to the molecular genetic basis of congenital heart disease *(7–9)*. Krantz and colleagues *(7)* identified two patients with congenital heart disease and no apparent liver disease who were found to have *JAG1* mutations. The first patient had tetralogy of Fallot and butterfly vertebrae, and, after karyotyping, was found to have a 20p12 deletion encompassing *JAG1*. The second patient had branch pulmonary artery stenosis, and, on closer inspection, typical facial features of Alagille syndrome, posterior embryotoxon, and mild hepatic alterations. Her family history was significant for four generations of presumably affected individuals. The mother (with similar features of the proband) and the proband were found to share a protein truncating mutation. More recently, Eldadah and colleagues *(8)* reported an extensive pedigree with apparently isolated heart disease, including tetralogy of Fallot and PPS. The affected members of this family did not have hepatic involvement, and were found to have a unique missense mutation. Finally, Le Caignec and colleagues *(9)* reported a family with eight affected members with typical types of cardiac defects seen in Alagille syndrome (posterior embryotoxon and deafness); the affected members of this family had a missense mutation of *JAG1* but no hepatic manifestations. These reports suggest that *JAG1* mutations are etiological for a subset of patients with congenital heart disease, and should be considered, particularly in cases of familial right-sided defects. Studies are ongoing in our laboratory to identify the cardiac population at risk for *JAG1* mutations in the absence of hepatic or familial disease.

1.3. Additional Vascular Manifestations of JAG1 Mutations

Additional extracardiac vascular anomalies have been reported in the literature in patients with Alagille syndrome, including cases with abdominal aortic coarctation, renal and visceral arterial stenoses, intracranial arterial anomalies, and Moyamoya. A recent retrospective analysis found that 9% (25/268) of a large cohort with Alagille syndrome had either extracardiac vascular anomalies or events *(10)*. Vascular accidents accounted for 34% of the mortality in this cohort, exceeding the reported mortality from either congenital heart (21%) or hepatic (10%) disease in this series. The findings of extracardiac vascular anomalies are consistent with the embryonic pattern of expression of *JAG1* in mice and humans *(11,12)*. Thus, additional extracardiac vascular anomalies are common in this disorder and present a significant risk for mortality and morbidity.

1.4. JAG1 and Mutations in Alagille Syndrome

JAG1 consists of 26 exons and encodes the Jagged1 protein, a cell-surface protein that functions as one of five ligands for the four human Notch receptors. The Notch signaling pathway has been implicated in several human diseases *(13)* and is critical to developmental cell-fate decisions *(14)*. The Jagged1 protein has a single-pass transmembrane domain, a small intracellular domain, and a larger extracellular domain that consists of a signal peptide; a highly conserved region, known as the DSL region (DSL stands for Delta, Serrate, and Lag-2, the name of the Notch ligands in *Drosophila* and *Caenorhabditis elegans*); 16 epidermal growth factor-like repeats; and another conserved region, called the cysteine-rich region.

To date, more than 300 Alagille syndrome patients have been screened for *JAG1* mutations. Approximately 60 to 70% of the mutations seem to arise *de novo*, whereas the rest are transmitted in a family. Although published reports find a *JAG1* mutation in 65 to 70% of those patients screened, recent studies in our laboratory now identify a mutation in more than 90% of patients with a definitive clinical diagnosis of Alagille syndrome *(15–17)*. The mutations in *JAG1* include total gene deletions (3–7% of mutations) and intragenic mutations. The intragenic mutations are protein truncating (frameshift and nonsense mutations account for ~70% of mutations), splicing (~10%), and missense (~10%) mutations. Thus, Alagille syndrome seems to result from haploinsufficiency of Jagged1 protein. The mutations are distributed across the entire gene, with no significant hot spots. Therefore, screening this large gene presents a technical challenge.

1.5. Testing for JAG1 Mutations

Because of the enormous clinical variability of patients with *JAG1* mutations, identifying the cardiac patient with a *JAG1* mutation or a microform of Alagille syndrome is important to offer appropriate testing and genetic counseling to families. Although additional research to help identify the at-risk cardiac patient is still underway, currently, suspicion for a *JAG1* mutation should be raised when a family history of right-sided cardiac defects or transient hepatic dysfunction is reported, even if the patient at hand does not meet the complete clinical criteria for Alagille syndrome. Clinical genetic testing for *JAG1* mutations by sequencing the entire coding region is now available. The techniques by which whole gene deletions (FISH) or coding mutations (CSGE) are identified in our laboratory are described in detail in this chapter. *JAG1* is composed of 26 exons that occupy 35,000 kb of genomic DNA on chromosome 20 in band 20p12. The total gene deletions can be detected by cytogenetic or molecular cytogenetic techniques (FISH), and, in practice, FISH using a bacterial artificial chromosome (BAC) probe that contains *JAG1* is a straightforward assay for deletions. A second probe is used that serves as a control to positively identify chromosome 20, and the control probe can be fluorescently labeled in one color, with the *JAG1*-containing probe labeled in a second color to facilitate screening (**Fig. 1**).

The majority of Alagille syndrome-associated *JAG1* mutations are intragenic mutations, and these can be identified by analyzing the sequence of amplified regions of *JAG1* for sequence variation. It is possible to sequence the 26 exons of *JAG1* to look for mutations, but this approach is quite expensive as a first pass. In our laboratory, we use the technique of CSGE to provide a relatively rapid and sensitive screening technique to identify sequence variations. CSGE is a method for screening heteroduplex DNA molecules. The method uses an

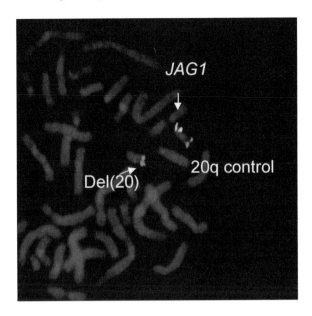

Fig. 1. Metaphase spread showing FISH using a probe containing the *JAG1* gene (that maps to the short arm of chromosome 20 at band 20p12), and a control probe that maps to the bottom of the long arm of chromosome 20. The chromosome on the right is normal, with one *JAG1* signal and one control signal, whereas the chromosome on the left has the control probe, but not the *JAG1*-containing BAC.

acrylamide gel matrix that includes 1,4 *bis* (acrolyl) piperazine (BAP) to crosslink, with ethylene glycol and formamide as mildly denaturing solvents. This environment enhances the differences in mobility shown by sequence mismatches in DNA heteroduplexes, so that variations as small as single nucleotide polymorphisms can be detected *(18)*. We screen a group of 25 patients at one time, and analyze the gene exon by exon. DNA from any patient whose DNA demonstrates a gel shift on electrophoresis is then sequenced for that exon to confirm the sequence (**Fig. 2**). CSGE scanning provides a powerful, cost-efficient method to scan genes with high sensitivity and specificity. However, we have found that CSGE identifies mutations in approx 70% of patients. As a follow-up to CSGE scanning, patients with a definitive diagnosis of Alagille syndrome, in whom no mutation is identified by CSGE, are targeted for further analysis, which is either direct sequencing of the 26 exons from genomic DNA, or sequencing of the 5.5-kb Jagged1 messenger RNA, which has been made into more stable cDNA.

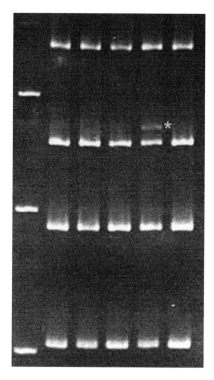

Fig. 2. Example of band with aberrant mobility on CSGE gel. Multiplex analysis of *JAG1* exons 13, 14, 15, and 21 (from top to bottom). First lane contains molecular weight markers, followed by PCR samples from five patients with Alagille syndrome. Note the aberrant band in exon 14 (*) in the fourth patient.

2. Materials
2.1. *Fluorescence* In Situ *Hybridization*

1. BACs are purchased from Children's Hospital Oakland Research Center. RP11-829A12 is an 183,891-bp BAC that contains the *JAG1* gene. The control BAC, RP11-15M15, maps to 20q.
2. Luria Bertani (LB) broth: NaCl (10 g), tryptone (10 g), yeast extract (5 g), dH$_2$O (1 L).
   Adjust pH to 7.0. Autoclave the LB broth and allow it to cool to room temperature. Using good aseptic technique, add 20 µg/mL of chloramphenicol (*see* **Note 1**).
3. LB agar: NaCl (10 g), tryptone (10 g), yeast extract (5 g), agar (10 g), dH$_2$O (1 L).
   Adjust pH to 7.0 Autoclave the LB Agar and allow it to cool to 45°C in a water bath. Using good aseptic technique, add 20 µg/mL of chloramphenicol. Pour 20 to

25 mL of agar into 60-mm plates and allow the agar to completely solidify (*see* **Notes 1** and **2**).
4. Fix solution: methanol (75 mL), acetic acid (25 mL), dH$_2$O (250 mL), 1–2 trays of ice cubes.
5. 2X sodium saline citrate (SSC) (0.3 *M* NaCl, 0.003 *M* Na Citrate, pH 7.0) and 0.05% Tween-20: 2X SSC (50 mL), Tween-20 (25 mL).
6. 0.4% SSC: 2X SSC (200 mL), sterile dH$_2$O (48.8 mL).

2.2. Mutation Detection

2.2.1. Polymerase Chain Reaction

1. 2 m*M* dNTP mix: 100 m*M* dATP (10 mL), 100 m*M* dCTP (10 mL), 100 m*M* dTTP (10 mL), 100 m*M* dGTP (10 mL), sterile dH$_2$O (460 mL).

2.2.2. Conformation-Sensitive Gel Electrophoresis

1. 40% Acryl:BAP: Acrylamide 40% solution (500 mL), BAP (2.02 g), sterile dH$_2$O (5 mL).
   Stir for 30 to 40 min, filter through a 0.2-µm nylon filter, and store at 4°C in the dark. Make fresh monthly (*see* **Note 3**).
2. 20X TTE: trizma base (108 g), taurine (36 g), EDTA (2 g).
   Dissolve in 200 mL of dH$_2$O by stirring on low heat. Adjust the volume to 500 mL and filter through a 0.22-µm nylon filter. Store at room temperature.
3. Loading dye: 30% Glycerol, 0.25% Bromophenol blue, 0.25% Xylene Cyanol FF, in 0.5X TTE buffer.
4. Staining buffer: 0.5X TTE, 0.1 mL/mL Ethidium bromide (10 mg/mL) (*see* **Note 4**).
5. 15% gel solution: 40% Acryl:BAP (75 mL), 20X TTE buffer (5 mL), deionized formamide (30 mL), ethylene glycol (20 mL), sterile dH$_2$O (68 mL), TEMED (114 mL), 10% ammonium persulfate (APS) (2 mL) (*see* **Note 5**).

2.2.3. cDNA Sequencing

1. Complete media: RPMI-1640 (389 mL), fetal bovine serum (100 mL), L-glutamine (200 m*M*) (10 mL), penicillin/streptomycin (100X) (1 mL) (*see* **Note 6**).
2. Cycloheximide media: Cycloheximide (50 mg), complete media (50 mL) (*see* **Note 7**).
3. Diethylpyrocarbonate (DEPC)-treated water: water is treated with 0.1% v/v DEPC and autoclaved to inactivate ribonuclease (RNase) in solution.

3. Methods

3.1. Fluorescence In Situ Hybridization

1. Streak LB agar plate (containing 20 µg/mL of chloramphenicol) with the *Escherichia coli*-containing BAC RPII-829A12 (this BAC contains the *JAG1* gene). Incubate overnight at 37°C.

2. A single colony from the plate is used to inoculate 10 mL of LB broth containing 20 µg/mL of chloramphenicol. Incubate at 37°C overnight.
3. Take 1 mL of the overnight broth and inoculate 100 mL of LB broth containing 20 µg/mL of chloramphenicol. Incubate at 37°C overnight. The remaining 9 mL can be frozen in 30% glycerol at –80°C for future use.
4. Centrifuge at 5858*g* for 15 min at 4°C.
5. Isolate DNA (Purgene DNA Isolation Kit, Gentra).
   a. Add 3 mL of cell lysis solution and mix well.
   b. Incubate at 80°C until cells are lysed (*see* **Note 8**).
   c. Cool the sample to room temperature.
   d. Add 2 mL of protein precipitation solution and vortex. Incubate on ice for 5 min and vortex until white precipitate forms.
   e. Centrifuge at 805*g* for 10 min.
   f. Pour supernatant into a clean 15-mL tube containing 3 mL of 100% isopropanol.
   g. Gently rock the tube back and forth until you see strands of white DNA.
   h. Using a sterile glass rod, transfer the DNA to a clean tube.
   i. Add 3 mL of 70% ethanol.
   j. Centrifuge at 805*g* for 1 min.
   k. Drain for 30 min. Make sure all ethanol has evaporated.
   l. Add 500 µL of DNA hydration solution.
   m. Incubate overnight at room temperature. Add sterile dH$_2$O if the DNA it does not go into solution well (*see* **Note 9**).
6. Determine the DNA concentration by running on a 1.5% agarose gel with a quantitative DNA marker. Polymerase chain reaction (PCR) can be performed to confirm that Jagged 1 is present in the BAC DNA (*see* **Subheading 2.2.1.**).
7. Probes can be fluorescently labeled with a commercially available Nick Translation Kit (32-801300; Abbott).
8. Place clean slides into fix solution for 1 min.
9. Use a Pasteur pipet to mix the cell pellet.
10. Remove slide from fix solution and allow slides to drain briefly at a 45° angle.
11. Hold slide over steam from a hot water bath for 3 s.
12. Hold pipet parallel to slide and place six drops from the cell pellet evenly along the slide.
13. Place slides on a slide warmer at 45°C to evaporate any excess fluid.
14. After most of fluid has evaporated, hold the slide over steam for 3 s, and then either incubate the slide overnight at room temperature or incubate the slide in an oven at 90°C for 1 h.
15. Place slides on the slide warmer at 45°C.
16. Add 10 µL of probe (RPII-829A12, *JAG1*) and 10 µL of a control (RPII-15M15, maps to 20q) in several drops. Probes should be labeled with different fluorochromes.
17. Place a coverslip (22 × 40 mm) on the slide, without creating air bubbles between the slide and the coverslip. If there are air bubbles, press gently on the coverslip.
18. Incubate slides on a hot plate at 75°C for 3 min.

19. Seal the coverslip to the slide by generously adding rubber cement around the edges of coverslip.
20. Incubate overnight in a humidified chamber at 37°C.
21. Remove slides from the chamber and remove rubber cement and coverslip (do not let slides dry out).
22. Incubate slides in 0.4% SSC for 2 min at 73°C.
23. Wash slide in 2X SSC/0.05% Tween at room temperature for 30 s to 1 min.
24. Remove slide, and allow it to drain briefly (do not allow slide to dry).
25. Add 10 μL of DAPI (Abbott), a counterstain that permits visualization of the chromosome, in several drops along the center of the slide.
26. Place a coverslip (24 × 50 mm) on the slide without creating air bubbles. Press gently on the slide if there are any air bubbles.
27. Visualize using a fluorescent microscope.

3.2. Mutation Detection

3.2.1. Polymerase Chain Reaction

1. **Table 1** has a list of primers, $MgCl_2$ concentrations, and PCR cycles for screening all 26 exons of the *JAG1* gene.
2. Place 5 μL of patient DNA [25 ng/μL] into a sterile 0.5-μL PCR tube.
3. Add the following to the PCR tube containing the patient DNA. PCR reaction:
   a. 11.2 μL-X sterile dH_2O.
   b. 2.5 μL 10X buffer.
   c. X (1 μL or 1.5 μL) 25 mM $MgCl_2$ (**Table 1**).
   d. 2.5 μL dNTP mix.
   e. 2.5 μL Dimethylsulfoxide.
   f. 0.5 μL 20 μM Forward primer (**Table 1**).
   g. 0.5 μL 20 μM Reverse primer (**Table 1**).
   h. 0.3 μL Amplitaq gold.
4. Vortex the tube and centrifuge briefly.
5. Place the samples into a thermocycler, programmed according to **Table 1**.
6. To determine whether amplification has been successful, DNA bands can be visualized by running the samples on a 1.5% agarose gel stained with ethidium bromide and illuminated with UV light (*see* **Note 10**).
7. PCR products can be used for CSGE, or purified for sequencing.

3.2.2. Confirmation-Sensitive Gel Electrophoresis

1. Heating PCR products at 98°C for 5 min and then at 68°C for 30 min creates heteroduplexes.
2. Assemble plates as follows:
   a. Wash glass plates with hot tap water, rinse with dH_2O and ethanol, and dry with lint-free tissue paper.
   b. Gel slick (*see* **Note 11**) should be added occasionally to large plates to prevent the gel from sticking during disassembly. Add gel slick, wipe it evenly across the plate, and let dry. Once dry, buff the gel slick off.

Table 1 Primer Pairs for CSGE

Exon	Forward primer sequence	Reverse primer sequence	Exon size (bp)	Product size (bp)	[MgCl₂]	Annealing temperature
Jag1 exon 01	5' CAG CGG CGA CGG CAG CAG CAC C 3'	5' AGA GGA CGG CTG GGA GGG A 3'	81	204	1.5 mM	62°C/30 s
Jag1 exon 02	5' CGC CAC CTC TAT ACT CGA AG 3'	5' CCA GGC GCG GGT GTG AG 3'	306	469	1 mM	50°C/1 min
Jag1 exon 03	5' GTG GGG TAT TCT GGG AGG 3'	5' GCA AGA GGT GGC AGA AAT 3'	51	254	1 mM	50°C/1 min
Jag1 exon 04	5' GGC TGC AAT GTG AAT ATT A 3'	5' TCC CAC CCC ACC TGA GAT A 3'	255	452	1 mM	50°C/1 min
Jag1 exon 05	5' GGA ATT TGC AGA CTT TAA TGC AA 3'	5' CAC AAT AAA GTC AGT TCC TC 3'	61	229	1 mM	50°C/1 min
Jag1 exon 06	5' ATG AGC CTT GGG AGT CTA C 3'	5' AAA CCC ACA CAG CAT TCA A 3'	131	388	1.5 mM	50°C/1 min
Jag1 exon 07	5' GGC TAG AAA CAT GGT GGG T 3'	5' ATC TTT GGA AGC TAT TTT C 3'	120	295	1.5 mM	50°C/1 min
Jag1 exon 08	5' GGA GGT AAC GGT GTG CAG GCA TC 3'	5' ACC TCT CCC CAG CGT GGT ATC TT 3'	114	236	1 mM	60°C/20 s[a]
Jag1 exon 09	5' GGA TCT AAT TGT CAG ATG GAT 3'	5' CCA CAC GCT CGT CTT CTG 3'	115	256	1 mM	50°C/1 min
Jag1 exon 10	5' TTC CAA GGT GGG GGA GAT 3'	5' CCT GAC CAC TCC CTC TCA AA 3'	114	300	1.5 mM	55°C/1 min
Jag1 exon 11	5' CAC CCA GCG TAA TAA CCT T 3'	5' CTA GTG TCG CAC AAA TCT 3'	47	262	1.5 mM	50°C/1 min
Jag1 exon 12	5' TGA AGC CCT GTG TTT GTG GAA TAC 3'	5' GAA AAG TAA AGG GAA GCG GAA GAG GAG 3'	174	354	1 mM	60°C/1 min
Jag1 exon 13	5' GTT TTA CTC TGA TCC CTC 3'	5' CAA GGG GCA GTG GTA GTA AGT 3'	151	273	1 mM	50°C/1 min
Jag1 exon 14	5' GAA TGC CGC ATC TGT GGG TG 3'	5' AGG CTG GGG AGC ACT GGT C 3'	165	263	1 mM	60°C/20 s[a]
Jag1 exon 15	5' AGG AGG GAG GAG CCA TGA AAA CTG C 3'	5' CAA CAT GAC CCA TAC ATC CCA GAG 3'	114	250	1.5 mM	54°C/30 s
Jag1 exon 16	5' GCC TGT CGT GAA TGG TCC TGG A 3'	5' CCA CAG AAG ACA GAG GGA AG 3'	124	231	1 mM	55°C/1 min
Jag1 exon 17	5' GCT ATC TCT GGG ACC CTT 3'	5' CCA CGT GGG GCA TAA AGT T 3'	114	192	1 mM	50°C/1 min
Jag1 exon 18	5' CCT CCA GAC TGT TTC TGG ATA 3'	5' GCA AGT CCC CAA GGG TGT CA 3'	117	244	1 mM	50°C/1 min
Jag1 exon 19	5' GGC TAA GAC CGC TTT CCC TGT T 3'	5' ACG ATA GTG GAT GAG TGC TGG CTT 3'	28	128	1 mM	60°C/1 min
Jag1 exon 20	5' CAT GTG AGT GAT TGG CAG C 3'	5' CAG CTG GAG GAG AGA GAT C 3'	86	298	1 mM	55°C/1 min
Jag1 exon 21	5' CAT TGC CAC ACA CCA TCA GTC 3'	5' CGC TCA CCC CAG AAG ACC CAT 3'	114	209	1.5 mM	60°C/20 s[a]
Jag1 exon 22	5' CAA AGA ATT GAA CCC CGA TCC 3'	5' GCT GGC AGC TTA GCA GGC ATG 3'	110	250	1 mM	50°C/1 min
Jag1 exon 23	5' ATG GCT GCC GCA GTT CA 3'	5' CAC CAT TCA AAA AAA AAA CAA AGG 3'	234	409	1 mM	50°C/1 mi
Jag1 exon 24	5' GCC TCA AAG AGA ACA TCT CAG 3'	5' AAC CGA ACT GCC TTG CCA TCG 3'	132	262	1 mM	55°C/1 min
Jag1 exon 25	5' GCA GAC ACA GAT TGT CGA 3'	5' CCC TCG ACC TGA TGG CTT TA 3'	156	378	1.5 mM	56°C/30 s
Jag1 exon 26	5' TCT TGG AGA GTT AAT TGG TTT TGT GC 3'	5' GAC AGT TTA AAG AAC TAC AAG CCC TCA GA 3'	455	525	1 mM	50°C/1 min

Cycle: initital, 94°C/5 min; 36 cycles of (denature, 94°C/1 min; annealing, 50°C/1 min; and extension, 72°C/30 s); and hold, 72°C/10 min.
[a]Cycle: Initital, 94°C/5 min; 36 cycles of (denature, 94°C/20 s; annealing, 60°C/20 s; and extension, 72°C/20 s); and hold, 72°C/3 min.

c. Place 1-mm spacers between the plates, flush on each side.

d. Place tape around the edges of the glass to prevent leaking. Clamps can also be placed along the edges to help prevent leaking.

e. Add the 15% gel solution between the plates with a 25-mL pipet. Do not create air bubbles. Tap lightly on the glass to remove any air bubbles (*see* **Note 12**).

f. Insert comb and add excess gel to the sides of the comb to prevent gel shrinkage. Make sure comb is pushed all the way in and use a clamp to hold the comb in place (*see* **Note 13**).

g. Let the gel polymerize for 2 h before use or for 30 min before wrapping for overnight storage at 4°C. For overnight storage, place paper towels soaked with dH$_2$O along the comb and wrap with plastic wrap to keep the gel from drying out.

h. Remove the tape from around the gel. Gently remove the comb from the gel without damaging the wells.

3. Attach plates to gel apparatus and add running buffer (0.5X TTE).

4. Rinse wells with running buffer, using a 20-mL syringe.

5. Prerun gel at 40 W for 15 min.

6. Rinse wells again with running buffer (*see* **Note 14**).

7. Mix 2 µL of PCR product with 1 µL of loading buffer.

8. Quickly load samples, using gel-loading tips to prevent diffusion of samples into the wells (*see* **Note 15**).

9. Run gel at 40 W for 6 to 8 h.

10. Detach the plates from apparatus and pry the plates apart, leaving the gel on the smaller plate.

11. Pour staining buffer on the gel (still attached to the plate) and soak for 10 min. Pour dH$_2$O on the gel and let soak for 10 min. Drain gel.

12. Apply a piece of Whatman 3 paper to the gel and remove the gel from the plate. Gel is now attached to paper.

13. Visualize the bands on the gel with a UV lamp (*see* **Note 10**). Take a photograph of the gel.

14. Purify PCR products from the samples with multiple bands and submit for sequencing (*see* **Note 16**).

3.2.3. cDNA Sequencing

1. Split cells (lymphoblastoid cell line or fibroblast cell line) into two flasks. Add fresh complete media until the volume reaches 20 to 25 mL.

2. Remove the complete media from one flask, with a pipet, being careful not to remove any cells (*see* **Note 17**). Remove as much media as possible without disturbing the cells. Add 25 mL of cycloheximide media. Do not do anything to the second flask (it will be a negative control).

3. Incubate for 6 hours.

4. Centrifuge at 453*g* for 10 min.

5. Remove the supernatant and add 1 mL of TRIzol®. Mix well and transfer to 1.5-mL tubes.

6. Freeze tubes at –80°C. To isolate RNA (*see* **Note 18**), thaw frozen samples at room temperature for 5 min.
7. Add 200 µL of chloroform and shake tubes vigorously.
8. Incubate at room temperature for 2 to 3 min.
9. Centrifuge at 4°C for 15 min at 13,400g.
10. Transfer the colorless upper layer to a new tube and add 500 µL of isopropanol to each tube. Incubate at room temperature for 10 min.
11. Centrifuge at 4°C for 10 min at 13,400g.
12. RNA should be in pellet form. Carefully remove supernatant. Add 1 mL of 75% ethanol to tube. Use DEPC-treated water to dilute ethanol.
13. Vortex the sample.
14. Centrifuge at 4°C for 5 min at 5100g.
15. Carefully remove supernatant and allow the tubes to air-dry for 10 to 15 min. Make sure that all ethanol has evaporated before proceeding to the next step.
16. Add 50 µL of DEPC-treated water to dissolve pellets.
17. Store RNA at –80°C.
18. RNA is reverse transcribed into cDNA using reverse transcription (RT)-PCR (Invitrogen, Superscript First-Strand Synthesis System for RT-PCR).
19. PCR can be performed on the cDNA for sequencing.
20. **Table 2** has a list of primers, $MgCl_2$ concentrations, and PCR cycles for screening all five regions of the *JAG1* cDNA.
21. Place 2 µL of cDNA into a sterile 0.5-µL PCR tube.
22. Add the following to the PCR tube containing cDNA.
    PCR reaction:
    a. 14.2 µL-X sterile dH_2O.
    b. 2.5 µL 10X buffer.
    c. X (1 µL or 1.5 µL) 25 mM $MgCl_2$ (**Table 2**).
    d. 2.5 µL dNTP mix.
    e. 2.5 µL Dimethylsulfoxide.
    f. 0.5 µL 20 µM Forward primer (**Table 2**).
    g. 0.5 µL 20 µM Reverse primer (**Table 2**).
    h. 0.3 µL Amplitaq gold.
23. Place the samples into a thermocycler, programmed according to **Table 2**.
24. Bands can be visualized by running the samples on a 1.5% agarose gel stained with ethidium bromide and illuminated with UV light.
25. PCR products should be purified and submitted for sequencing.

4. Notes

1. It is important to let the LB Broth or agar cool before adding the chloramphenicol.
2. Store LB Agar plates inverted at 4°C. Plates are inverted to prevent moisture from accumulating on the agar surface.
3. **Caution:** acrylamide is a neurotoxin and BAP is irritating to the eyes and skin, so handle with care.
4. **Caution:** ethidium bromide is a carcinogen.

Table 2
PCR Primers for cDNA Screening

Region	Forward primer sequence	Reverse primer sequence	[MgCl$_2$]	Annealing temperature	Exons per region	Product size (bp)
A	5' CGC TCT TGA AAG GGC TTT TGA AAA GTG GTG 3'	5' CAT CCA GCC TTC CAT GCA A 3'	1 mM	50°C/1 min	exons 1–3 and part of exon 4	800
B	5' CAC TTTT GAG TAT CAG ATC CGC GTG A 3'	5' CGA TGT CCA GCT GAC AGA 3'	1.5 mM	58.8°C/1 min	Part of exon 4 through exon 13	1200
C	5' CGG GAT TTG GTT AAT GGT TAT 3'	5' GGT ACC AGT TGT CTC CAT 3'	1.5 mM	55°C/1 min	Part of exon 12-part of exon 18	1000
D	5' GGA ACA ACC TGT AAC ATA GC 3'	5' GGC CAC ATG TAT TTC ATT GTT 3'	1.5 mM	55°C/1 min	exon 18 –23 and part of exon 24	825
E	5' GAA TAT TCA ATC TAC ATC GCT T 3'	5' CTC AGA CTC GAG TAT GAC ACG A 3'	1 mM	52°C/30 sa	part of exon 24 through exon 26	756

Cycle: initial, 94°C/5 min; 36 cycles of (denature, 94°C/30 s; annealing, 50°C/1 min; and extension, 72°C/30 s); and hold, 72°C/10 min.
aCycle: initial, 94°C/5 min; 36 cycles of (denature, 94°C/30 s; annealing, 52°C/30 s; and extension, 72°C/30 s); and hold, 72°C/10 min.

5. Add TEMED and APS immediately before pouring the gel. Adding TEMED and APS will cause the gel to polymerize. Do not add TEMED and APS before you are ready to pour the gel.

6. Make complete media fresh weekly and store at 4°C. L-Glutamine degrades over time.

7. Make cycloheximide media fresh for each use.

8. Solution will appear clear when cells are lysed. You may need to vortex the cells a few times during incubation.

9. If the sample has a hazy appearance, do not dilute the sample. You can place samples at –80°C overnight and centrifuge to clarify the solution.

10. **Caution:** UV light can be damaging to eyes and skin.

11. Gel slick is a glass-plate coating that prevents gels from adhering to electrophoresis plates.

12. Air bubbles make it difficult to visualize band shifts.

13. Comb must be clamped down to prevent them from shifting as the gel polymerizes. If the comb shifts, the wells will not form properly and the samples will not run correctly.

14. It is critical that wells be clean so that the PCR products run into the gel at the same time.

15. It is important that all samples enter the gel at the same time. Diffused samples can appear band shifted.

16. PCR products from samples with blurry bands should also be purified and sequenced. A blurry appearance of bands could be two bands very close together.

17. Lymphoblastoid cells will settle in the bottom of the flask.

18. Make sure to work in an area that is RNase free. Also make sure that the tubes and pipets are RNase-free. If you are not careful, RNase can degrade your RNA. Areas and equipment can be treated with RNase Away spray (Gentra) to remove any RNase contamination.

References

1. Watson, G. H. and Miller, V. (1973) Arteriohepatic dysplasia: familial pulmonary arterial stenosis with neonatal liver disease. *Arch. Dis. Child.* **48**, 459–466.

2. Alagille, D., Odievre, M., Gautier, M., and Dommergues, J. P. (1975) Hepatic ductular hypoplasia associated with characteristic facies, vertebral malformations, retarded physical, mental, and sexual development, and cardiac murmur. *J. Pediatr.* **86**, 63–71.

3. Li, L., Krantz, I. D., Deng, Y., et al. (1997) Alagille syndrome is caused by mutations in human Jagged1, which encodes a ligand for Notch1. *Nat. Genet.* **16**, 243–251.

4. Oda, T., Elkahloun, A. G., Pike, B. L., et al. (1997) Mutations in the human Jagged1 gene are responsible for Alagille syndrome. *Nat. Genet.* **16**, 235–242.

5. McElhinney, D. B., Krantz, I. D., Bason, L., et al. (2002) Analysis of cardiovascular phenotype and genotype-phenotype correlation in individuals with a JAG1 mutation and/or Alagille syndrome. *Circulation* **106**, 2567–2574.

6. Yuan, Z. R., Kohsaka, T., Ikegaya, T., et al. (1998) Mutational analysis of the Jagged 1 gene in Alagille syndrome families. *Hum. Mol. Genet.* 7, 1363–1369.

7. Krantz, I. D., Smith, R., Colliton, R. P., et al. (1999) Jagged1 mutations in patients ascertained with isolated congenital heart defects. *Am. J. Med. Genet.* **84**, 56–60.

8. Eldadah, Z. A., Hamosh, A., Biery, N. J., et al. (2001) Familial tetralogy of Fallot caused by mutation in the Jagged1 gene. *Hum. Mol. Genet.* **10**, 163–169.

9. Le Caignec, C., Lefevre, M., Schott, J. J., et al. (2002) Familial deafness, congenital heart defects, and posterior embryotoxon caused by cysteine substitution in the first epidermal-growth-factor-like domain of jagged 1. *Am. J. Hum. Genet.* **71**, 180–186.

10. Kamath, B. M., Spinner, N. B., Emerick, K. M., et al. (2004) Vascular anomalies in Alagille syndrome: a significant cause of morbidity and mortality. *Circulation* **109**, 1354–1358.

11. Loomes, K. M., Underkoffler, L. A., Morabito, J., et al. (1999) The expression of Jagged1 in the developing mammalian heart correlates with cardiovascular disease in Alagille syndrome. *Hum. Mol. Genet.* **8**, 2443–2449.

12. Jones, E. A., Clement-Jones, M., and Wilson, D. I. (2000) JAGGED1 expression in human embryos: correlation with the Alagille syndrome phenotype. *J. Med. Genet.* **37**, 658–662.

13. Gridley, T. (2003) Notch signaling and inherited disease syndromes. *Hum. Mol. Genet.* 12 Spec No 1, R9–13.

14. Artavanis-Tsakonas, S., Rand, M. D., and Lake, R. J. (1999) Notch signaling: cell fate control and signal integration in development. *Science* **284**, 770–776.

15. Spinner, N. B., Colliton, R. P., Crosnier, C., Krantz, I. D., Hadchouel, M., and Meunier-Rotival, M. (2001) Jagged1 mutations in alagille syndrome. *Hum. Mutat.* **17**, 18–33.

16. Ropke, A., Kujat, A., Graber, M., Giannakudis, J., and Hansmann, I. (2003) Identification of 36 novel Jagged1 (JAG1) mutations in patients with Alagille syndrome. *Hum. Mutat.* **21**, 100.

17. Wathen, D. M., Moore, E. C., Kamath, B. M., et al. (2005) Jagged1 (*JAG1*) mutations in alagille syndrome: increasing the mutation detection rate. *Hum. Mutat.* (in press).

18. Ganguly, A. (2002) An update on conformation sensitive gel electrophoresis. *Hum. Mutat.* **19**, 334–342.

14

Array Analysis Applied to Malformed Hearts

Molecular Dissection of Tetralogy of Fallot

Silke Sperling

Summary

Microarray technology as a method for large-scale gene expression analysis has entered into widespread use in the field of cardiovascular research. This chapter summarizes the application of arrays to study gene expression profiles of congenital heart diseases, in particular the molecular portrait of tetralogy of Fallot.

The sections of this chapter correspond to the several distinct steps of microarray experiments. A general introduction to the method, and information on the selection of arrays and preparation of labeled complementary DNA samples are given. A specific focus of the chapter is the experimental design and data analysis.

Key Words: Microarray; cDNA array; experimental design; gene expression profiling; tetralogy of Fallot; congenital heart diseases.

1. Introduction

Recently, complementary DNA (cDNA) microarray technology has entered into widespread use to understand gene expression, and the technology is tantalizing in the possibilities it presents. In light of this excitement, some perspective is in order, to ensure well-designed and accomplished experiments. This chapter summarizes the application of cDNA arrays to study gene expression profiles of congenital heart disease (CHD) focusing on tetralogy of Fallot (TOF).

CHDs are the clinical manifestation of anomalies in heart development, which is a complex process requiring the precise integration of cell type-specific gene expression and morphological development; both are intertwined in their regulation by transcription factors. Although studies of heart development in fish, frog, mice, chicken, flies, and worms have begun to unravel how

From: *Methods in Molecular Medicine, vol. 126: Congenital Heart Disease: Molecular Diagnostics*
Edited by: M. Kearns-Jonker © Humana Press Inc., Totowa, NJ

morphogenesis and hierarchies of developmental control are exerted, the basic mechanism for CHD in human is still incompletely defined. The rarity of large CHD human families and the incomplete penetrance of CHD as a phenotype have limited the usefulness of linkage analysis in identifying causative genes. The genetics of CHD points to the existence of powerful disease modifiers because wide phenotypic spectra are seen in patients harboring identical disease alleles.

The application of cDNA arrays as a large-scale technology for the simultaneous analysis of thousands of genes permits the identification of specific gene expression profiles of the various stages of cardiac development. Moreover, the comparison of gene expression patterns between human normal and congenital malformed hearts or among different types of CHDs will identify differentially expressed genes that may point to the molecular mechanisms involved in normal and CHD states, and perhaps provide new insights for the discovery of novel molecular targets for diagnostics and therapeutics.

Any microarray experiment involves several distinct stages. First, there is the design of the experiment. The researcher must decide on the source of RNA to be hybridized to the arrays, on the set of genes to be represented on the arrays, and on the number of replicative hybridizations to be performed. Second, the wet-lab experiments, including RNA isolation, labeling, and array hybridization, follow. Third, the array data are processed and analyzed to select differentially expressed genes, to identify patterns within the data, and to interpret the resulting molecular portraits. The sections of this chapter correspond roughly to these three steps and focus on specific considerations for the molecular dissection of TOF in humans. Regarding the recent developments of commercially available gene expression analysis arrays, this chapter provides an overview on the general technique, with hands-on information, and explains, in detail, the specific considerations for the analysis of CHDs.

Generally, cDNA arrays are a measurement tool with cDNA (the probes) of known sequence immobilized in an orderly arrangement of tens to hundreds of thousands of unique DNA molecules. Labeled cDNA samples (the targets) are simultaneously hybridized to the array and the signal intensity from the bound target is quantified. There are many unknown quantities in this process; however, the basic principle is as follows: for a given sequence spotted on the array, the quantity of the corresponding transcript of the sample hybridized is measured using the intensity of the fluorescence or radioactive signal, which should be proportional to the quantity of the corresponding transcript. Finally, the obtained transcript quantities for each gene within each sample are bioinformatically and statistically analyzed with respect to the hypothesis that drive the experiment. The main advantage of the application of cDNA arrays compared with other quantitative methods, such as real-time polymerase chain

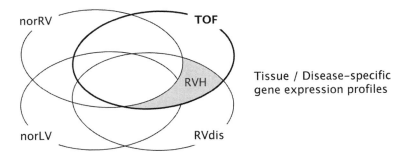

Fig. 1. Molecular dissection of tetralogy of Fallot (TOF). Schematic representation of molecular portraits for the normal right and left ventricle (norRV and norLV) as well as for the diseases stages of TOF and a variety of cardiac malformations (RVdis) sharing the feature of right ventricular hypertrophy in response to pressure overload in the TOF cases. The characteristic changes of gene expression in each tissue and diseases can be extracted by comparing the molecular portraits.

reaction (PCR), is the simultaneous analysis of thousands of genes within very small samples. Using large-scale arrays, we are able to analyze more than two-thirds of the entire set of human transcripts with samples as small as 8 μg of total RNA for one assay *(1)*.

The concept for the analysis of gene expression profiles in the setting of TOF in human is outlined in **Fig. 1**. This concept focuses on the study of disease-specific transcriptome changes in patients with TOF and on the dissection of the molecular portrait corresponding to the primary dys-development and the molecular portrait associated with the secondary hemodynamic changes because of the heart malformation. For such a study, the analysis of the transcriptome of the right ventricle (RV) of patients with TOF, as well as of patients showing a variety of cardiac malformations but sharing the common cardiac adaptation feature of the RV (RV hypertrophy [RVH]), should be envisaged. To further distinguish the diseased from the normal ventricular portrait, normal samples of at least the RV should be profiled as well.

2. Materials

2.1. Patient and Sample Collection

To allow for the selection of a balanced patient population enabling the separation of disease- or tissue-specific expression patterns, we collected 150 samples of human ventricular and atrial cardiac tissue. For the storage of all general, clinical, and sample collection information, we set up a relational database with an Internet interface. The overall clinical characterization included 250 features of hemodynamical, morphological, and therapeutical information. The sample collection and laboratory information section contained surgical or interventional conditions (e.g., patient temperature and cardiac arrest) of the sample retrieval as well as timing and cardiac localization.

2.2. DNA Microarrays

In our study we used "Human Unigene Set-RZPD 2" cDNA arrays (nylon membrane arrays) from the German Resource Center for Genome Research, Berlin, Germany.

Other sources of premade human DNA arrays are GeneChips® (Affymetrix, Santa Clara, CA), BD Atlas Arrays (BD Biosciences Clontech, Palo Alto, CA), ResGen (Invitrogen, Hunstville, AL), Agilent (Agilent Technologies, Palo Alto, CA), sciTRACER Cardio Vascular 725 (Scienion, Berlin, Germany), and several other resources. Custom-made arrays are also available from some of these suppliers.

2.3. RNA Isolation, Labeling, Hybridization, and Signal Detection

We used TRIzol® reagent for RNA isolation, $pd(T)_{12-18}$ oligonucleotides for reverse transcription to cDNA, and α-^{33}P-dCTP for labeling. For signal detection, we scanned our arrays using a Fuji Film Bas-1800 reader (Fuji photo film).

Finally, the material for labeling, hybridization, and signal detection strongly depends on the arrays used, and the majority of array suppliers purchase the material along with their arrays. For example, the oligonucleotide arrays GeneChip or cDNA arrays sciTRACER are hybridized with biotin-labeled or Cy3/Cy5-labeled targets, respectively.

2.4. Data Analysis Tools and Array Databases

A selection of software packages for the analysis of array data follows:

1. SAM Software, Stanford University (Stanford, CA http://www-stat.stanford.edu/~tibs/SAM).
2. R, Bioconductor project, http://www.bioconductor.org.
3. TM4, TIGR Institute for Genomic Research (Rockville, MD, http://www.tigr.org/software/tm4).
4. GeneSpring, Silicon Genetics (Redwood City, CA, http://www.silicongenetics.com).

Public repositories for array data follow:

5. GEO—Gene Expression Omnibus, National Center for Biotechnology Information (Bethesda, MD, http://www.ncbi.nlm.nih.gov/geo).
6. ArrayExpress, European Molecular Biology Laboratory–European Bioinformatics Institute (Cambridge, UK, http://www.ebi.ac.uk/arrayexpress).

3. Methods
3.1. Selection of Samples

The questions that can be answered by the array experiment mainly depend on the sample selection regarding the studied phenotype and cardiac localization of the obtained sample. Focusing on the analysis of TOF, we compared samples from patients with TOF with samples from a variety of CHD cases also sharing the feature of RVH caused by pressure overload as the cardiac adaptation to their aberrant disease state. In addition, we compared these diseased hearts with normal hearts. For our study, we chose right ventricular samples of the CHD patients and samples from all four cardiac chambers as well as the interventricular septum of normal hearts. Furthermore, we profiled right atrial samples of patients with single atrial or ventricular septal defects (*see* **Note 1**). In general, to consider known confounding factors, such as age and gender, the number of collected samples needs to widely exceed the number of samples finally chosen for the experiment. Moreover, all clinical features should be assembled in a detailed and sufficiently searchable way. The selected patient populations should represent a tight range of those factors on which the analysis will focus (in our study TOF, RVH, and tissue specificity) and a wide range of all other clinical factors known or unknown as confounding factors, for which no stringent selection can be achieved, e.g., because of natural sample limitation (*see* **Note 2**).

3.2. Selection of cDNA Array

The various types of cDNA arrays currently available for gene expression profiling differ mainly in their basic source for the DNA probes on the array and in the array platform. Either each probe is individually synthesized on a rigid surface (usually glass) *(2)*, or presynthesized probes (oligonucleotides or PCR products) are attached to the array's platform (usually glass or nylon membranes) *(3,4)*. Although the *in situ* probe synthesis method requires sophisticated and expensive robotic equipment, the method of attaching presynthesized cDNA probes (usually 100–5000 bases long) to a solid surface, such as glass or nylon membrane, is affordable for academic research laboratories, and many institutions have developed core facilities for the in-house manufacture of custom glass slide cDNA arrays.

For our genome-wide array study of CHD in human, we used the nylon membrane Human Unigene Set 2 arrays from the RZPD (http://www.rzpd.de). In total, 61 arrays were used, each represented by 3 Hybond N+ membranes containing PCR products (600–1200 bases long) of 74,695 different IMAGE clones, spotted in duplicate, representing 34,000 Unigene clusters and approx 20,000 genes annotated by Ensembl.

3.3. Experimental Design

Statistics is often thought to concern only the analysis of observational or experimental data. However, experimental design is one of the oldest subfields of statistics. The experimental design affects many things: the analysis that will be possible, the question that will be answerable, and the quality of the results *(5)*. Although a good design does not guarantee a successful experiment, a suitably bad design guarantees a failed experiment, no results, or useless results. Many experimental designs for gene expression profiling experiments are possible. However, no matter what the purpose of the experiment, a sufficient number of measurements must be obtained for statistical analysis of the data, either through multiple measurements of homogeneous samples (replication) or through multiple sample measurements (e.g., across subjects or time). This is because many genes will show considerable changes in expression levels between two experimental conditions, without the changes being significant. These false-positive results arise from chance occurrences caused by uncontrolled biological variance as well as experimental and measurement errors. Experimental errors include variations in the sample retrieval procedure (surgical probes vs catheter biopsies can lead to different cell sample types), and the treatment and handling of RNA during extraction and subsequent processing. For example, if large frozen samples are reduced to smaller pieces for the RNA isolation procedure, this should be done without thawing, because a change of gene expression profiles could be caused if samples encounter a temperature shift, even for a short time. In addition, the protocols for RNA isolation and cDNA preparation should be standardized for all samples and should preferably be performed by a single person, e.g., cDNA preparation either with random or oligo d(T) priming. On the other hand, biological variance is sometimes more difficult to control (*see* **Subheading 3.1.**). On top of these sources of errors, the quality of DNA array data can vary depending on the type of array and the array manufacturing methods and quality.

With these considerations in mind, we used the experimental design presented in **Subheading 3.1.** for our gene expression-profiling study. Our study consisted of 55 cardiac samples and 1 control sample that were hybridized to 61 array sets, each consisting of 3 array subsets, thus, all together, we had 183 arrays. Except for the control sample, the gene expression profile of each sample was measured only once. The smallest statistical analysis group consisted of four different samples and two measurements per gene, because those were represented in duplicates on the arrays.

On the biological side, we classified our samples according to the disease state, tissue type, gender, and age. On the experimental side, our selected gene set was represented on three different arrays and, for manufacturing reasons, we had to use two different lots of array sets produced from PCR products of different production dates. Furthermore, the hybridizations were performed in two different hybridization ovens. To minimize the influence of the experimental errors, we put together groups of four samples that were hybridized simultaneously in the same oven at one time. Two hybridization sessions were carried out per week. Each sample received a hybridization group number, which allowed for later statistical analysis of any of the factors. Considering the fact that each sample was hybridized three times (one array subset each time), we randomly distributed the different hybridizations through the overall experimental time of 14 consecutive weeks to avoid a possible influence of training time. The same researcher performed all procedures of our experiment, and all solutions were prepared in advance for the entire experimental period. In addition, a large control RNA batch was intermittently used as an experimental hybridization control. An example of our hybridization groups for a 3-wk period is given in **Table 1**.

3.4. RNA Isolation, cDNA Synthesis, Labeling, Hybridization, and Signal Detection

Our procedure used for radioactive labeling and nylon membrane arrays is described as follows. Total RNA of all cardiac tissues and control HEK 293 cells was extracted using TRIzol reagent, according to the standard protocol. Labeling was performed by reverse transcription of 8 µg of total RNA with AMV-reverse transcriptase in the presence of $pd(T)_{12-18}$ and α-^{33}P-dCTP (*see* **Note 3**). Unincorporated nucleotides were removed using ProbeQuant G-50 micro columns, and cDNA was added to the hybridization solution, together with salmon sperm DNA, placenta DNA, and $pd(A)_{40}$ (*see* **Note 4**). Hybridizations were performed at 65°C for 16 h. After washing, arrays were exposed for 24 h to phosphor-imaging plates and scanned subsequently to obtain signal intensities (*see* **Note 5**).

3.5. Data Processing and Further Analysis

Before one can determine the differential gene expression profiles between two samples or conditions obtained, one first needs to ascertain that the data are comparable. That is, one should use a method to normalize the data sets for sources of experimental and biological variations, such as those discussed in **Subheading 3.3.** However, with few exceptions, the sources of these variations have not been measured and characterized within the experiment. Normalization methods attempt to correct for the following variables:

Table 1
Experimental Design[a]

Disease	Tissue type	Sex	Age	Array subset	Array batch	Hyb-group	Week
ASD	RA	m	y	1	1	1a	1
ASD	RA	m	o	1	1	1a	1
VSD	RA	m	y	1	1	1a	1
Normal	RA	f	o	1	1	1a	1
RVdis	RV	m	y	1	1	1b	1
RVdis	RV	m	y	1	1	1b	1
TOF	RV	m	y	1	1	1b	1
Normal	RV	m	o	1	1	1b	1
RVdis	RV	m	y	1	2	2a	1
TOF	RV	m	o	1	1	2a	1
TOF	RV	f	y	1	1	2a	1
Normal	RV	m	o	1	2	2a	1
Normal	RA	f	o	1	1	2b	1
Normal	RV	m	o	1	1	2b	1
Normal	LV	m	o	1	1	2b	1
Normal	IVS	m	o	1	1	2b	1
ASD	RA	m	y	2	1	3a	2
ASD	RA	m	o	2	1	3a	2
VSD	RA	m	y	2	1	3a	2
Normal	RA	f	o	2	1	3a	2
ASD	RA	f	y	2	1	3b	2
ASD	RA	f	o	2	1	3b	2
TOF	RA	m	o	2	1	3b	2
control				2	1	3b	2
RVdis	RV	m	y	2	1	4a	2
RVdis	RV	m	y	2	1	4a	2
TOF	RV	m	y	2	1	4a	2
Normal	RV	m	o	2	1	4a	2
Normal	RA	f	o	2	1	4b	2
Normal	RV	m	o	2	1	4b	2
Normal	LV	m	o	2	1	4b	2
Normal	IVS	m	o	2	1	4b	2
ASD	RA	f	y	3	1	9a	5
ASD	RA	f	o	3	1	9a	5
TOF	RA	m	y	3	1	9a	5
control				3	1	9a	5
Normal	RA	f	o	3	1	9b	5
Normal	LA	f	o	3	1	9b	5
Normal	RV	f	o	3	1	9b	5

(continued)

Table 1 *(continued)*

Disease	Tissue type	Sex	Age	Array subset	Array batch	Hyb-group	Week
Normal	LV	m	o	3	1	9b	5
ASD	RA	m	y	3	1	10a	5
VSD	RA	m	y	3	1	10a	5
RVdis	RV	m	y	3	1	10a	5
RVdis	RV	f	o	3	1	10a	5
RVdis	RV	f	o	3	1	10b	5
RVdis	RV	f	y	3	1	10b	5
TOF	RV	f	o	3	2	10b	5
Normal	RV	f	o	3	1	10b	5

[a]Excerpt of experimental schedule for our array study. Hyb-group, hybridization group; a or b, assignment for the hybridization oven used; f, female; m, male; o, old (≥7 years); y, young (<7 years); ASD, atrial septal defect; VSD, ventricular septal defect; RVdis, a variety of CHDs having right ventricular hypertrophy is common; RA, right atrium; IVS, interventricular septum.

1. Number of cells and different cell types in the sample.
2. RNA isolation and labeling efficiency.
3. Hybridization efficiency.
4. Signal measurement sensitivity.

The most widely used data normalization method is the normalization by global scaling *(6)*. Here, the sum of the measurements of each array is simply scaled to a constant sum. This scales the total signal on all arrays to a value of one, with the advantage that each individual measurement is expressed as a fraction of the total signal, in other words, as the fraction of total messenger RNA (mRNA).

Because our hybridizations were performed on arrays from two different production batches, which significantly affected the measurements, we corrected the influence of the production as follows. We considered two virtual reference hybridizations, defined by the spot-wise medians of 10 hybridizations from the respective array batch. These two sets of hybridizations were performed with samples from patients as well as with control samples sharing equal phenotype profiles. The logarithms of ratios between the intensities of each hybridization of interest and those of the respective batch-specific virtual reference hybridization were shifted, such that the median over the 40% of spots with highest average log intensity became zero. Finally, the obtained log-ratio values were averaged over duplicate spots per clone, resulting in values of "normalized" expression levels. To limit the analysis to meaningful data that did not show consistently low intensity or low variance across the samples, all further statistical analysis was performed on the normalized expression levels of 8069 selected genes, whose intensities were among the 15% highest in at least four samples, and whose natural log-ratios had a standard deviation across the samples of at least 0.5 (*see* **Note 6**).

The statistical analysis follows normalization and array data preprocessing. As a road map, the statistical analysis can be essed between a control (normal tissue) and experimental situation (disease tissue) is addressed. The second level is multiple genes, where clusters of genes are analyzed in terms of common functionalities, interactions, coregulations, and so on. Finally, the third level attempts to infer and understand the underlying gene and protein networks that ultimately are responsible for the pattern observed. One approach commonly used in the literature (at least in the first wave of publications) is a fold-change approach, in which a gene is declared to have significantly changed if its average expression level varies by more than a constant factor, typically two, between the treatment and control conditions. Inspection of gene expression data suggest, however, that such a simple "twofold rule" is unlikely to yield optimal results. First, it depends on well data normalization, because a factor of two can have quite different significance and meaning in different regions of the spectrum of expression levels, in particular, at the very high and very low ends. Moreover, this approach does not account for the influence of major confounding factors that can hardly be completely balanced by the sample selection in a disease study.

Therefore, we used linear models, incorporating the factors age, gender, disease, and tissue type, as a statistical framework for identifying genes that are affected in particular phenotypes *(7)*. We subjected the normalized expression levels of each clone to a linear model of the following form: $y_{hijk} = \mu + A_h + S_i + T_j + D_k + \varepsilon$, where A_h is the effect of age h, S_i the effect of the patient's gender, T_j the effect of tissue j, and D_k the effect of disease status k. Thus, we obtained a *p* value quantifying the statistical significance of differential expression for each gene and each phenotype comparison of interest. Estimating the rates of falsely significant genes with a permutation approach further assessed the reliability of the obtained results *(8)*. An overview of the numbers of differentially expressed genes obtained for the phenotype of TOF, the feature of RVH in response to pressure overload, and the comparison of atria and ventricle, is given in **Table 2**.

Most, if not all, genes act in concert with other genes. What DNA microarrays are really investigating are the patterns of expression across multiple genes and phenotypes.

We hierarchically clustered all known genes that seemed significantly differential ($p < 0.01$) in at least one of our overall comparisons (**Fig. 2**; $-\log_{10}$ (P)

Table 2
Overview of Differentially Expressed Genes ($p < 0.01$)^a

	Data set	TOF in RV	RVH in RV	A vs V
Clones	8069	324	198	438
Estimated false discovery rate		14%	25%	12%
Unigene cluster	6059	264	154	315
Known genes	1880	86	49	100

^{a}Total numbers of cDNA clones differentially expressed in different phenotype comparisons together with the represented number of Unigene clusters and known genes. The estimated false discovery rate is given. A, atrial; RVH, right ventricle hypertrophy; TOF, tetralogy of Fallot; V, ventricular.

color-coded). This overview allows for a comparison between the transcriptional portraits of each of these genes in the different phenotypes.

Furthermore, array data can be used to discriminate among different known or previously unknown cell types or conditions, which is addressed by many powerful techniques for class prediction and class discovery.

To see which class distinctions among our cardiac tissue samples are most pronounced in terms of gene expression profiles, we applied the class discovery method, ISIS *(9)*. This is an unsupervised algorithm that is designed to detect groups of samples with distinctive gene expression patterns. Within our data, the most outstanding binary class distinction identified, irrespective of sample annotations, was exactly the distinction between atria and ventricle samples.

Finally, one of the central challenges within the analysis of array data is to cope with the enormity of data sets. Examining a spreadsheet of gene names and expression ratios and significance values often provides little insight into the interesting trends or patterns that may exist within the data.

To provide a global view of the association of functional gene categories with particular phenotypes, we used the statistical method of correspondence analysis after assigning our genes to the gene ontology categories (AmiGO, http://www.godatabase.org) according to the annotation in LocusLink database (http://www.ncbi.nlm.nih.gov/LocusLink).

In addition to these analysis methods, several software packages for the analysis and visual display of array data are freely or commercially available (for selection, *see* **Subheading 2.4.**).

4. Notes

1. Different developmental origins of the heart have to be taken into account when selecting the samples. Furthermore, the comparison of biopsies obtained by car-

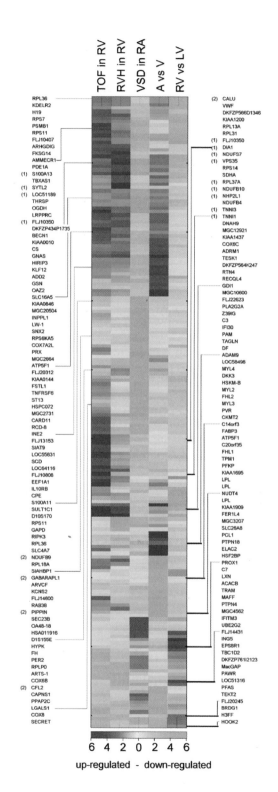

up-regulated - down-regulated

diac catheterization with samples obtained by surgical procedures should be avoided, because the cell-types within these samples could differ significantly regarding the proportion of endocardial and myocardial cells.

2. Having confounding factors in mind, we screened our sample population for additional clinical factors in advance. For example, we selected only patients with normal sinus rhythm, because cardiac arrhythmia is known to dramatically change the myocardial gene expression profiles. On the other hand, little is known about changes of the transcriptional portrait regarding low oxygen saturation, heart rate (newborn and young children have a higher heart rate than adults), or tissue temperature at the time of sample collection (most cardiac surgeries take place in a state of low body temperature vs normal body temperature during cardiac catheterization). For example, the oxygen saturation is influenced by various disease factors, which can never be matched completely in an observational study. Therefore, to enable the separation of disease- and tissue-specific expression patterns, the selected patient populations for the different phenotypes represented a range of these factors, rather than having been selected stringently for one or another factor. Finally, the statistical analysis regarding oxygen saturation as well as body temperature independent of the underlying diseases did not show a significant number of differentially expressed genes within our study.

3. In cases of very little sample material, the preparation of total RNA instead of mRNA is advisable. mRNA labeling can be achieved by the use of $pd(T)_{12-18}$ in the reverse transcription reaction. If mRNA is available, it is suggested that random hexamers, which are slightly more efficient be used (*see also* **Note 4**).

4. The $pd(A)_{40}$ was added to the hybridization solution to bind polyA stretches that could occur within spotted probes (PCR products of 600–1200 bases) and could lead to unspecific signals, especially in the presence of targets labeled using pd(T). The radioactivity should be within the first half-life of the isotope.

5. When using radioactively labeled probes, the hybridization and exposure time should be kept as stable as possible during the time period of the different experiments. We managed to have a variance of 15 min for both.

6. The smallest statistical analysis group consisted of four samples.

Fig. 2. (*opposite page*) Overview of *p* values and expression levels for different phenotype comparisons. Shown are annotated genes with $p < 0.01$ in at least one comparison. Gene names are listed. Each comparison is represented by one column, and each gene by one row. The $-\log_{10}(P)$ of each gene in the particular comparison is color-coded in yellow to red for upregulated and yellow to green for downregulated genes. For example, a value of 2 stands for $p = 0.01$ and is color-coded in red if the gene is upregulated. The differentially expressed genes confirmed by real-time PCR are indicated with "(1)" if tested for TOF in RV and "(2)" if tested for ventricular septal defects (VSD) in the right atrium. V, ventricular; A, atrial.

Acknowledgments

This work was supported by the Max Planck Society for the Advancement of Science. Among many colleagues that have provided me with input, help, and support I thank Bogac Kaynak. I express my gratitude for the intellectual support of Anja von Heydebreck, who has contributed in many ways to this work.

References

1. Kaynak, B., von Heydebreck, A., Mebus, S., et al. (2003) Genome-wide array analysis of normal and malformed human hearts. *Circulation* **107,** 2467–2474.
2. Fodor, S. P., Rava, R. P., Huang, X. C., Pease A. C., Holmes, C. P., and Adams, C. L. (1993) Multiplexed biochemical assays with biological chips. *Nature* **364,** 555–556.
3. Maier, E., Meier-Ewert, S., Ahmadi, A. R., Curtis, J., and Lehrach, H. (1994) Application of robotic technology to automated sequence fingerprint analysis by oligonucleotide hybridisation. *J. Biotechnol.* **35,** 191–203.
4. Bowtell, D. and Sambrook, J. (ed.) (2003) *DNA Micorarrays: A Molecular Cloning Manual.* Cold Spring Harbor, New York.
5. Kerr, M. K. (2003) Experimental design to make the most of microarray studies, in *Functional Genomics: Methods and Protocols* (Brownstein, M. J. and Khodursky, A. B., eds.), Humana, Totowa, NJ, pp. 137–147.
6. Beibarth, T., Fellenberg, K., Brors, B., et al. (2000) Processing and quality control of DNA array hybridization data. *Bioinformatics* **16,** 1014–1022.
7. Jin, W., Riley, R. M., Wolfinger, R. D., White, K. P., Passador-Gurgel, G., and Gibson, G. (2001) The contributions of sex, genotype and age to transcriptional variance in Drosophila melanogaster. *Nat. Genet.* **29,** 389–395.
8. Storey, J. D. and Tibshirani, R. (2003) SAM thresholding and false discovery rates for detecting differential gene expression in DNA microarrays, in *The Analysis of Gene Expression Data: Methods and Software* (Parmigiani, G., Garrett, E. S., Irizarry, R. A., and Zeger, S. L. eds.), Springer, New York.
9. von Heydebreck, A., Huber, W., Poustka, A., and Vingron, M. (2001) Identifying splits with clear separation: a new class discovery method for gene expression data. *Bioinformatics* **17,** 107–114.

15

DNA Mutation Analysis in Heterotaxy

Stephanie M. Ware

Summary

Heterotaxy refers to the abnormal arrangement of internal organs in relation to each other. It is characterized by complex cardiac malformations that are thought to result from abnormal left–right patterning in early embryonic development. Mutations in four genes have been identified in human heterotaxy. *ZIC3*, a zinc finger transcription factor, causes X-linked heterotaxy. *EGF-CFC, ACVR2B*, and *LEFTYA* are all members of a transforming growth factor-β signal transduction pathway that is critical for proper left–right development. Point mutations have been identified in each of these genes using polymerase chain reaction-based mutation analysis strategies. *ZIC3* mutation screening will be used to illustrate the methods for molecular sequence data acquisition and examination. These techniques are applicable to any gene of interest and will be useful for further evaluation of candidate genes for heterotaxy.

Key Words: Left–right asymmetry; molecular sequence data; point mutation; candidate gene; *ZIC3*; heterotaxy; nodal signal transduction pathway; ARMS assay; RFLP.

1. Introduction

Heterotaxy is a clinical phenotype that results from a partial or complete failure of appropriate patterning of the left and right sides during early embryogenesis *(1,2)*. Research in a number of different model organisms has identified genes important in initiating and maintaining left–right asymmetry in the early embryo *(3–5)*. Loss of these genes results in complex cardiovascular malformations. To date, point mutations in four genes have been identified in patients with heterotaxy: *ZIC3, EGF-CFC, ACVR2B*, and *LEFTYA (6–11)*. In addition, deletions of the *ZIC3* locus have been identified using fluorescence *in situ* hybridization *(12)*. Analysis of these genes is currently available only on a research basis, although *ZIC3* mutation screening should be clinically available in the near future. Using *ZIC3* as an example, this chapter discusses the design of oligonucleotide primers for sequence analysis, PCR

From: *Methods in Molecular Medicine, vol. 126: Congenital Heart Disease: Molecular Diagnostics*
Edited by: M. Kearns-Jonker © Humana Press Inc., Totowa, NJ

amplification and purification, analysis of sequence data, and design of controls.

2. Materials

1. Sample genomic DNA.
2. 10X polymerase chain reaction (PCR) buffer: 500 m*M* KCl, 100 m*M* Tris-base, pH 8.3, 1.5 m*M* MgCl$_2$.
3. Taq DNA polymerase.
4. dNTPs (dCTP, dATP, dGTP, and dTTP).
5. Oligonucleotide primers.
6. Agarose and gel electrophoresis equipment.
7. 10X Tris-acetate-EDTA running buffer.
8. Ethidium bromide.
9. PCR purification kit.
10. PCR thermocycler equipment.
11. Restriction enzymes and buffers.

3. Methods
3.1. Preparation of Genomic DNA

There are a variety of methods and kits available for preparation of genomic DNA. Most commercially available kits work well to generate substrates for PCR. We currently use the Gentra Puregene DNA extraction kit for preparation of DNA from cells, blood, tissues, or Ficoll, according to the manufacturer's instructions.

3.2. Design of Oligonucleotide Primers

The open reading frames of *ZIC3*, *EGF-CFC*, *ACVR2B*, and *LEFTYA* have been screened for point mutations *(6–11)*. The design of oligonucleotide primers is critical to the success of the PCR amplification reactions and subsequent screening.

3.2.1. Identification of the Intron–Exon Boundaries of the Gene of Interest

Information on intron–exon boundaries can be obtained from a number of the publicly available databases for many genes. The information in these databases is annotated on a regular basis and it is therefore worthwhile to periodically check for updates. **Fig. 1** shows an example of a search for *ZIC3* on the University of California, Santa Cruz genome browser.

1. Go to http://genome.ucsc.edu/ and click on the genome browser link.
2. On the human genome browser gateway page, enter *ZIC3* (or your gene of interest) in the box marked "position." A menu of search results will be displayed.

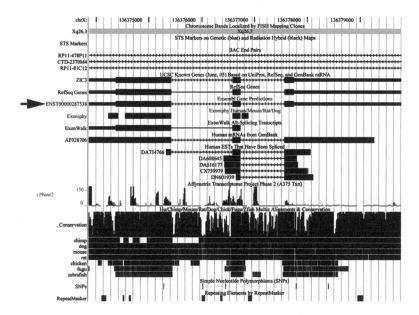

Fig. 1. University of California, Santa Cruz Genome Browser web page. The three exons and two introns of *ZIC3* are shown in black boxes and lines, respectively. The location on the X chromosome is given. Links to additional information can be found in the columns at the left. A link to Ensembl (arrow) is useful for obtaining sequence data with introns and exons demarcated.

3. Click on any human *ZIC3* listing to get to the page shown in **Fig. 1** (*see* **Note 1**).
4. Click on "Ensembl gene predictions" (**Fig. 1**, arrow) followed by "genomic sequence from assembly" to view the genomic sequence with intron–exon boundaries demarcated *(13–15)*.

3.2.2. Selection of Primers

Figure 2 shows information from Ensembl for *ZIC3* and illustrates the location of oligonucleotide primers within the sequence.

1. For exons of fewer than 400 bp, such as exon 2 and 3 of *ZIC3*, oligonucleotide primers are designed to flank the exon (*see* **Note 2**).
2. For exons larger than 400 bp, design overlapping primer sets (*see* **Fig. 2**, exon 1) (*see* **Note 2**).
3. Design oligonucleotide primers of 18 to 22 bases with a GC base content close to 50%.

3.2.3. Oligonucleotide Primers for X-Linked Heterotaxy (see **Note 3**)

Oligonucleotide primers can be purchased from a variety of commercial sources and do not require any additional purification steps for use with PCR. Primers used for *ZIC3* sequence analysis are listed in **Table 1** (*see* **Note 4**).

```
CCCTCTGCAG GAGACTCTTG CAGTGACGGA AAGTTGCAGC CCCTGGTAGC
GCCTTGGGGG TCTCCCCGCA GTGTCCAACC GCCGCCACCC CTTTCCGACT
ACGGCACTTC GGAGATCTCC TCCTTCGCCG GTACCCTCTC TCACTTCGGC
CGGATCGCCT GTGCCCAGAA CGTCCCACCC ATGACGATGC TCCTGGACGG
AGGCCCGCAG TTCCCTGGGC TGGGAGTGGG CAGCTTCGGC GCGCCGCGCC
ACCACGAGAT GCCCAACCGT GAGCCGGCAG GCATGGGGCT GAATCCCTTC
GGGGACTCAA CCCACGCCGC CGCCGCCGCC GCCGCCGCCG CTGCCTTCAA
GCTGAGCCCT GCCGCGGCGC ACGATCTATC TTCAGGCCAG AGCTCGGCTT
TCACGCCGCA GGGTTCGGGC TACGCCAACG CCCTGGGCCA CCATCACCAC
CACCATCACC ATCATCACCA CACCAGCCAG GTGCCCAGCT ACGGTGGCGC
TGCCTCTGCC GCCTTCAACT CAACGCGCGA GTTTCTGTTC CGCCAGCGCA
GCTCCGGGCT CAGTGAGGCG GCCTCGGGTG GCGGGCAGCA CGGGCTCTTC
GCCGGCTCGG CGAGCAGCCT GCATGCTCCA GCTGGCATCC CCGAGCCCCC
TAGCTACTTG CTGTTTCCCG GGCTGCATGA GCAGGGCGCT GGGCACCCGT
CGCCCACAGG GCACGTGGAC AACAACCAGG TCCACCTGGG GCTGCGTGGG
GAGCTGTTCG GCCGTGCTGA CCCATACCGC CCAGTGGCCA GCCCGCGCAC
GGACCCCTAC GCGGCCGGCG CTCAGTTTCC TAACTACAGC CCCATGAACA
TGAACATGGG AGTGAACGTG GCGGCCCACC ACGGGCCCGG CGCCTTCTTC
CGTTATATGC GGCAGCCTAT CAAGCAGGAG CTGTCGTGCA AGTGGATCGA
CGAGGCTCAG CTGAGCCGGC CCAAGAAGAG CTGCGACCGG ACCTTCAGCA
CCATGCATGA GCTGGTGACA CATGTCACCA TGGAGCATGT GGGGGGGCCCG
GAGCAGAACA ACCACGTCTG CTACTGGGAG GAGTGCCCCC GGGAGGGCAA
GTCTTTCAAG GCGAAGTACA AACTGGTCAA CCACATCCGA GTGCACACGG
GCGAGAAGCC CTTCCCATGC CCCTTCCCGG GCTGCGGGAA GATCTTTGCC
CGTTCTGAGA ACCTCAAGAT CCACAAGAGG ACCCACACAG GTAAGGGAAA
AAAGCAGGCG GGCGTGGGTT CCACTGGCGA TACCCGTCA CGCAGCGGAC
TTAGAGCGCG AGGGAGAGAG GTGGCGGCCA GGGAAGGGG CGACGCCCCG

ACCGCCGGGA GCTCAGTCTC CTGCTGCTTG CCTCTGAGAA ACTCCGGCGC
TGACCGTATT TTACCCCCCT TGGGTTTTTG CCTTTTGCAG GTGAGAAACC
TTTCAAATGT GAATTTGAAG GCTGTGACAG ACGCTTTGCC AACAGCAGCG
ACCGTAAGAA GCACATGCAT GTGCATACCT CGGACAAGCC CTATATCTGC
AAAGTGTGCG ACAAGTCCTA CACGCACCCG AGCTCCCTGC GCAAACACAT
GAAGGTAATT ACCTCTTTAT TAGCGGTCGG CGGTTTGTAA ACACTCGGCC
CGACGCCGGG CCGCGGAACG GAAGCGCCCG CGCTGCCAAC CCTCTGTCTT
CCACGTTAAA TCCGATTTGC TCCAGCAGTG ACACCTTGAA CCCATTTTGG

CTCGAATTCT GCTCTTGTTT TTGCTTGCAC ATTGCCAGTT GGAATTATAT
TCATTATAAT ATATACATGT TAATTTTAGG TTCATGAATC TCAAGGGTCA
GATTCCTCCC CTGCTGCCAG TTCAGGCTAT GAATCTTCCA CTCCACCCGC
TATAGCTTCT GCAAACAGTA AAGATACCAC TAAAACCCCT TCTGCAGTTC
AAACTAGCAC CAGCCACAAC CCTGGACTTC CTCCTAATTT TAACGAATGG
TACGTCTGAG GACAAACACA AACCCTGTTA ATTATAGAAT GGACCAAATA
CATTTTTAAA AGAAAACTGA GACCAATCAG ATGGAAATGG AGTTTTAAGG
```

F–ig. 2. Partial sequence information for *ZIC3*. Exons (bold) and partial sequence from introns are shown. The oligonucleotide primers used for sequence analysis are underlined. Note that exon 1aR and 1cF are the same primer in opposite orientations (*see* **Table 1**).

Table 1
Oligonucleotide Primers for *ZIC3* Exon Amplification by PCR[a]

Amplicon	Primer pair	Annealing temperature (°C)	Product size
Exon 1a	1aF 5' TCTTGCAGTGACGGAAAGTT 3'		
	1aR 5'TTCATGTTCATGGGGCTGTA 3'	56	839
Exon 1b	1bF 5' GCGCACGATCTATCTTCAGG 3'		
	5' CCGCATATAACGGAAGAAGG 3'	53	546
Exon 1c	1cF 5' TACAGCCCCATGAACATGAA 3'		
	1cR 5' TCTCCCTCGCGCTCTAAGT 3'	56	483
Exon 2	2F 5' GCTGCTTGCCTCTGAGAAAC 3'		
	2R 5' ACGTGGAAGACAGAGGGTTG 3'	56	334
Exon 3	3F 5' GCTCTTGTTTTTGCTTGCAC 3'		
	3R 5' CATTTCCATCTGATTGGTCTCA 3'	56	329

[a]F, forward; R, reverse.

3.3. PCR Amplification

For each patient genomic DNA sample, five PCR reactions are performed, using the primers listed in **Table 1**. The reaction conditions are given in **Table 2** (*see* **Note 5**).

Make a master mix according to **Table 2**, with a sufficient quantity for all patient samples, and aliquot 48 μL per tube. Add 2 μL of sample DNA (50 ng/μL) to each tube. The general PCR thermocycling program is given in **Table 3** (*see* **Note 5**).

A 5-μL aliquot from each sample can be removed and run on a 2% agarose gel to monitor PCR amplification. The remaining 45 μL is purified for subsequent sequencing.

3.4. Purification of PCR Products

PCR products are purified using Qiagen QIAquick PCR purification kit according to the manufacturer's instructions (*see* **Note 6**). The DNA is now ready to be submitted for sequencing.

3.5. Sequence Analysis

There are a variety of software programs available for purchase to perform mutation analysis on sequence traces. This section will describe the basic goals of sequence analysis and give instructions for analysis without sequence analysis software (*see* **Note 7**).

Table 2
PCR Mix

10X PCR buffer (100 mM Tris-base, pH 8.3; 500 mM KCl; and 1.5 mM MgCl$_2$)	5 µL
dNTPs (200 µM each)	4 µL
Oligonucleotide primers, 100 pmol/µL each	0.2 µL each
Taq DNA polymerase	0.2 µL (1 U
H$_2$O	38.4 µL

Table 3
PCR Thermocycling Program

Step	Temperature (°C)	Time	Procedure
1	94	3 min	Initial denaturation
2	94	30 s	Denaturation
3	*See* **Table 1**	30 s	Annealing of primers
4	72	45 s	Extension
5			Repeat 34 times from **step 2**
6	72	10 min	Final extension
7	4°C	forever	

1. Scan the sequence trace for each sample to determine the quality of the sequence.
2. Copy the sequence text and paste into the BLAST two-pair nucleotide alignment page (http://www.ncbi.nlm.nih.gov/blast/bl2seq/bl2.html).
3. Run a two-way alignment using human *ZIC3* (accession number NM_003413) and the sequence output data (*see* **Note 8**).
4. Confirm any mismatches by visualization of the sequence trace (*see* **Fig. 3**).
5. If a nucleotide mismatch is identified, translate the sequence containing the mismatch in all six frames. Paste sequence into the box provided at http://us.expasy.org/tools/dna.html, and submit. The results can be compared with the ZIC3 amino acid sequence to determine whether the mutation results in a silent, nonsense, or missense change.
6. If a sequence software program is not used, the exon–intron boundaries must be analyzed for each exon, to determine whether splice site mutations are present.

3.6. Design of Controls

For missense amino acid changes, control samples must be analyzed to determine whether the change represents a polymorphism (>1% of control samples). The two most commonly used methods are restriction fragment length polymorphism (RFLP) analysis and amplification refractory mutation system (ARMS) assay.

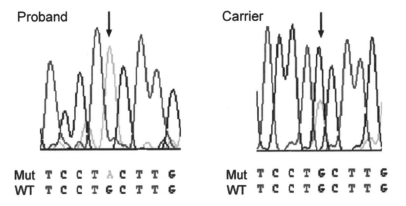

Proband   Carrier

Mut T C C T A C T T G   Mut T C C T G C T T G
WT   T C C T G C T T G   WT   T C C T G C T T G

Fig. 3. Sequence data from a proband and his carrier mother. A nonsense *ZIC3* mutation results from a G-A nucleotide substitution (arrow). Note that the hemizygous male has only the mutant allele. The carrier mother is heterozygous. Although her sequence trace shows both G and A alleles, the wild-type "G" assigned by the sequence trace misses the mutation, illustrating the importance of careful visual sequence analysis.

3.6.1. Restriction Fragment Length Polymorphism

1. Determine whether the mutation has created or deleted a restriction site by using a program such as Webcutter (http://www.firstmarket.com/cutter/cut2.html) to identify restriction sites in both the wild-type and mutant sequence.
2. Perform PCR for the exon of interest and purify the fragment, as described previously (*see* **Note 9**).
3. Cut purified DNA with the restriction enzyme and analyze by agarose gel electrophoresis, using standard molecular biology techniques *(16)*.
4. Ethnically matched controls should be analyzed.

3.6.2. ARMS Assay

In the event that no restriction site has been altered by the mutation, ARMS assay analysis can be performed on controls. This technique uses primers incorporating either the mutation or wild-type nucleotide as the last base of the oligonucleotide primer.

1. Generate a wild-type and mutation oligonucleotide primer that differ only at the most 3'-base. The same reverse primer can be used with both wild-type and mutation forward primers.
2. Perform PCR. Each DNA sample should have one reaction performed with wild-type primers and one performed with mutation primers (*see* **Note 10**).
3. Purify PCR reactions and analyze by gel electrophoresis, using standard molecular biology techniques.

4. Notes

1. This page provides information about the structure and alignment of *ZIC3*. Links to additional databases provide information about intron–exon structure, comparative sequence analysis between species, bacterial artificial chromosomes containing the sequence of interest, protein structure, and more.

2. The primers should be a minimum of 50 bp outside of the exon, so that all coding sequence will be visible on the sequence trace. To ensure that high-quality sequence can be obtained from the entire coding region, exons larger than 400 to 500 bp should be divided into segments. The length that can be screened in a single sequence trace will depend on both the architecture of the genomic DNA region as well as the sequencing facility.

   Publicly available primer design programs include Net Primer (http://www.premierbiosoft.com/netprimer/netprlaunch/netprlaunch.html), Primer 3 (http://frodo.wi.mit.edu/cgi-bin/primer3/primer3_www.cgi), and Prophet (the National Institutes of Health program, now discontinued but still very useful). There are also commercially available primer design programs, including Primer Premier (http://www.premierbiosoft.com/products/price_list/price_list.html) and Oligo (www.oligo.net). In addition to oligonucleotide length and GC content, these programs will identify primers without significant secondary structure or hairpin loop formation, and will usually eliminate annealing between primers that can result in primer–dimer formation.

3. Primers for PCR amplification of the open-reading frames of *EGF-CFC*, *ACVR2B*, and *LEFTYA* are published *(9–11)*. These genes were all screened initially by single-stranded conformation polymorphism (SSCP) analysis, and abnormalities were confirmed by direct sequencing. SSCP, denaturing high-performance liquid chromatography (DHPLC), and direct sequence analysis all use PCR amplification of exons as an initial step. The choice of procedure depends on the scale of the mutation screening, the available equipment, and technical expertise. Direct sequencing is attractive because of its widespread commercial availability and its increasing affordability. However, the cost of DHPLC remains substantially below direct sequencing (after the initial equipment costs and training) and is a better choice for screening of very large genes or large sample numbers. Both SSCP and DHPLC are screening tools and require direct sequencing to confirm abnormalities.

4. Exon 1a is the most problematic to amplify. If multiple bands amplify, the fragment of interest can be cut from the agarose gel and purified before sequencing. A 20-μL reaction gave better results than a 50-μL reaction.

5. The annealing temperatures are determined empirically. Thermocycling programs using a gradient of annealing temperatures were used to establish the temperature that maximizes the product and minimizes nonspecific products. In general, for difficulties with amplification, any component of the reaction mixture can be altered. Changing the annealing temperature or altering the magnesium chloride content will often increase specificity. If these modifications are not effective, we have generally found that it is most efficient and cost effective to try at least

one primer redesign before significantly attempting to further optimize reaction conditions.

6. Higher throughput purification can be achieved using a 384- or 96-well plate format. Purification is performed using a vacuum manifold. Multichannel pipetters are useful for both PCR reaction set up and purification.

7. "N" is the sequence designation assigned when no nucleotide call can be made. In genes on the autosomes, mutations result in heterozygosity at a nucleotide position, read as "N" on the sequence trace. It is important to evaluate all "N" designations because this may simply reflect poor sequence quality within a region. It is also important to look at all sequence traces (or know how your sequence analysis software functions), because heterozygous positions can fail to be designated as "N" (*see* **Fig. 3**, carrier). In males with *ZIC3* mutations, a nucleotide mismatch will be observed. In these patients, "N" usually implies poor sequence results.

8. This method will fail to align two regions of exon 1a of the *ZIC3* gene. Both the polyhistidine and polyalanine tracts must be aligned manually because of failure of BLAST two-pair alignment.

9. If the mutation site is very near one end of the amplicon, new primers may need to be designed, such that restriction digestion of the product results in two readily visible bands after gel electrophoresis.

10. The ARMS assay is predicated on failure of amplification when a mismatch between the last (most 3') base of the primer and genomic DNA exists. In reality, the amplification may be robust and occur even with this mismatch. Therefore, it is very important to optimize reaction conditions to ensure both proper amplification and failure of amplification in known samples before screening additional probands or controls.

Acknowledgments

I thank Jianlan Peng, Trang Ho, Laura Molinari, Brett Casey, Jeff Towbin, and John Belmont for their contribution to the *ZIC3* mutation analysis. This work was supported by the National Institutes of Health grants HL67355 and HD41648.

References

1. Aylsworth, A. S. (2001) Clinical aspects of defects in the determination of laterality. *Am. J. Med. Genet.* **101,** 345–355.

2. Ware, S. M. and Belmont, J. W. (2004) *ZIC3, CFC1, ACVR2B,* and *EBAF* and the visceral heterotaxies, in *Inborn Errors of Development: The Molecular Basis of Clinical Disorders of Morphogenesis* (Epstein, C. J., Erickson, R. P., and Wynshaw-Boris, A., eds.), Oxford University Press, New York, pp. 300–314.

3. Hamada, H., Meno, C., Watanabe, D., and Saijoh, Y. (2002) Establishment of vertebrate left–right asymmetry. *Nat. Rev. Genet.* **3,** 103–113.

4. Bisgrove, B., Morelli, S., and Yost, H. (2003) Genetics of human laterality disorders: insights from vertebrate model systems. *Ann. Rev. Genomics Hum. Genet.* **4,** 1–32.

5. Tabin, C. J. and Vogan, K. J. (2003) A two-cilia model for vertebrate left–right axis specification. *Genes Dev.* **17,** 1–6.
6. Gebbia, M., Ferrero, G. B., Pilia, G., et al. (1997) X-linked situs abnormalities result from mutations in ZIC3. *Nat. Genet.* **17,** 305–308.
7. Megarbane, A., Salem, N., Stephan, E., et al. (2000) X-linked transposition of the great arteries and incomplete penetrance among males with a nonsense mutation in ZIC3. *Eur. J. Hum. Genet.* **8,** 704–708.
8. Ware, S. M., Peng, J., Zhu, L., et al. (2004) Identification and functional analysis of ZIC3 mutations in heterotaxy and related congenital heart defects. *Am. J. Hum. Genet.* **74,** 93–105.
9. Bamford, R. N., Roessler, E., Burdine, R. D., et al. (2000) Loss-of-function mutations in the EGF-CFC gene CFC1 are associated with human left–right laterality defects. *Nat. Genet.* **26,** 365–369.
10. Kosaki, K., Bassi, M. T., Kosaki, R., et al. (1999) Characterization and mutation analysis of human LEFTY A and LEFTY B, homologues of murine genes implicated in left–right axis development. *Am. J. Hum. Genet.* **64,** 712–721.
11. Kosaki, R., Gebbia, M., Kosaki, K., et al. (1999) Left–right axis malformations associated with mutations in ACVR2B, the gene for human activin receptor type IIB. *Am. J. Med. Genet.* **82,** 70–76.
12. Ferrero, G. B., Gebbia, M., Pilia, G., et al. (1997) A submicroscopic deletion in Xq26 associated with familial situs ambiguus. *Am. J. Hum. Genet.* **61,** 395–401.
13. Birney, E., Andrews, D., Bevan, P., et al. (2004) Ensembl 2004. *Nucleic Acids Res.* **32(Database issue),** D468–470.
14. Clamp, M., Andrews, D., Barker, D., et al. (2003) Ensembl 2002: accommodating comparative genomics. *Nucleic Acids Res.* **31,** 38–42.
15. Hubbard, T., Barker, D., Birney, E., et al. (2002) The Ensembl genome database project. *Nucleic Acids Res.* **30,** 38–41.
16. Sambrook, J., Fritsch, E. F., and Maniatis, T. (1989) *Molecular Cloning, A Laboratory Manual,* Cold Spring Harbor Laboratory Press, NY.

16

Use of Denaturing High-Performance Liquid Chromatography to Detect Mutations in Pediatric Cardiomyopathies

Amy J. Sehnert

Summary

This chapter describes the use of denaturing high-performance liquid chromatography as a high-throughput method to detect genetic mutations in pediatric cardiomyopathies. An overview of the classification, incidence, and etiologies of the major cardiomyopathies is provided, with emphasis on the special circumstances of the pediatric patient. During the past 15 yr, the genetic bases of inherited dilated, hypertrophic, and restrictive cardiomyopathy have been elucidated. As the list of known and candidate cardiomyopathy genes continues to grow and our ability to screen for genetic mutations improves, the cause of cardiomyopathy will be identified in a larger percentage of cases. This outcome is highly relevant to children with cardiomyopathy as well as those at risk for developing the disease because of their family history.

Key Words: Cardiomyopathy; DCM; HCM; RCM; genetic mutations; DHPLC.

1. Introduction
1.1. Classification of Cardiomyopathies

Cardiomyopathies are the leading cause of heart failure, arrhythmias, and sudden cardiac death, and are the leading indication for heart transplantation *(1)*. Three major classes of cardiomyopathies, dilated cardiomyopathy (DCM), hypertrophic cardiomyopathy (HCM), and restrictive cardiomyopathy (RCM), are defined by clinical criteria established by the World Health Organization *(2)*. Patients with DCM show thin-walled, enlarged ventricles with systolic dysfunction. Patients with HCM show a thick-walled, hypercontractile heart of increased mass, which may exhibit abnormal relaxation. Patients with RCM show normal or nearly normal ventricular size, wall thickness, and systolic function, with restrictive ventricular filling pressures and atrial enlargement *(1,3,4)*. Cardiomyopathies may occur at any time from fetal life through old

From: *Methods in Molecular Medicine, vol. 126: Congenital Heart Disease: Molecular Diagnostics*
Edited by: M. Kearns-Jonker © Humana Press Inc., Totowa, NJ

age and are either primary (caused by an intrinsic heart muscle abnormality), or secondary (caused by ischemia, valve abnormalities, congenital heart disease, systemic disorders, infections, or toxins). In this chapter, we focus on the special case of primary cardiomyopathies in children.

1.2. Incidence and Causes of Pediatric Cardiomyopathies

The incidence of primary cardiomyopathy in children younger than 18 yr old in the United States is 1.13 per 100,000. Almost half of all cases are ascertained in infants younger than 1 yr of age, in which group, the incidence is 8.34 per 100,000. A second peak occurs during adolescence *(5)*. DCM accounts for 51% of pediatric cardiomyopathies, and HCM accounts for 42% of cases. Less common forms, such as RCM and arrhythmogenic right ventricular dysplasia (ARVD) account for only a minor fraction of cases (<5%). Overall, the cause remains unknown in two-thirds of children presenting with primary cardiomyopathy, and the mortality rate is 13% within 2 yr of diagnosis *(5,6)*. When a cause is assigned for DCM, it is most likely caused by a neuromuscular disorder (i.e., X-linked muscular dystrophy), myocarditis, or familial inherited disease. For HCM, the leading identified causes are familial inherited disease, inborn error of metabolism (i.e., disorders of glycogen metabolism or oxidative phosphorylation), and malformation syndrome (i.e., Noonan syndrome) *(5,6)*. In general, familial cardiomyopathies represent an important diagnostic category that may go unrecognized if cardiovascular symptoms are absent or mild in a child undergoing routine clinical examination. Specifically documenting whether a family history of cardiomyopathy and/or sudden cardiac death exists is an essential component of pediatric care.

1.3. Genetic Basis of Familial Cardiomyopathies

Familial cardiomyopathies are largely caused by autosomal-dominant mutations in structural proteins of the cytoskeleton (i.e., lamin A/C and sarcoglycan), cardiac sarcomere (i.e., myosin heavy and light chains, troponins, and tropomyosin), sarcoplasmic reticulum (i.e., ryanodine receptor and phosholamban), and energy-regulating pathways (i.e., adenosine 5'-monophosphate-activated protein kinase) *(1,3,4,7)*. HCM occurs in 1 in 500 adults, of which, 80% of cases are caused by a genetic mutation *(8)*. DCM occurs in 1 in 2500 adults, and it is currently estimated that approx 30 to 40% of cases are genetic. For these reasons, annual clinical screening is currently recommended for offspring in families with any form of primary cardiomyopathy to look for evidence of disease *(9)*. Both the discovery of mutations in inherited forms of cardiomyopathy and the burden of disease screening have made genetic diagnosis in pediatric patients an important endeavor.

1.4. Detecting Genetic Mutations in Cardiomyopathies

Hundreds of mutations in more than 20 genes have now been identified as the cause of DCM, HCM, RCM, and ARVD, and more disease genes and mutations remain to be discovered (*1,3,4,11*, and Sehnert, unpublished data). Currently, the bulk of mutation screening in known and candidate genes is conducted in research laboratories by investigators interested in cardiac genetics. In this setting, a variety of methods are used to detect genetic variations (polymorphisms and mutations) in human DNA samples. This chapter describes the use of denaturing high-performance liquid chromatography (DHPLC) as a high-throughput method for screening cardiomyopathy genes for mutations. It highlights examples from the cardiomyopathy literature and our own experience (*12–33* and Sehnert, unpublished data).

2. Materials

1. Polymerase chain reaction (PCR) machine.
2. DHPLC equipment and column.
3. Computer and vendor software.
4. Source DNA.
5. *Taq* polymerase.
6. Oligonucleotide primers.
7. HPLC-grade water.
8. HPLC-grade acetonitrile.
9. 2 *M* triethlyammonium acetate (TEAA).
10. Shrimp alkaline phosphatase.
11. Exonuclease I.
12. Gene-sequencing capability.

3. Methods

The use of DHPLC for mutation detection requires investment in a commercially available system or access to a core facility that offers such capability (*see* **Note 1**). The methods described in the chapter present the principle of DHPLC technology, and provide a practical guide to optimize PCR conditions for DHPLC analysis, interpret results, and process samples for gene sequencing.

3.1. DHPLC: How It Works

Originally developed to facilitate evolutionary studies of the Y-chromosome, DHPLC has subsequently been validated and used as a highly sensitive method to detect variations in more than 300 genes that cause a variety of diseases, including cancers, and neurological, hematological, metabolic, autoimmune, and cardiovascular disorders, and others (*34–38*). DHPLC offers a nonbiased method to screen DNA for single base changes as well as small

Table 1
Cardiomyopathy Genes Analyzed by DHPLC

Disease gene(s)	Gene symbol	Refs.
HCM		
β-Myosin heavy chain	*MYH7*	*12–15*
Myosin-binding protein C	*MYBPC3*	*16*
Cardiac troponin T	*TNNT2*	*13,14,17,18*
Cardiac troponin I	*TNNI3*	*17,18*
α-Tropomyosin	*TPM1*	*17–19*
α-Cardiac actin	*ACTC*	*17*
HCM with WPW syndrome		
AMP-activated protein kinase	*PRKAG2*	*18,20,21*
Noonan syndrome (HCM)		
Protein-tyrosine phosphatase nonreceptor-type 11	*PTPN11*	*22–27*
DCM		
Sarcoglycan	*SGCD*	*28*
Lamin A/C	*LMNA*	*29–31*
ARVD		
Cardiac ryanodine receptor 2	*RYR2*	*32*
Mitochondrial genome	mtDNA	*33,38*

DHPLC, denaturing high-performance liquid chromatography; HCM, hypertrophic cardiomyopathy; WPW, Wolff–Parkinson–White; AMP, adenosine 5'-monophosphate; ARVD, arrhythmogenic right ventricular dysplasia; mtDNA, mitochondrial DNA.

insertions or deletions *(39,40)*. The method is ideal for detecting heterozygous missense changes that are characteristic of the autosomal-dominant cardiomyopathies *(3,4,39,40)*. **Table 1** shows a list of cardiomyopathy genes previously subjected to DHPLC analysis, including references.

DHPLC relies on a reusable, novel matrix column, and an ion-pairing reagent (TEAA) that bridges negatively charged DNA molecules to the stationary phase *(36,37,39)*. Using this technique, mixed PCR products from normal (homozygous) and test subject DNA are denatured (heated) and reannealed (cooled). In the presence of sequence variations, the heating and cooling step allows heteroduplexes and homoduplexes to form (**Fig. 1A**). Heteroduplexes and homoduplexes are then fractionated under partially denaturing conditions on the heated column of hydrophobic beads. The altered denaturation and migration properties of heteroduplex products provide the basis for detecting sequence variations (**Fig. 1B**; *see* **Note 2**). The optimal temperature for DHPLC analysis is determined using software computation programs *(41)*. The high-

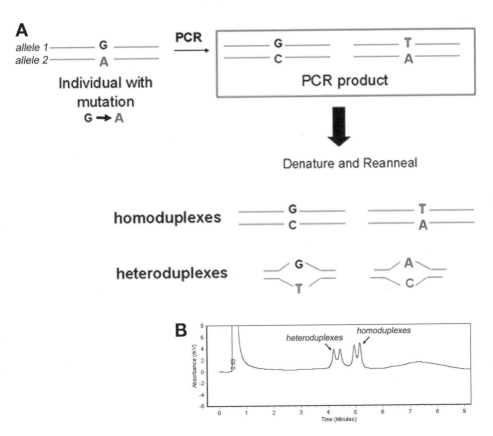

Fig. 1. Homoduplex and heteroduplex formation. (**A**) shows the double-stranded PCR products amplified from template DNA containing a single base G → A substitution in sample from a heterozygous individual. When the PCR products are denatured and reannealed, homoduplexes and heteroduplexes are formed, as shown in the line drawings. Altered denaturation and migration properties of the homoduplexes and heteroduplexes result in different elution times off of the DHPLC column, as shown in (**B**). Heteroduplexes elute off first. Data shown is taken from the Transgenomic mutation standard run in our lab. Absorbance, ultraviolet absorbance.

throughput nature of the method is achieved by combining multiple samples for simultaneous analysis.

3.2. Amplify Target Sequence

Autosomal-dominant transmission is the most common mode of inheritance of DCM, HCM, RCM, and ARVD (*1,3,4*). The vast majority of causative mutations are single base substitutions within exons that result in missense

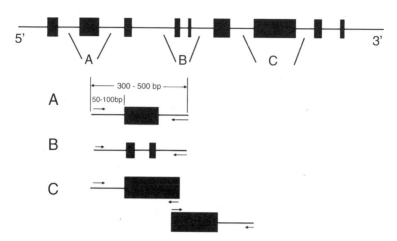

Fig. 2. Design PCR fragments for DHPLC. Genomic structure of a hypothetical gene with nine exons (black, filled boxes) is shown. Ideal fragments for DHPLC analysis are 200- to 500-bp long. (**A**) Shows the most typical fragment design including one exon with flanking intron sequence (50–100 bp on either side of the exon). (**B**) Shows a fragment spanning two small exons with an intervening intron. (**C**) Shows a large exon scanned in two overlapping fragments that were independently amplified by PCR. Small arrows indicate the PCR primers.

changes, or changes at exon–intron boundaries that alter gene splicing *(3)*. It is, therefore, typical to begin to scan a candidate gene for variations by targeting gene fragments that contain an exon sequence with some flanking intron (**Fig. 2A**). Selected portions of 5'-upstream and 3'-downstream sequences can also be included, as well as the entire genomic sequence, depending on gene structure, the size of introns, and the purpose of the project. Many primers have been selected and are published (**Table 1**) and/or are available online at: http://insertion.stanford.edu/dhplc_genes1.html *(38)*.

3.2.1. Analyze the Sequence

Once a candidate gene or genes have been selected for analysis, the first step is to gather as much information as possible from the literature and human genome databases regarding the sequence and structure of the genes (*see* **Note 3**). At this time, it is also relevant to note the presence of verified single-nucleotide polymorphisms (SNPs) and their location within the sequence of interest. When possible, sequences containing uninformative SNPs can be eliminated from target fragments to minimize the variations that would be detected by DHPLC. On the other hand, if knowledge of a particular SNP allele frequency is important to the project, then fragments can be designed to include SNP bases.

Next, determine the number of fragments to be analyzed per gene, based on the length of the coding and noncoding regions. Although the DHPLC method is capable of detecting mutations in long fragments (i.e., 1000–1500 bp), the ideal fragment size is 200 to 500 bp *(36,37,39)*. In most cases, fragments for DHPLC analysis contain a single exon with flanking intron (i.e., 50 to 100 bp of intron sequence on each side, **Fig. 2A**). Occasionally, it is possible to screen a fragment that contains two exons and an intervening intron (**Fig. 2B**). Sometimes it becomes necessary to scan large exons in two or more overlapping fragments (**Fig. 2C**). Before designing PCR primers, it is important to look at the melting profile of each given sequence (*see* **Note 4**). Ideally, temperatures should vary slightly across the fragment to allow partial melting, but not by more than 15°C *(39,41)*. This process is reiterated as necessary to achieve the best possible melt profiles for sequences that span the gene of interest.

3.2.2. Design Primers

Once the sequence fragments are approximated using the steps given in **Subheading 3.2.1.**, specific primers can be designed. Many software and on-line resources are available to assist in primer picking using selected constraints (i.e., http://frodo.wi.mit.edu/cgi-bin/primer3/primer3_www.cgi). In general, primers with a melting temperatur between 55°C and 58°C and within 1°C of each other are desirable. During the process of sequence analysis and primer design, one can examine the affect of modifications to improve the melt profile, such as adding a GC-clamp to the ends of primers. High-purity oligonucleotide primers should be used (we recommend high-purity, salt-free oligonucleotides from MWG Biotech, Highpoint, NC). Depending on the fragment being amplified, it may be necessary to reiterate primer design to arrive at an optimal pair. Technical support is also available from the DHPLC vendors to troubleshoot and assist with primer design for difficult fragments.

3.2.3. Extract DNA

Extract DNA from blood or tissues using standard molecular methods to produce a high-quality template for PCR (i.e., Qiagen genomic-tip system).

3.2.4. Optimize PCR conditions

Perform PCR on 50 to 100 ng of template DNA using a standard thermocycler and a touch-down program (94°C for 4 min followed by cycling at: 94°C for 30 s, annealing temperature for 1 min, and 72°C for 1 min; the annealing temperature is reduced from 60°C to 55°C in 0.5°C increments with each cycle, followed by 20 to 30 cycles at 55°C; and a final extension at 72°C for 10 min). Run a test PCR for each primer pair to examine the strength and quality of the product by gel electrophoresis, and confirm its sequence before proceeding to DHPLC. For best results on small fragments (100 to 500 bp), we recommend using a 9:1 ratio of Ampli*Taq* Gold® (Applied Biosystems) to *Pfu* Turbo (Stratagene) with the Ampli*Taq* Gold buffer. To allow adequate sample for gel electrophoresis (8–10 µL), DHPLC (20–30 µL), and sequencing (5–10 µL), we amplify in 50-µL PCR volumes with primers, dNTPs, buffer, MgCl^{2+}, and *Taq* polymerase. A pure PCR product is critical to good DHPLC results. Alter PCR conditions as needed to meet this end (*see* **Note 5**). Once the PCR conditions are optimized, amplify the fragments for DHPLC analysis from template DNA, including a control sample.

3.3. Denature and Reanneal PCR Product

After PCR, combine equal amounts of the product from each test sample with the control product (i.e., 15–20 µL each), then denature and reanneal the mixed sample. The mixture of samples can also be approached through sample pooling (i.e., three or more samples combined together). In the case of cardiomyopathies, in which most mutations are heterozygous in nature, it is also reasonable to screen individual samples without mixing, as long as it is understood that this will not detect homozygous changes. To denature, heat samples to 95°C for 8 min, then gradually decrease the temperature by 2°C/min down to 21°C.

3.4. Perform DHPLC

3.4.1. Select Operating Temperatures

Select operating temperatures for DHPLC analysis based on the melt profile for each fragment. Ideal temperatures are calculated using system software or programs such as the one at http://insertion.stanford.edu/dhplc.html. It is highly recommended that each fragment be run at two or three different temperatures to ensure detection of all polymorphisms in a fragment. The operating temperatures typically vary by 1 to 2°C, and sometimes more, depending on the sequence.

3.4.2. Run Samples

DHPLC is an automated method (*36,37*). Running buffers can be purchased or prepared according to manufacturer's directions using volumetric flasks and HPLC-grade water (*see* **Note 6**). Buffer A is a 0.1 *M* TEAA solution, Buffer B contains 0.1 *M* TEAA with 25% acetonitrile. Wash solutions of 8% acetonitrile and 75% acetonitrile are used for the injection syringe and DHPLC column, respectively. A 96-well plate format and autosampler allow for long runs once the conditions are specified and entered in a table on the computer. In general, use a 10-µL volume for each DHPLC injection and test each fragment at a minimum of two operating temperatures. Run a mutation standard at the beginning of each run and blank injections before and between samples. When possible, include positive-control samples for selected fragments. Start by using running buffer gradients selected by the system software. The buffer gradients can be adjusted, if necessary, to improve detection for any given fragment. Consult vendor manuals and technical support for detailed operating instructions and troubleshooting information.

3.4.3. Interpret Results

Once samples have been run, review the data using the system software. Analyze the peaks for their quality (cleanliness and amplitude) and informative value (presence of homoduplex and heteroduplex peaks). Example traces are shown in **Fig. 3**. Be aware that a variety of trace morphologies may be encountered and that these may also vary between runs for the same fragment. Every effort should, therefore, be taken in the process of PCR to generate consistent, high-quality products for analysis. Newer instruments offer software that can perform automated peak analysis and classification to aid high-throughput analysis. Each application needs to be customized at the beginning of the project and confirmed by sequencing to achieve the most reliable and repeatable results.

3.5. Examine Suspect Fragments for Sequence Variations

Purify PCR products from fragments that show heteroduplexes for direct sequencing using standard methods (i.e., add shrimp alkaline phosphatase [Roche Molecular Biochemicals] and exonuclease I [New England Biolabs]; heat to 37°C for 35 min, then to 95°C for 15 min). Perform automated DNA sequencing and analyze sequence traces for variations using appropriate software (**Fig. 3**).

4. Notes

1. DHPLC instrumentation is commercially available from two major manufacturers, the Transgenomic WAVE™ (Omaha, NE) and Varian Helix HPLC (Palo Alto, CA). We found that the quality and condition of the column, technical support provided by the vendor, and routine system maintenance were critical to successful operation of the WAVE instrument.
2. Samples are injected into a flow path with TEAA and acetonitrile. The hydrophobic portion of TEAA interacts with hydrophobic beads in the column, and the negatively charged phosphate backbone of partially denatured PCR products interact with the positively charged ammonium groups of TEAA. At increasing concentrations of acetonitrile, the TEAA to DNA attraction is reduced, and products are eluted off of the column such that heteroduplexes with the mismatched

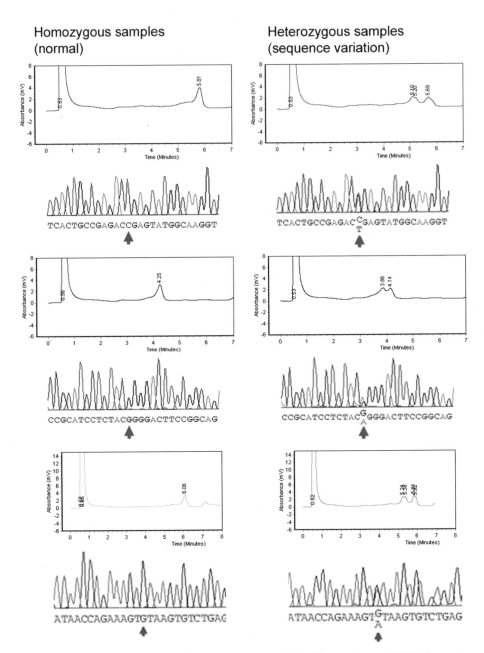

Fig. 3. DHPLC spectra and sequence traces. This figure shows DHPLC spectra above the corresponding sequence traces for three PCR fragments (top to bottom). Results from homozygous (normal) samples are on the left, and results from heterozygous samples (containing a sequence variation) are on the right. Normal samples show a single elution peak, whereas heterozygous samples show a separation of the elution peaks. This indicates the presence of heteroduplexes in the sample. Arrows below sequence traces point to base changes confirmed in these fragments.

bases elute off first and homoduplexes elute off next (**Fig. 1B**). As fragments pass through the UV detector, absorbance is measured and data are sent to the computer for analysis (http://www.transgenomic.com/).

3. We routinely used the University of California at Santa Cruz website (http://genome.ucsc.edu/) as a primary source for sequence information and related links.

4. The melting curve of the fragment can be examined using DHPLC system software or melting curve calculators available on-line (i.e., http://insertion.stanford.edu/melt.html or http://web.mit.edu/osp/www/melt.html).

5. We found that subamplification of small fragments from a long-range PCR product (6 to 8 kb amplified with SuperMix High Fidelity *Taq* polymerase [Invitrogen]) yielded specific, strong products for DHPLC. A potential limitation is that this requires an additional round of PCR.

6. Prepare buffers using volumetric flasks provided by the vendor. To prevent bacterial growth in Buffer A, add 250 µL of HPLC grade acetonitrile to 1 L of buffer. Use clean, glass wide-mouth bottles with screw caps for operation and storage of buffers. DO NOT autoclave water or bottles used for DHPLC buffers because small metal fragments may damage the column.

Acknowledgments

The author thanks Renee Reijo Pera, PhD, who shared her DHPLC equipment for studies of pediatric cardiomyopathies, the patients who participated, and their families. I also acknowledge the technical expertise of Matthew Bensley, who performed the majority of our mutation detection experiments. This work was supported by grants from the National Institutes of Health (K08HL004068), the Greenberg Foundation Young Investigator Award in Cardiovascular Genetics, and the University of California at San Francisco Pediatric Clinical Research Center (to AS).

References

1. Towbin, J. A. and Bowles, N. E. (2002) The failing heart. *Nature* **415,** 227–233.
2. Richardson, P., McKenna, W., Bristow, M., et al. (1996) Report of the 1995 World Health Organization/International Society and Federation of Cardiology Task Force on the definition and classification of cardiomyopathies. *Circulation* **93(5),** 841–842.
3. Fatkin, D. and Graham, R. M. (2002) Molecular mechanisms of inherited cardiomyopathies. *Physiol. Rev.* **82(4),** 945–980.
4. Seidman, J. G. and Seidman, C. (2001) The genetic basis for cardiomyopathy: from mutation identification to mechanistic paradigms. *Cell* **104(4),** 557–567.
5. Lipshultz, S. E., Sleeper, L. A., Towbin, J. A., et al. (2003) The incidence of pediatric cardiomyopathy in two regions of the United States. *N. Engl. J. Med.* **348(17),** 1647–1655.
6. Nugent, A. W., Daubeney, P. E., Chondros, P., et al. (2003) The epidemiology of childhood cardiomyopathy in Australia. *N. Engl. J. Med.* **348(17),** 1639–1646.

7. Arad, M., Maron, B. J., Gorham, J. M., et al. (2005) Glycogen storage diseases presenting as hypertrophic cardiomyopathy. *N. Engl. J. Med.* **352(4)**, 362–372.
8. Richard, P., Charron, P., Carrier, L., et al. (2003) Hypertrophic cardiomyopathy: distribution of disease genes, spectrum of mutations, and implications for a molecular diagnosis strategy. *Circulation* **107(17)**, 2227–2232.
9. Maron, B. J., McKenna, W. J., Danielson, G. K., et al. (2003) American College of Cardiology/European Society of Cardiology clinical expert consensus document on hypertrophic cardiomyopathy. A report of the American College of Cardiology Foundation Task Force on Clinical Expert Consensus Documents and the European Society of Cardiology Committee for Practice Guidelines. *J. Am. Coll. Cardiol.* **42(9)**, 1687–1713.
10. Ahmad, F. (2003) The molecular genetics of arrhythmogenic right ventricular dysplasia-cardiomyopathy. *Clin. Invest. Med.* **26(4)**, 167–178.
11. Mogensen, J., Kubo, T., Duque, M., et al. (2003) Idiopathic restrictive cardiomyopathy is part of the clinical expression of cardiac troponin I mutations. *J. Clin. Invest.* **111(2)**, 209–216.
12. Blair, E., Redwood, C., de Jesus Oliveira, M., et al. (2002) Mutations of the light meromyosin domain of the beta-myosin heavy chain rod in hypertrophic cardiomyopathy. *Circ. Res.* **90(3)**, 263–269.
13. Ackerman, M. J., VanDriest, S. L., Ommen, S. R., et al. (2002) Prevalence and age-dependence of malignant mutations in the beta-myosin heavy chain and troponin T genes in hypertrophic cardiomyopathy: a comprehensive outpatient perspective. *J. Am. Coll. Cardiol.* **39(12)**, 2042–2048.
14. Van Driest, S. L., Ackerman, M. J., Ommen, S. R., et al. (2002) Prevalence and severity of "benign" mutations in the beta-myosin heavy chain, cardiac troponin T, and alpha-tropomyosin genes in hypertrophic cardiomyopathy. *Circulation* **106(24)**, 3085–3090.
15. Van Driest, S. L., Jaeger, M. A., Ommen, S. R., et al. (2004) Comprehensive analysis of the beta-myosin heavy chain gene in 389 unrelated patients with hypertrophic cardiomyopathy. *J. Am. Coll. Cardiol.* **44(3)**, 602–610.
16. Van Driest, S. L., Vasile, V. C., Ommen, S. R., et al. (2004) Myosin binding protein C mutations and compound heterozygosity in hypertrophic cardiomyopathy. *J. Am. Coll. Cardiol.* **44(9)**, 1903–1910.
17. Van Driest, S. L., Ellsworth, E. G., Ommen, S. R., Tajik, A. J., Gersh, B. J., and Ackerman, M. J. (2003) Prevalence and spectrum of thin filament mutations in an outpatient referral population with hypertrophic cardiomyopathy. *Circulation* **108(4)**, 445–451.
18. Mogensen, J., Bahl, A., Kubo, T., Elanko, N., Taylor, R., and McKenna, W. J. (2003) Comparison of fluorescent SSCP and denaturing HPLC analysis with direct sequencing for mutation screening in hypertrophic cardiomyopathy. *J. Med. Genet.* **40(5)**, e59.
19. Van Driest, S. L., Will, M. L., Atkins, D. L., and Ackerman, M. J. (2002) A novel TPM1 mutation in a family with hypertrophic cardiomyopathy and sudden cardiac death in childhood. *Am. J. Cardiol.* **90(10)**, 1123–1127.

20. Oliveira, S. M., Ehtisham, J., Redwood, C. S., Ostman-Smith, I., Blair, E. M., and Watkins, H. (2003) Mutation analysis of AMP-activated protein kinase subunits in inherited cardiomyopathies: implications for kinase function and disease pathogenesis. *J. Mol. Cell. Cardiol.* **35(10)**, 1251–1255.

21. Vaughan, C. J., Hom, Y., Okin, D. A., McDermott, D. A., Lerman, B. B., and Basson, C. T. (2003) Molecular genetic analysis of PRKAG2 in sporadic Wolff-Parkinson-White syndrome. *J. Cardiovasc. Electrophysiol.* **14(3)**, 263–268.

22. Kosaki, K., Suzuki, T., Muroya, K., et al. (2002) PTPN11 (protein-tyrosine phosphatase, nonreceptor-type 11) mutations in seven Japanese patients with Noonan syndrome. *J. Clin. Endocrinol. Metab.* **87(8)**, 3529–3533.

23. Tartaglia, M., Kalidas, K., Shaw, A., et al. (2002) PTPN11 mutations in Noonan syndrome: molecular spectrum, genotype-phenotype correlation, and phenotypic heterogeneity. *Am. J. Hum. Genet.* **70(6)**, 1555–1563.

24. Froster, U. G., Glander, H. J., Heinritz, W. (2003) Molecular genetic mutation analysis of the PTPN11 gene in the multiple lentigines (LEOPARD) syndrome. *Hautarzt* **54(12)**, 1190–1192.

25. Legius, E., Schrander-Stumpel, C., Schollen, E., Pulles-Heintzberger, C., Gewillig, M., and Fryns, J. P. (2002) PTPN11 mutations in LEOPARD syndrome. *J. Med. Genet.* **39(8)**, 571–574.

26. Schollen, E., Matthijs, G., and Fryns, J. F. (2003) PTPN11 mutation in a young man with Noonan syndrome and retinitis pigmentosa. *Genet. Couns.* **14(2)**, 259.

27. Musante, L., Kehl, H. G., Majewski, F., et al. (2003) Spectrum of mutations in PTPN11 and genotype–phenotype correlation in 96 patients with Noonan syndrome and five patients with cardio–facio–cutaneous syndrome. *Eur. J. Hum. Genet.* **11(2)**, 201–206.

28. Love, D. R. (2004) Limb girdle muscular dystrophy: use of dHPLC and direct sequencing to detect sarcoglycan gene mutations in a New Zealand cohort. *Clin. Genet.* **65(1)**, 55–60.

29. Taylor, M. R., Fain, P. R., Sinagra, G., et al. (2003) Natural history of dilated cardiomyopathy due to lamin A/C gene mutations. *J. Am. Coll. Cardiol.* **41(5)**, 771–780.

30. Taylor, M. R., Robinson, M. L., and Mestroni, L. (2004) Analysis of genetic variations of lamin A/C gene (LMNA) by denaturing high-performance liquid chromatography. *J. Biomol. Screen.* **9(7)**, 625–628.

31. Arbustini, E., Pilotto, A., Repetto, A., et al. (2002) Autosomal dominant dilated cardiomyopathy with atrioventricular block: a lamin A/C defect-related disease. *J. Am. Coll. Cardiol.* **39(6)**, 981–990.

32. Tiso, N., Stephan, D. A., Nava, A., et al. (2001) Identification of mutations in the cardiac ryanodine receptor gene in families affected with arrhythmogenic right ventricular cardiomyopathy type 2 (ARVD2). *Hum. Mol. Genet.* **10(3)**, 189–194.

33. Stanford Genome Technology Center. (2004) Available at: http://insertion.stanford.edu/mtDNA.html. Accessed at UCSF.

34. Underhill, P. A., Jin, L., Lin, A. A., et al. (1997) Detection of numerous Y chromosome biallelic polymorphisms by denaturing high-performance liquid chromatography. *Genome Res.* **7(10)**, 996–1005.

35. Underhill, P. A., Shen, P., Lin, A. A., et al. (2000) Y chromosome sequence variation and the history of human populations. *Nat. Genet.* **26(3),** 358–361.
36. Premstaller, A. and Oefner, P. J. (2003) Denaturing high-performance liquid chromatography. *Methods Mol. Biol.* **212,** 15–35.
37. Frueh, F. W. and Noyer-Weidner, M. (2003) The use of denaturing high-performance liquid chromatography (DHPLC) for the analysis of genetic variations: impact for diagnostics and pharmacogenetics. *Clin. Chem. Lab. Med.* **41(4),** 452–461.
38. Stanford Genome Technology Center. (2004) Available at: http://insertion.stanford.edu/dhplc_genes1.html. Accessed at UCSF.
39. Oefner, P. and Underhill, P. (1998) DNA mutation detection using denaturing high-performance liquid chromatography (DHPLC), in *Current Protocols in Human Genetics* (Dracopoli, N. C. K. B., Moir, D. T., Morton, C. C., Seidman, C. E., Seidman, J. G., and Smith, D. R., eds), John Wiley and Sons, New York, pp. 7.10.1–7.2.
40. Xiao, W. and Oefner, P. J. (2001) Denaturing high-performance liquid chromatography: a review. *Hum. Mutat.* **17(6),** 439–474.
41. Jones, A. C., Austin, J., Hansen, N., et al. (1999) Optimal temperature selection for mutation detection by denaturing HPLC and comparison to single-stranded conformation polymorphism and heteroduplex analysis. *Clin. Chem.* **45(8 Pt 1),** 1133–1140.

Index